P

M

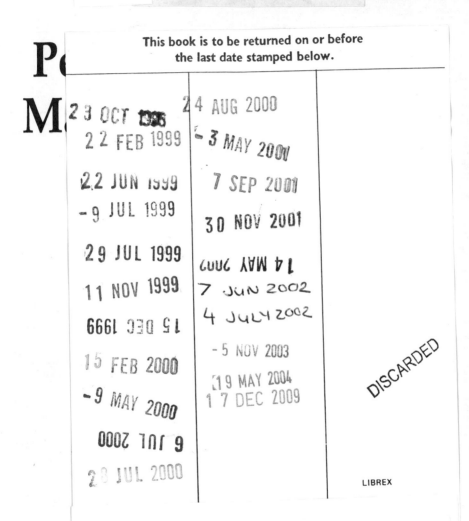
The Library, Ed & Trg Centre   KTW
Tunbridge Wells Hospital at Pembury
Tonbridge Rd, Pembury
Kent TN2 4QJ
01892 635884 and 635489

A member of the Hodder Headline Group
LONDON · SYDNEY · AUCKLAND
Co-published in the USA by Oxford University Press Inc., New York

First published in Great Britain in 1998 by
Arnold, a member of the Hodder Headline Group
338 Euston Road, London NW1 3BH
http://www.arnoldpublishers.com

Co-published in the USA by
Oxford University Press Inc.,
198 Madison Avenue, New York, NY 10016

British Library Cataloguing in Publication Data
A catalogue record for this book is available from the British Library

Library of Congress Cataloging-in-Publication Data
A catalog record for this book is available from the Library of Congress

ISBN 0 340 69254 5

Publisher: Clare Parker
Production Editor: Rada Radojicic
Production Controller: Priya Gohil
Cover Designer: Terry Griffiths

Composition in 10/12pt Palatino by Photoprint, Torquay, Devon
Printed and bound in Great Britain by J W Arrowsmith Ltd, Bristol

Contents

List of contributors   v
Foreword: mapping the territory   vii

Chapter 1   Pain lashes out: a personal story of pain   1
Judith Thwaite

Chapter 2   The pains of living with an artificial limb   18
Claire L. Carter

Chapter 3   Talking about pain   26
Marion V. Smith

Chapter 4   Effective pain management: is empathy relevant?   46
Judith H. Watt-Watson

Chapter 5   Cultural dimensions of pain   66
Bryn D. Davis

Chapter 6   Researching pain: paradigms and revolutions   84
Bernadette Carter

Chapter 7   Psychotherapy, fetal memory and pain   98
Chris Sparks

Chapter 8   Counselling in the management of chronic pain   109
Beatrice Sofaer

Chapter 9   Pain: a feminist perspective?   118
Angela Cotton

Chapter 10   Suffering, emotion and pain: towards a sociological understanding   127
Eileen Fairhurst

Chapter 11   Pain management: training and education issues   142
J. Edmond Charlton

Chapter 12   Organizing acute pain management   153
Ramon Carlo Pediani

Chapter 13   Developing best practice through comparison and sharing   171
Judith Ellis

Chapter 14   The prevention of chronic pain   186
Richard G. Potter

Chapter 15   Child assent, consent and the refusal of painful procedures   195
Marilyn Persson and David Bunting

Chapter 16   Children and their experience of pain   206
Bernadette Carter

Chapter 17   Young people and acute pain   231
              Marjorie L. Gillies

Chapter 18   Pain in later life   243
              Trevor M. Corran and Beatrice Melita

Chapter 19   Fibromyalgia and pain   264
              Angela R. Vale

Chapter 20   Shoulder pain in hemiplegia   278
              Christine Elizabeth Brown

Chapter 21   Constructive management of cardiac pain   294
              Michael Lappin

Chapter 22   The pain of withdrawing from illicit heroin use   306
              Stephen Cromey

List of contributors

Christine Elizabeth Brown SRN, BSc (Hons)
Senior Research Nurse, G Grade, Cheadle, Cheshire, UK

David Bunting RN, BHSc
Consultant Liaison Nurse Practitioner, Starship Children's Health, Auckland, New Zealand

Bernadette Carter PhD, PGCE, RNT, BSc (Hons), RSCN, RGN
Senior Lecturer in Health Care Studies, Manchester Metropolitan University, Elizabeth Gaskell Campus, Manchester, UK

Claire L. Carter BA (Hons), MInst AM
Divisional Administrator, West Yorkshire Police, Drighlington, West Yorkshire, UK

J. Edmond Charlton MB BS, FRCA
Consultant in Pain Management and Anaesthesia, Royal Victoria Infirmary, Newcastle upon Tyne, UK

Trevor M. Corran MA (Clin Psych)
Clinical Psychologist, Private Practice, Leading Pathways, Dandenong, Victoria, Australia

Angela Cotton RMN, BSc (Hons)
Lecturer in Health Care Studies, Manchester Metropolitan University, Elizabeth Gaskell Campus, Manchester, UK

Stephen Cromey RMN, BSc (Hons)
Community Psychiatric Nurse, Wigan Community Drug Team, Wigan, UK

Bryn D. Davis PhD, BSc (Hons), RGN, RMN, RNA
School of Nursing Studies, University of Wales, College of Medicine, Cardiff, UK

Judith Ellis MSc, BSc (Hons), RSCN, RGN, PGCE, RNT
Senior Lecturer/Practitioner (Paediatrics), Preston Acute Hospitals NHS Trust, University of Central Lancashire, Lancashire, UK

Eileen Fairhurst
Department of Health Care Studies, Manchester Metropolitan University, Manchester, UK

Marjorie L. Gillies MSc, RGN, RSCN, DipN
Research Fellow, Department of Child and Adolescent Psychiatry, University of Glasgow, Glasgow, UK

Michael Lappin BSc (Hons), RGN, SEN
Development Leader, Elderwell Unit, Ladywell Hospital, Salford, UK

Beatrice Melita
Clinical Psychologist, National Ageing Research Institute, Victoria, Australia

Ramon Carlo Pediani RGN, DipN, BSc (Hons)
Clinical Nurse Specialist for Acute Pain Control, Blackpool Victoria Hospital, Blackpool, Lancashire, UK

Marilyn Persson RN
Pain Nurse Practitioner, Starship Children's Health, Auckland, New Zealand

Richard G. Potter MB BS (Lond), MRCGP
Principal in General Practice, Cheshire, and Research Fellow, Centre for Primary Health Care, University of Keele, UK

Marion V. Smith BA (Manc), M Phil (Cantab), PhD (Cantab)
Research Fellow, Department of Sociology and Social Anthropology, Keele University, Keele, UK

Beatrice Sofaer RN, BA, PhD, Dip Couns
Reader in Nursing, University of Brighton, and Counsellor, Pain Management Unit, Brighton Health Care NHS Trust, University of Brighton, Faculty of Health, Falmer, East Sussex, UK

Chris Sparks BA, AWMIP
Psychotherapist, Lancaster, UK

Judith Thwaite BA, Cert Educ, Dip Soc Stud, ACP
Writer, Congleton, Cheshire, UK

Angela R. Vale BSc (Hons), RGN
Ward Sister, Rheumatology, Buxton, Derbyshire, UK

Judith H. Watt-Watson RN, PhD
Associate Professor, University of Toronto, Faculty of Nursing, Toronto, Ontario, Canada

Foreword: mapping the territory

This book sets out to explore the geography of pain: to map some of the territory. Maps provide a representation of a landscape and, although they give you a good idea of what features you will find there and what sort of preparations to make, they do not actually let you see the landscape. Whilst they are beautiful in themselves, provide varying amounts of information (some useful, some not) and have often been meticulously researched, nearly all of the subjective beauty, wildness and emotional response that the landscape evokes for individuals is missing. People can agree as to what they think a landscape will look like on the basis of carefully reading a map, and from their own previous experiences of maps and the 'real world'. However, on arrival at the actual area of countryside, its contours, features and presence can still often surprise. Individuals respond differently to different landscapes – the high wild mountains may fill some people with a profound sense of joy, whilst others may be filled with an equally profound sense of terror. A map may impress the onlooker with its crazily winding and closely laced contour lines, but they may be unable to imagine standing on one of those small brown contour lines with a 2000-foot drop beneath them.

Just as maps convey a beautiful, highly functional representation of something which does exist, so do theoretical constructs about pain. Writing and researching pain changes it (regardless of the philosophical paradigm from which the research arises). The only person who can experience the full reality of *their* pain is the person themself. Any report of pain starts to take on a map-like quality. An overwhelming, all-consuming experience starts to become reduced and fragmented – the experience is reduced to 'bits' which can be coded, recorded and documented. The totality is lost.

Other people can never legitimately hope to share the individual's private landscape of pain. However, other people must learn to read the maps effectively. Reading maps requires sound knowledge and a level of imagination if interpretation is to be accurate. (We probably all recognize the map symbol for a church with a steeple – ᛒ – but when we look at the real church in the real landscape we do not expect it to look like a circle with a cross on it.)

This book aims to explore areas of the pain territory that can add to our understanding of people's pain. It explores conceptual and abstract issues such as language, culture and suffering, as well as specific issues related to managing the experience. Each contribution is informed by a wealth of experience and commitment to understanding pain. Each author draws on the literature provided by the early explorers who helped to make the first maps and had the courage to start exploring the territory of pain.

This book does not attempt to 'do everything' – it is not a whistle-stop tour of the landscape of pain. Rather, it encourages the reader to stop, think and look at specific features of the territory, some of which tend to get missed. The 'reader-explorer' will experience something of the personal landscape of pain by reading the chapters by two contributors who have been willing to share their personal experience.[1] These chapters are deliberately placed at the start of the book, as they are the key or the map legend that allows some of the more theoretical perspectives to be placed in context. These chapters help us to keep in focus the fact that it is *people* who *experience* pain. The contributions which follow challenge the reader to consider the nature and complexity of pain, and the equal complexity of so many elements that are an indivisible part of that experience. Conceptual issues are addressed through exploring language, empathy, culture, psychotherapy, counselling and the individual perspective. The means of managing the pain experience are considered by addressing issues related to the educational, organizational and quality aspects. The challenge of the prevention of pain and the ethical issues related to procedural pain are also explored. The territory of pain is explored from a life-continuum perspective as the experience is considered through children, young people and those in their later years. Finally, four different types of pain, and the special challenges that they provoke, are explored. These were not chosen for their representativeness of pain experience, but rather because they provide insight into other issues such as believing other people's pain, intervening appropriately, professional-lay interactions, the vulnerability of people in pain, and the more emotive aspects of pain.

Each contributor offers their own perspective on their own specific area of interest. Each takes a different way through the literature and provides a different map – a different representation of what they see to be the landscape of pain. The map of pain that the reader-explorer takes away with them from this book will be their own. I hope that this book will inform your map of the territory of pain.

Bernadette Carter
January 1998
Lancaster, UK

[1]Claire Carter is my sister. In reading Claire's chapter, I came to know her pain better. Despite being very close to her, there were parts of her story which I did not know, even if I had perhaps guessed them. She says in her chapter that it was painful to write – for me it was intensely painful to read.

For Jonathan
a *true* place in life, my 'herio'

'It is not down in any map: true places never are'
(Melville, H. (1951) *Moby Dick*)

Pain lashes out: a personal story of pain

Judith Thwaite

Introduction

A personal experience of pain must be just that – very personal. I have experienced a wide spectrum which I feel encompasses various types of pain. I am in my fifties, was diagnosed with follicular lymphoma in 1988, and after five relapses am currently in remission. I discovered the lymphoma one day as I was teaching. I rubbed my neck, and my fingers detected a small pea-shaped lump. I was not aware of any nasal, tooth or scalp infections and did not have a cold, which might have caused an enlargement of a lymph gland. When the swelling did not go down I was referred to a consultant. He hinted that I was making a fuss about nothing, but as my son, Mark, had died in 1971 of lymphosarcoma, I was not prepared to be patronized by someone who, whilst not backward about accepting my cheques and giving me regular appointments, was reluctant to do anything about it. It was my GP who encouraged me to demand a biopsy. After 5 months I was admitted to hospital where the gland was removed and examined. The consultant rang me and told me it was malignant. I felt devastated as I put down the phone. I was left with a word but no knowledge of the course of the disease or the prognosis. Like many cancer patients I began to search in my head for reasons why. I was a non-smoker, a vegetarian, walked for miles and was a regular distance swimmer. For a week, until I saw the consultant to have the stitches removed, I fed off my own and other people's fear. I imagined malignant cells spreading and contaminating every part of my body. Nights were especially difficult to cope with. I had no pain from the cancer, but I experienced so much pain of loss, fear and, after caring for my son, an anticipatory fear of dying without relief or dignity.

Pain is an umbrella term that encompasses such a wide variety of sensations that one person's grading on a scale of 0 to 10 could differ widely from that of another. I know that there are times when I can cope better with the same pain. At times of stress, nerves throughout my body set up a jangle of pain. A tooth that was filled last week decides it will stir like a sleeping giant and make its presence felt. Joints stiffen making it difficult to get upstairs. Fingers regularly explore my neck glands for any hint of enlargement and a return of the lymphoma. On a chemotherapy regime any extra pain seems almost too much to bear.

Even among these sensations, pain can be subdivided into categories. Intense physical pain, which is so acute that every other peripheral activity is wiped out, is all-absorbing, making it impossible to escape from it. You cry out for morphine hours before it is due. This is an all-encompassing pain, and no other sensation or feeling is important. All energy is taken up in trying to reduce it. The body seems to shut down all extraneous activity.

Generalized pain can be divided into a background pain, like an old glove that is well worn and familiar, and a dark refracted pain that pervades enough vital functions for the whole body to seem to be affected. The first type may be caused by an old injury that 'plays up', and the second could be triggered by chemotherapy causing so many side-effects that one becomes exhausted. Any chronic pain is bearable for a short period, but grinds down resistance if it is prolonged, especially if there does not seem to be a time limit, and if the cause, progression or outcome of the pain is unknown. Anticipatory pain is induced by fears of future pain or memories of past reactions to pain. These pains cannot be intellectualized for the pain is a body memory path awakened by certain sounds, smells or visual triggers. Mental pain can cause physical pain when one experiences so much that one's body cannot cope with the constant tension and stress. There are general strategies for coping with pain, but each person has to work out the best method to suit his or her constitution and personality. I intend to deal with each of these categories in order, although the different types of pain overlap.

Intense pain

There have been times when I have experienced so much intense pain that, if I had had the means to do so, I would have stopped it drastically – pills or shotgun, it would not have mattered which. For me, the worse pain is not after a serious accident, for after the incident the body's 'shut-down' mechanism can numb the first wave of pain so that, although there is pain, it is often not immediate. I would never have managed to get back to the house after being impaled through the foot if I had felt the pain which I subsequently suffered. By the time I was in a lot of pain, my very competent GP was on the scene. I then felt that both he and I were in control and had the facilities to do something. I no longer felt helpless. A time of intense pain, which jumps to the forefront of my mind, occurred after I came round from a gall bladder operation to find myself attached to various drains and tubes and was unable to move to relieve my back pain, which had me begging for morphine. I could not see an end to the pain. It did not get any easier for 24 hours, and those were the longest 24 hours I have ever experienced. No strategy worked, for to succeed in this you must be in some kind of control. I was too enveloped by pain even to acknowledge anything else. The pain was the centre of a boiling solar system, and I was spinning round it in a trajectory that I could do nothing about. It was far worse than the mess the wound was when it became infected, or the sight of the large haematoma or the releasing of stitches, even though I wondered if my innards would burst out through the gap. It obviously helps to feel that there is a positive friendly presence near your space. After four births, two stand out as painful and frightening. Jennifer Ann was born 6 weeks early. The consultant told me to go home and get my feet up, as I was only having slight contractions and the baby was not ready. The midwife insisted on performing an internal examination as, by size, I was ready. I was young and inexperienced, and very frightened. The baby was born with an explosion of amniotic liquor and died after 3 days. I never held her, and the only thing I have of her to save is a memory:

> One Small Suitcase (excerpt)
>
> I've nothing to put in for Jennifer Ann.
> Not a vest or a shoe
> not a photo or a hospital tag.
> She never touched anything of mine
> before she died – not even my hand.
> Never felt my arms round her
> just a ringlet of bone
> as she shot through
> six weeks early.
> I have her picture in my head
> but it has faded over the years.
> I can't share that with you.
>
> Reproduced with permission from the
> National Poetry Foundation (1996)

In 1974 I had become pregnant again. By then I had lost Jennifer Ann, Mark had died and I had had seven miscarriages. The baby I was carrying was my tenth pregnancy, and although I had adopted two boys, I had no natural live birth to show for my years of childbearing. I went into labour, was taken into hospital on my own, and a nurse at the foot of my bed asked a student if she had 'had any abnormal births'. When the answer was no, she said she would try to induce me before she went off, as I had a 'history'. I had been to natural childbirth classes with my husband, and was coping well before that. She did an internal examination to break the waters, and put me on a drip. I began to get strong contractions and begged them to call home. The contractions were so severe that I turned the drip off after they left, as there was no one in the ward. I was enmeshed in fear, pain and anxiety. I thought that those in power must know that the baby was having problems. I was not in control, and there was no one around to support me. Once my husband arrived I was able to concentrate on organizing pain by following strategies I had worked out previously. I felt in control, and although it was not an easy birth, I don't remember the birth itself as a bad memory, just the horror of being alone and in pain in what I felt was an alien place.

Of all Mark's procedures, the one he most hated – and I hear his screams still – was a bone marrow biopsy. Having had them myself I now know why. Perhaps the very thought of a drill and bit screwing into one's bone, and not a whiff of oblivion to boot, sets one's teeth on edge before the start. The great pressure required, and then the pulling out of marrow, causes pain not only at the site of the biopsy but also along the long bones of the leg. I have not yet had a biopsy in which the core has come out cleanly at the first attempt. To hang on until I think it is finished and then to know it will start all over again, and perhaps again and again after that, is something I also dread. After the first débâcle, when a new houseman tried to take the sample and made a total mess of it, I came to dread this procedure. I now insist that only the haematologist does it. When I wanted to know the differential readings between the first and second test, I was told that the first sample was not good enough for any readings. Now I wave away any learner – they can practise on a cow iliac. A doctor, on her first day at the hospital from Holland, asked me if I had 'night sweets'. She wheeled in the instrument trolley, but she did not inspire me with enough confidence to let her loose on me with a drill. I declined her offer. During subsequent biopsies I have had a friend sitting on one side, and I have asked her to write down my phrases and words which describe the pain.

Bone Marrow Biopsy

Curled up coil tight
pale knees to chest
knotted fists knuckle white
jaw clench-clamped, muscles tensed
waiting for the drill to bite.

The first sharp pain of metal thrust
fiery tip bores pinioned flesh
no resistance to its force
no protection from its lust.

Meets the hip bone, whines with effort
bites into the iliac hard
burns the lumbo sacral ligaments
push to marrow. Flesh? discard.

Pressure exploding down the long bone
mounting pressure, unuttered in-groan
as thick red lymphocytes are drawn.
Send them off in saline liquid
core and clots and marrow slides
to do a test for metastases
try to stem the spreading tide.

Unpublished poem by Judith Thwaite

Perhaps this is good feedback for the doctor, too. I am wary when I know the procedure will be painful and I need to have confidence in the doctor. I do not want the doctor to appear apprehensive, but on the other hand neither do I want an insensitive person who assures me that 'it is nothing'. How much pain one feels does depend on the positive or negative vibes one receives from those around one, be they professional carers or family and friends. I have built a good relationship with the hospital Professor of Oncology and his senior registrar. I respect their expertise, but question them and insist that my own expertise is in listening to and interpreting signs from a body which I have got to know quite well after 50 years. I do not wish to see a different person at every appointment. Rather I choose to wait and see someone I know.

Generalized pain or background pain

It is possible to adapt to pain and learn to push one's pain threshold higher. Children in poor families used to tolerate tight shoes and boots, as there was no cash to replace them. They had to wear shoes and they had to live with pinched feet. After all, Chinese women suffered bound feet. Soldiers bore constant pain in the trenches. If one cannot do anything about it, one has no option but to bear it. If there is no one else who can do anything about it, pain becomes tolerable or one goes under. My uncle used to yell if my aunt took out a splinter, and when he had a carbuncle it was a major incident. He came back from the war with foot rot, along with many of his comrades. He had endured months in what to most people would have been intolerable conditions. Men around him were dying, so his pain was relative. He also had to cope with his pain day after day, so his choices were rather limited. This general pain is more like a nagging toothache, an arthritic pain that has to be lived with because it will always be there, but which sometimes flares up to heights that are incompatible with normal tasks.

Whatever triggers these surges, be it a physical or an emotional cause, the results are exhausting. After chemotherapy and the learned effect on my body of violent raspberry cyclophosphamide pills from a small brown bottle, I now feel nauseous at the sight of those bottles. It is a learned response. I used to have homeopathic remedies in the same type of bottle and had no response to them at all. In fact, I felt that they were beneficial, but could detect no immediate effect. Since the bottles became synonymous in my mind with bad side-effects, despite trying to rationalize the reactions, my stomach churns, even now, at the handling of any small brown bottle.

It always astonished me that my mother keeps a smile even though she is in constant pain from harnessed knees aching and fiery with arthritis. Now I know that it takes a special effort to make sure one does not become criss-crossed with facial pain lines. Sometimes it is a great effort to keep that smile. Of course there are times when background pain is pushed over the edge into chronic pain, with no natural relief.

Continuous chronic pain

Many types of pain are bearable if one knows that there is an end to them. It is the pain with no relief that is so debilitating. Once one can understand why and how the pain is caused, it is not so frightening. Even if painkillers reduce the pain, it is hard to cope with if one is not sure of its cause. I had chest pain. Nothing could be heard with a stethoscope, and my own GP was on holiday. I was experiencing difficulty breathing, and can only describe it as a 'dry drowning'. If it had eased at all I would have been prepared to let time work, but each day I was having problems. I insisted on an X-ray, after which I was sent post-haste to the hospital as glands in my chest had enlarged to such an extent that my lungs looked like chicken shanks. I am normally against taking any pills unless it is absolutely necessary, but at that time I would have taken anything to ease my breathing. If I had been told that a side-effect would be that I would turn green, I would still have gulped them down like an ostrich. Fortunately I obtained relief fairly quickly, and in any case my breathing was not as laboured once I knew treatment was under way. It is the typical dental surgery syndrome – as soon as you sight the surgery, toothache has a tendency to ease.

Chemotherapy induces much generalized pain. Pain which is difficult to pinpoint is often referred pain from other parts of the body. The reason it is so difficult to cope with is that one often does not feel ill before the treatment, but one knows that as soon as the toxic drip has been going for a few minutes one's body will react badly to it. There will often be nausea and dizziness. After particularly aggressive chemotherapy, with so much vomiting that community nurses were coming in morning and evening, and with visits from the Macmillan nurse, my electrolyte balance became very disturbed, causing tremors, shaking and an inability to rest or sleep. One evening I wrote with difficulty a letter to my children, and left a message on my friend's answerphone, as I did not think I would survive the night. I have experienced much worse acute pain, but I could not understand what was happening to my own body.

After Mark died, I knew no pain could ever be as bad as losing a child. I had experienced the depths of despair, and for 2 years coped not only with my pain but also with his. When it was discovered that I had non-Hodgkin's lymphoma in 1988 it was almost a *déjà vu* situation. How many times had I wished that it was me who had his illness – but I had wished for it to be me instead of – not as well as – him. I tried to tell myself that if Mark had coped, then I should too, and how much more frightening it must have been for a child. I had the disadvantage of having walked the road before with the discovery that it was a cul-de-sac.

I was surprised that after surgery when lymph glands were removed from the right side of my neck I was not in any physical pain. Mental pain was at a high, however, and this was highlighted every time friends called.

Like many cancers, the pain comes once one is on chemotherapy. The treatment regime varies according to the kind of cancer, sometimes the peccadilloes of the doctor, and the stage that the cancer has reached. One has to learn to tolerate regular searches by phlebotomists to find veins. If this is straightforward it does not last too long and one knows that it will soon be over. However, most patients range from those who are well and for whom the appointment is a check-up after many 'all-clears', to those who are in the middle of treatment and are not only very anxious about further treatment effects, but also how the last treatment has affected the day's blood count.

If the blood count is too low, there will be no chemotherapy until it recovers – a mixed blessing. Many regard cancer as an alien invader, and delaying treatment means that it will be spreading out of control throughout the body, unseen and invidious. No matter how often visits result in an 'all-clear', there is always apprehension. One can never be blasé about cancer. Mental homeostasis, once shaken after the first diagnosis, is always fragile. Given that there is apprehension if not fear, it is surprising that so many blood samples have a first time hit rate. I have experienced days when, after three attempts, I have had to soak my arm in hot water to bring a vein to the surface. Many of us have elusive veins, and after many months or even years of treatment they collapse quickly. I dread the foraging for a 'hit', especially when a nerve is touched in the process.

With the existence of so many more invasive treatments it seems trite even to mention blood tests. Odd ones are not even retained in the memory, but when so much hinges on the results of such tests in cancer hospitals, one wakes up wondering apprehensively whether by evening one will be knocked to the floor again.

Pain is heightened when one is feeling frightened and also when, in the middle of treatment, one is feeling vulnerable and ill.

Mental pain

There is conflicting evidence as to whether some diseases may be caused by stress. After 8 years as a cancer patient and also working with cancer patients, I am convinced that some cancers are triggered by trauma or a prolonged period of tension. The fear of dying experienced by patients with terminal disease can cause pain and disease in the body. This can be an illusory pain at first but, like migraine, it takes on a pathology of its own. Pain can be caused by seeing someone one loves in great pain, and this too is relative. When my 8-year-old son was dying in hospital, another mother – a nurse no less – was hysterical in the corridor as her child had been diagnosed as a diabetic. I would have liked to have swapped the prognosis I had been given for Mark. At the time I found that mother's reactions, among a group of parents of terminally ill children, insensitive. Years later, when my daughter was hospitalized with viral pneumonia, I too was focused only on her, unable to find space to be aware of other parents' fears when my own child was critically ill.

Thank God it is not possible to relive the acuteness of pain. Like memory, it dims with time. When my 8-year-old son lay on the narrow hospital bed in a large children's hospital, pain was tearing my whole body. It was difficult to breathe or to be aware of peripheral stimuli. Everything focused on a whirling of pain. There was no fear – there was no space for it. My own body was reduced to a head and hands. I wanted to hold my son and suffuse him with energy and warmth. Even after 2 years of bone marrow biopsies and chemotherapy, and the effort it took to keep going, I just could not believe that he was dead.

The effort of trying to turn off a tap of energy results in a physical sag, so that the body has no more vitality left in it than a piece of chewed string. Rarely at that time did one see children die in television hospital dramas. Invariably, science would swoop in at the eleventh hour in the form of Doctor Kildare. There was nothing waiting in the wings for Mark. Why was only one nurse standing mute behind me, instead of rushing forward with resuscitation – and she an agency nurse? Perhaps she was not well qualified. Perhaps she did not know the drill. In the light of day these questions were irrelevant, but if one is alone with one's child and he stops breathing, it is difficult to accept. The fact that one knows he is very ill is immaterial. I had been by my son's side all through his illness, had lived in his room, held him through treatments, swapped beds with him when the hospital bed was too hard for his tender bones, slept with one ear tuned to his every breath, rated staff on a scale of 1 to 10 when they gave him his injections, and now I was just expected to turn off, and go and sit in the children's playroom until a stranger washed him and put a white chrysanthemum in his clasped hands.

Pain lashes out in anger, shock and despair.

In 1971 there was no counselling, but only a young houseman telling me he was sorry my son had passed away. Such euphemisms are patronizing. I needed to understand – why now? Perhaps to be told that he could not be resuscitated because his vital functions had broken down would have helped. One cannot just stop all the force that was essential to keep everything going. Perhaps that is why many who lose family members channel this energy into fundraising, forming support groups for others or taking on a big negligence case. I was offered a cup of tea before being turned out for my taxi to King's Cross, leaving him behind. It was not enough. Yes, the pain has dulled, although it is like a scab – easily knocked off. It was certainly years before I could even think of time with Mark prior to his stay in hospital – back to happier times. I mastered the ability to remember on two levels. The clinical superficial level talking to medical staff never allowed any probe to do more than scratch and disturb the surface of memory. In this mode I was able to communicate intellectually about treatment and drugs. In fact, I had read so extensively on leukaemia and lymphosarcoma that my GP called me to the surgery to discuss presenting symptoms that he had observed in another child.

Later, I fostered two brothers who were haemophiliacs, and became adept at ringing up Wards to order 10 packs of Factor VIII to be thawed prior to our arrival. I became a master of the facial veneer. On the other hand, it was years before I could even write about Mark, and even now it brings on physical effects, notably the feeling of an imminent explosion in my throat. Buried grief does take its toll.

These days television programmes are more realistic – children die in them, and expectations are not so high. We are not back to the years of naming all children with the same name because of poor survival rates, but we are not cushioned by a Hollywood interpretation of a children's ward. Pain is dulled but not forgotten, for those beaten neural paths are as deeply trodden as the ancient terrace paths that can still be seen from aircraft centuries after their use.

Memories are not in such sharp focus, but they will not be wiped out until, or unless, long-term memory is affected. Even Mark's face is not so clear, although I often catch a glimpse of him on another child's lips.

Delayed pain

During one course of treatment when my white cell count was down to 1000, I stepped back on some old timber in the garden. A 6 inch nail went through my shoe, through the ball of my foot and came out at the top, so that I was impaled on the plank. I fell into an area overgrown with nettles and briars and had difficulty in pulling free. I could feel blood in my shoe, but shock acted as a barrier to the transmission of pain messages. I managed to walk back 75 yards to the house and telephone the surgery to say that I needed a tetanus jab. My daughter drove me to the surgery, and by that time, after I had been able to recreate the scenario in my head, the pain had become intense. I was still able to hold a planned meeting at the house that evening, although I could not put my foot to the floor. By the next day painkillers had no effect on the pain. I was alone in the house, and in between periods of hallucinatory wanderings I called the hospital and talked to my oncologist. He said that I should come in immediately. Owing to the severe pain in my leg, I had to slither down the stairs. Toxic shock caused the hallucinations, and drips and 7 days of transfusions confined me to a hospital bed. I did say that I hoped I was not receiving blood from a meat-eater, as I was vegetarian. My white cell count dropped down to 300, and for a few days I was in a great deal of pain. Obviously drips had to be put up immediately and therapy started on a 'guesstimate' until the laboratory report came back, but as I knew that antibiotics were passing into me, not chemo drugs, I had great faith that each hour would bring an improvement. My low white cell count did sound very low to me, so I asked the senior registrar how low it would have to dip before I 'kicked the bucket'. His reply that 'he did not think I would drop off my perch yet' made me laugh, and after the visit of the medical photographer, who came to record my foot for posterity, I wrote a poem about it. The staff were hoping to include that poem and their article in the *British Medical Journal*.

I had a positive attitude to this treatment, and could cope with the pain despite having to have cannulas inserted four times in my wrist, forearm and hand, as the veins kept collapsing. It is very important to me that I remain a person and not a number in a hospital situation. Hospital staff get very touchy if one dares to voice this view. They think that it is an indictment of the hospital or of their care.

In the first booklet, entitled PATCHWORK (mentioned later), which is an acrostic for Poetry At The Christie Hospital, there was a poem which included the following lines:

> I won't be a number
> I'll make them know my name.

Although there had been months of discussion with the management, as they had the proof manuscript for weeks, they banned the booklet because of these words. It was my poem, and I was devastated at first, as I thought that patients should be encouraged to work through the different stages. One experiences reactions of grief, loss, aggression and anger when one first hears that one has a terminal illness. This is why support groups flourish, because no one censors members' thoughts or forces them to adopt a 'chocolate-box' response. Now I am pleased that I have joined the ranks of other poets banned for their beliefs. After many more talks we brought out the second issue without any restrictions, and have now produced 20 editions which are distributed all over the UK as well as abroad, and contributors range in age from 8 to 90 years, with poems from both patients and carers. I was the winner of the North West of England Whitbread Volunteer Action Award for the booklet and other voluntary work that I do. The voice of the patient and carer has not been gagged, and both are free to express their pain or joy in print.

The fear of losing one's identity is very strong, in direct proportion to the amount of pain experienced. When pain takes over, one's ability to control both oneself and the immediate environment deteriorates. In other professions, such as the police and education, clients or service users (the politically correct term seems to change) are vulnerable, but nowhere is one as vulnerable as in hospital. All professionals have their jargon which excludes the client, and if one was detained in custody it would be easier to get representation. In hospital – you complain – the bedpan could just be an hour or two getting to you. You also have to take on trust that medication is correct or that nothing untoward happens if you are under anaesthetic. A friend of mine had read a report of work at the John Radcliffe Hospital in Oxford, where it was shown that patients on the operating table recover faster if positive affirmations are repeated, even though they are under anaesthesia. She asked that the staff be positive while she was on the table, rather than discussing their plans for the weekend. When I had to have the right axillary lymph nodes removed to check that the lymphoma had not changed in character, I added a codicil to the consent form when I noticed the small print on the reverse. I wanted no other procedures carried out, especially by students practising internal examinations. I felt that, as it is my body, I had a right to do this. I realize that in a busy ward, often short-staffed, it is difficult to treat patients as individuals, but whereas the removal of lymph nodes is a 'piddly' operation on that day's list, it is very traumatic for the patient. Other treatment may hinge on the outcome after laboratory tests.

Strategies for coping and the positive aspects of empowerment

There are strategies to lessen pain or to reduce its effects, and affirmations to enable one to feel more in control. Of course, these will vary with each person.

It makes me feel in control if I ask questions. While I recognize the expertise of the consultant, I think of him or her as a facilitator to enable me to get well – not as a god. The doctor has knowledge of various treatments at his or her disposal, just as I have knowledge of my field. I am of equal worth to anyone in the hospital. My IQ does not drop by 30 points just because I push through the double doors. If the doctor refers to me by a first name, I reciprocate. When I was diagnosed with cancer, I would look at myself in the mirror or catch sight of my reflection in a shop window and know that I looked like exactly the same person from the outside, but something which I could not control was growing inside. I felt that I could neither see it nor stop it. I anticipated that I would reach a stage when my young daughters who were 12 and 13 years old then would find it difficult to talk to me about it. I was determined to discuss things with them rationally whilst I was still fairly fit. My way of coping is to laugh, and for 90 per cent of the time I can use the power of laughter, even though it may sometimes be black humour. I asked my daughters if they thought I would look good in a Tina Turner wig. They would cry at first, or have nightmares about me dying, and they would creep into my bed at night. Night-time was the most difficult time for me, too. Despite reassuring them, I would wonder if I would be with them at Christmas and for their next birthday, or around for them during GCSEs and A levels. I knew those early-hour imagination projections were doing me no good. I applied to go to the Bristol Cancer Help Centre. It was the best move I ever made. The week was assigned to healing sessions (which I would like to think did some good, but am still not sure about), relaxation, music and art therapy, visualization sessions, biofeedback, foot massage and sessions explaining aromatherapy and Bach flower remedies. We were each assigned a personal counsellor and had long sessions with the doctor. I had been asked on my first visit to the cancer hospital if I would like to receive counselling. I was pleased to say 'Yes'. I am still waiting 8 years on. When I asked again, I was told that they thought I did not need it as I seemed well balanced. They did not anticipate that perhaps I was just practised at putting on an artificial front. What Bristol achieved for me was threefold. It enabled me to talk about fears that I could not express to close family or friends, who were full of admiration at how well I was 'coping'. Having once invented this persona, I could not destroy it. It also gave me strategies for coping in the early hours of the morning. I need not lie there in fear, trying to cry silently so as not to disturb anyone. Now I could visualize my own healing. I was not a passive body to which things were happening. I was in charge of me and I could, by mind control, influence the outcome. I could control pain by escaping somewhere else. Well, that was the idea. Usually it worked.

The most long-lasting effect was that I had control of my treatment. One of the statements made at Bristol was that all treatment is negotiable. This body is mine, and I do not have to have anything done to it that I do not want. I have exercised this option on occasion when I have felt the strength of the drugs has been gauged too high for me. I decide if the strength needs to be reduced, because only I can tell the effects on my body.

The counsellor at Bristol encouraged me to take a good look at my lifestyle. I could see that I had been an earth-mother figure all my life. The eldest of five,

I learned while young to care for others, and that continued all my life. I was a staunch supporter of many voluntary groups, on the committees of many groups to support my children, belonged to PTAs, Scouts, Brownies, ran foster groups, etc. I did not resent this involvement. In fact, within a few months of being diagnosed with cancer, I put my name forward as a parent governor at my daughters' comprehensive school. I decided that it would be a sort of talisman to guard me if I was elected. I topped the poll by a very large majority. I intend to serve my 4 years. This is a sign, I thought. I shall survive that long at least. I became chairman.

With so many people drawing on me and teaching on supply, I knew when I stood back to reassess my lifestyle that I had left no space in the schedule for myself. What did I really want to achieve, now that I had to telescope my ambitions into a more compacted life? I had no intention of abandoning every dream. I decided that I wanted to spend more time writing and painting. Within weeks of my stay at Bristol I had booked on to a residential course for writers at an Arvon Centre at Heptonstall. I was very green and apprehensive.

I discovered that I could use writing as a tool to fight and cope with pain. I could not eliminate it, but perhaps I could make it more tolerable. My first published poem was about vulnerability. Soon after diagnosis I had felt as if I was bound to a wheel gathering speed down a slope and unable to pull off. Words were and are important for me to come to terms with pain and fear. I found that, as the hospital had such a large catchment area, people in the out-patients department were packed back to back, with not much communication between them. I felt very isolated. I decided to try to break down this barrier by putting up notices to encourage others who might enjoy writing to contact me. About five individuals replied before the notices were removed, and one of them, an art lecturer and a patient at the hospital, offered help in getting a group started. It was a great goal. We soon discovered that it was impracticable to hold writing groups at the hospital.

People came from too far away, and one of the stress factors of out-patients is the long wait that involves sitting in rows in out-patients and on the ward, hanging around for treatment, and never knowing at what time one would be called or what state one would be in afterwards. We decided to begin a booklet that would consist mainly of poetry and journal entries, to be open to anyone whose life was or had been affected by cancer.

It was already apparent that carers are under a tremendous amount of stress, too. Had I not had 3 days of stress migraines after every bone marrow biopsy or lumbar puncture that Mark experienced? I had used words then to try and write out the pain. Nothing seemed to halt the crashing lights and vomiting once the early signs of pain above the eye and tense neck muscles began. Only an injection could halt the constant sickness. The pattern was only interrupted by acupuncture from a trained acupuncturist GP who saw me regularly and gradually tapered off the visits. After 30 years of the most horrendous pain, when I was sure that I must have a brain tumour because the pressure in my head was so great, I was clear of migraine. I am a great believer in the power of words, both written and spoken. If you can speak about pain and fear, there is relief in that.

Lying in a 4-bed ward with only flimsy curtains separating one patient from another, I cringe at the dialogue I hear. *'Hello Betty. How are we?'*. *'I'm all right, thank you doctor.'* They are obviously not all right. They are in for treatment. Hospital staff do seem to adopt the 'Royal We' and expect an affirmative response. If I am not well, I refuse either to see a houseman or be seen in a communal ward for an out-patient clinic appointment. It is distressing to have to form relationships when one is ill. Obviously in emergencies this is not a priority, but during a long-term illness there should be continuity. I will not discuss my vaginal thrush with the world and his dog on the other side of a curtain. I have heard really painful internal procedures, causing a patient to cry out, just behind a cotton drape. It makes everything so much worse if one has no privacy. In this situation I walk out, saying that every patient is entitled to expect privacy.

Unfortunately, at the large cancer hospital I attend, the Patient Satisfaction Committee, which is probably a paper response to the Patients' Charter, has no patient representative on it. Patients are not even allowed to have the name and telephone number of the community health representative who has been nominated to be the voice of patients. How can there be genuine feedback if stooges have to speak for patients? Can policemen speak for prisoners, or lecturers for students?

Pain reduction techniques

I have long felt that some pain can be eased by using various techniques. When I am writing I can be so totally immersed in work that I am unaware that my leg is twisted, my hand is clenched, or that I have lower back pain spasms caused by being thrown across a taxi when its near side was opened up like a tin of baked beans.

The same principle applies when one is lying in bed feeling terrible and a visitor pops round the door. It is possible to put some pain on the back boiler and relegate it to background pain.

Dr Robin Phillips from the epidemiology unit at Bristol University is working on a link between pain and poetry in research sponsored by the World Health Organization. His team has shown that either reading or writing poetry reduces the need for painkillers. It may be a while before doctors hand out a haiku or a ballad to patients instead of distalgesics but, although when I am in a lot of pain I cannot be distracted by any external factor, just above that level being absorbed in writing can alleviate pain. One thing I find difficult in long-term illness is the linkage factor. Not only does one link certain objects, such as bottles, to pain, but places too. I was determined to break this link when I had to have a core biopsy in the theatre. I had discovered a lump on the right breast, and various opinions suggested that it could be a lipoma, primary breast carcinoma or a return of lymphoma.

I would like to have had the nerve to treat it solely with complementary medicine, but as there was talk of a lumpectomy I decided to go ahead with surgery. I wanted a fine-needle biopsy, but was persuaded that this would not show a clear enough sample for histology. After talking it through, I opted for a tru-cut biopsy and was booked in. There would be no general anaesthetic, so I asked if a friend could be admitted to the operating theatre, not to hold my hand, but merely to be a friendly presence. The surgeon agreed, and Annabelle sat just inside the door. I took in my own collection of poetry and organized where the green cloths would be so that they would not impede my holding the book, as I intended to read through the book aloud during the procedure. I managed this with one hand. It was very reassuring to read my own poetry and, apart from the odd gasps, to read non-stop. It took eight cores before the surgeon obtained a suitable one. The theatre staff were a bit bemused, but supportive. At the end the surgeon said, '*Well I have never heard of anyone doing this before.*' '*Aren't you glad I'm not an opera singer.*' I replied. I would have found this very difficult to cope with because of the number of attempts. One relaxes after each extraction, and it is a blow to realize that one needs to tense up all over again. After a few attempts one begins to wonder whether the surgeon will ever manage to obtain any worthwhile sample. I felt that I imprinted my personality in the theatre. I exerted some control over how the procedure went, and was not a passive recipient of surgery. It is very important to me to be an individual. I do not want to lose my identity when I walk into a hospital. Most hospitals pay lip service to individuality, but in practice one is a damn nuisance if one refuses to go along quietly with the flow. Of course this applies to other large institutions that deal with the public, but perhaps health centres and hospitals can impose their system more easily, as the people they deal with are so vulnerable. Anyone who is frightened or in pain, or even anticipates that they may be in pain in the future, is going to think twice before antagonizing those who hold the power. One is not in a very strong position when hooked on a drip and reliant on the good nature of someone to come when one rings a bell.

I have been quite ill in hospital but, up to now, have been able to keep true to 'me'. After the third cannula insertion due to the drip seeping into tissues I had waited 3 hours after I was due to have another bag hooked on the drip. The houseman said that she was too tired after so many hours on duty and was going off. She would send someone from another ward. When a young white-coated lad came on the ward asking for me I insisted on checking his credentials, telling him that he could be someone off the street with delusions of grandeur. It cheers me up if, when I feel apprehensive, I am comfortable enough with myself to express these feelings.

I was able to laugh about the experience. Now I think back to it with amusement and not fear. Although I do gain help from complementary therapies, they are not usually of immediate benefit and are more effective during chronic rather than acute pain. For me, intense pain needs a more orthodox approach. I have been very lucky to live close to a hospital which is regarded as a centre of excellence. I know I can turn up there if I am in pain. At the day ward I am greeted by name by some staff, and to me that is important. In any large institution there are bound to be some staff who, whether by design or ignorance, seem to go out of their way to shuffle one into categories and ignore personal input. Sometimes it is hard work to ensure that this does not happen. I try to guard against it, and resist any efforts to reduce me to a number. This has certainly paid off at the hospital, and most of the staff and I have built up a mutual respect for each other. Fear and pain are often very closely inter-twined, and respect for a patient eases both. When I am at home I rely heavily on my GP, who is not only very supportive, but has an open mind to new ideas, will listen to me and is willing to explore complementary treatment. On occa-sions he came to see me during severe reactions to 'chemo' when he was off duty, so I was not seen by an unknown locum. He gave me his home telephone number at this time, and this had the effect of making me feel in control. I knew that if the pain was unbearable I could obtain help. I never used it. I was able to think – I'll just manage another hour (and then another) before I call. In this way I was able to get through. Had I not had that reassurance I would have called for help on some evenings, afraid that I could not cope during the night. I need to know as much about the disease and its accepted treatment as possible. I do not want a prognosis. I am not a library book needing a date stamp. I know I shall not make old bones, but so long as I have caring medics around me, like my GP and friendly staff at the surgery and hospital, I am confident that I can cope with the final time.

The high-street pharmacist I use has the computer software known as Patient Information Leaflets (PILs), which enables him to print out leaflets detailing a two-page spread of drug information, some illnesses and milder conditions that do not necessarily need a drug therapy. These leaflets were designed to be read by laymen, and are not interspersed with 'gobbledegook'. It is important to me to be able to use this and to feel that I can go in to see the pharmacist at any time and ask for information on a variety of treatments. He will tell me what is on the market to control sickness, for example, as well as the side-effects. When I had great problems with drug-induced cystitis, I despaired of resting for more than 3 minutes at a stretch, but he explained just what was happening and suggested remedies that I could try. He never pushes drugs on me, even suggesting types of food that could help. It is important to me to have a support system, and I feel that both my GP and my pharmacist are part of that system. I feel comfortable and confident with their help and advice. I need to feel that I am involved in any treatment – to accept it or not – and I need to feel that those treating me care about me as a person. Pain is easier to bear under these circumstances.

I do rely on techniques learned at the Bristol Centre – not all the time, but at times when I am fragile in mind or body. I am concerned about keeping 'me' going, and if this slews statistics – tough. Just as my daughter, who is asth-matic, has to concentrate on breathing during an attack, I use visualization to enable me to control pain and to get through long nights of 'chemo'. Visual-ization as practised at the Bristol Cancer Help Centre starts with a relaxation exercise, and when the body is in a relaxed state the mind is trained to find a place of peace and safety. Obviously this place is different for each person. With red hair and a fair skin, sunning on a tropical beach would be my idea of hell, but a wonderful place for some of my friends. Instead, I visualize either a spring meadow full of wild flowers or, if I feel more in need of clearing out illness, it could be a hilltop with warm winds filling me with health. I find water healing, both the sound of it and the feel of it, so I visualize standing beneath the warmth of a gentle waterfall on a hot day. I visualize it cleansing every part of me. Many tapes suggest that one envisages colour swirling through one's body, but for the life of me I cannot find a colour, apart from the sunlight, that remotely seems to heal. Green is supposed to be a healing colour, but the thought of swirls of green remind me only of a pea soup fog, and I associate yellow with the sulphurous clouds that used to hover above an Iron and Chemical Company I remember as a child. One has to find something that one is comfortable with. I listen to every tape before I expect to drop into a deep relaxation. I know of one facilitator who has a voice like a cracked cup, and by the time I have listened to that tape for 10 minutes every muscle is tense, and I spend the time debating the merits of strangulation or suffocation.

Self-hypnosis as I practise it is one step on from visualization. Both are reputed to ease physical discomfort, and research studies have shown that many ailments in which tension and anxiety are factors can be eased by them. Colitis, migraine, stomach ulcers and high blood pressure have been shown to be helped in this way.

My daughter finds her own version of self-hypnosis is helpful during an asthma attack. It is extremely frightening if she is on her own in a high-rise student flat in the midst of Manchester and she cannot breathe. She has been lucky that both at home and in the city she has had caring GPs. Both my daughters, being scientists (one a pharmacist and the other a microbiologist), tended to look askance at complementary medicine until they both suffered torticollis neck spasms. My first daughter was in such pain that I had to ring round and borrow a neck collar before I could help to dress her and get her to hospital. She was fitted with her own collar and sent off with very strong painkillers. An acupuncturist, who is also a GP, made a space in his busy schedule for her after 3 days when the pain had not eased. She accompanied me reluctantly, muttering words like 'mumbo-jumbo'. She could hardly bear him to remove the collar. He inserted one needle after finding the correct point, moved her neck whilst pressing an acupressure point, and the intense pain ceased instantly. She did not need the collar again. The words 'miracle cure' replaced 'mumbo-jumbo'. My other daughter thought it could be coincidence until, in the midst of degree finals, she also had neck spasm and could not even move her head to look at notes, let alone write, and she was in a lot of pain. Dr Cotton saw her on a Saturday, and although her case was more complicated and required needles at a number of points, she too obtained relief as soon as the treatment was finished. Many people from the Cancer Support Group that I attend have been treated by this practitioner, including a friend with prostate cancer that had spread to the bones. He was in the terminal stage, and was in a lot of pain which was not totally controlled allopathically. These drugs were making him like a zombie and causing gastric problems. Acupuncture enabled him to cut down on them, so that the latter part of his life was more bearable and dignified.

I obtain pain relief from shiatsu, moxibustion, homeopathy and reflexology, and despite orthodox scepticism I will use them not as total therapy but as complementary therapy. It does not worry me that all orthodox practitioners do not agree with me. If I find that regular visits to the Homeopathic Hospital enable me to be treated as a whole person, then I shall continue to visit. It does not help my total well-being when specialist hospitals will only focus on one part of me. All parts of me are interrelated.

Conclusions

We all cope with pain in different ways, and we have varying strategies to cope with it. Acute intense pain is all-encompassing. Reactions to it are almost reflexive. We cannot help but disregard any other sensations or feelings. Socializing and the use of accepted responses to pain are not much help when pain is intense. One can neither remember the stiff upper lip nor does one care. There is an imprinted response which is triggered. Only when the pain is easing can any learned reactions be used. Chronic intense pain that seems never-ending can result in feelings of '*I can't cope with this any more*'. Many of my friends have decided that they will not have any more chemotherapy because the side-effects are so bad and only serve to prolong life for a short time. They have made a decision that the treatment is not worth the pain. 'Quality not quantity' is their response if they are encouraged to have yet another course. The nagging familiar pain is easier to bear, especially if there is relief at times. Sometimes resting or lying in a hot bath provides some respite, or painkillers may do so. Unfamiliar pain is frightening just because of the fear of what it may indicate. Once it can be named it is often easier to bear. People react in different ways to pain and long-term illness. I chose an aggressive way to fight, but some would rather try to deny it or to accept it as their lot in a stoical way, while others throw in the towel in a negative response. There is no right or wrong way. Studies have shown that people who fight and those who deny survive longer. I feel that constant pain does accentuate the differences between personalities. I find it hard to overhear patients being browbeaten, but perhaps they would not be comfortable with my responses. I cannot say what is right for them – only what I think is right for me.

Only I know my own body. I can listen to it and I know the effect of drugs on it. I do not intend to relinquish the responsibility for it to others. Treatment is negotiable, and I hope that I can continue to control pain by any means I choose.

Further Reading

National Poetry Foundation 1996: *Clapping in the wings*. London: National Poetry Foundation.

Patchwork. A quarterly booklet of poetry for and by cancer patients. Obtainable from the Christie Hospital, Manchester.

The pains of living with an artificial limb

Claire L. Carter

Introduction

Up until the age of 21 years I lived a pretty active life. I attended university and, like many other students, participated in a range of outdoor activities such as rock-climbing and fell-walking, as well as a fairly varied indoor sports repertoire of squash and swimming and, less frequently, jogging. Having finished university, and prior to taking up a position as a police constable, I was on holiday in northern Scotland when, as a pedestrian, I was run down by a speeding motorcyclist. The foot pedal caught me at the rear of my left calf and severed my leg, leaving it attached by only an inch and a half piece of skin. After an emergency operation followed by a month in hospital, I then spent 5 months recuperating and getting used to an artificial limb. Six months after the accident I had a new job, was living on my own and was beginning to try to get on with my life.

Today, 14 years on, I live a normal existence and encounter only minor problems. I still go swimming, have been climbing and caving, and I regularly walk, although I now restrict the distance to 4 to 5 miles. I have walked up Snowdon, and indeed have climbed Mt Toubkal, the highest peak in North Africa, since the accident. However, long walks and other activities which are 'hard' on my leg create pain and discomfort and affect my working life to such a degree that I no longer consider that pushing myself to the point where my stump really suffers can be justified. This was a *personal* decision. Initially, I spent many years proving to other people and, if I am really honest, mainly to myself that I could do anything. It took me a long time to realize that I was still the same person inside and did not have to outdo more able people in order to be accepted.

In trying to write about my experiences it is worth explaining the different types of pain (both physical and emotional) that I experienced, the treatments and the nursing care I received and, importantly, how I felt, what helped me to get through the tough times and what sorts of things did not help at all. I found this chapter really difficult to write, and at times I did not want to finish it, as it has brought back some painful memories and emotions that I had previously buried.

I reiterate that this is a personal viewpoint and I cannot speak for other individuals, although I will occasionally refer to the other people I meet on my rare visits to the hospital for 'repairs' and other clinic appointments. I have written from a non-professional perspective, as I do not have a medical background. My own professional expertise is in management and my degree, which I gained just before the accident, is in geography. The title of this chapter, and the topic itself, may suggest that my life is dismal – this is *not* so. I believe that life does go on and can be lived to the full. I think I am a more understanding person as a result of the changes in my life, and hopefully, by sharing some of my thoughts and experiences, you (the reader) may be able to understand a little more about people like me.

Emotional memories and physical feelings

Pain is difficult to remember as an actual feeling. When the accident happened the pain was intense – I certainly knew all about it and it was very real. However, after a period of time healing starts and the level of pain decreases and whilst one knows it hurt, it is really difficult to remember the pain accurately. What I actually remember is all the other things linked with the pain, especially the level of fear relating to it. Perhaps it is like being bitten by a dog and being afraid of dogs for the rest of one's life. I am sure people do not remember the pain of the bite itself, but rather the fear that incident brings about. I am not sure why this is – perhaps it is the body's way of healing. Whatever it is, the emotional memories are intense and still affect me. Probably the best way to explain this point is for me to describe something that happened to me about 4 years ago.

I was going to bed one evening, had taken off my artificial limb and was sitting on the edge of the bed fiddling with the alarm clock or something trivial when I decided that I needed something from the other side of the room. I had completely forgotten that I had removed the leg, and set off to walk. I fell heavily on to the end of my stump. The pain I experienced can only be described as excruciating, I was shocked and frightened and – I suppose – became a little hysterical, screaming for help although I knew there was nothing anyone could do. Two points about this incident were frustrating. Because of the painful swelling and bruising, I had to resort to using crutches for 3 weeks. I found this difficult as I was busy at work, had a full diary of interviews to conduct, and was working in a department I had only recently joined.

The other point about this fall was that it took me straight back to the time I was in hospital, when I fell one night while trying to walk to the bathroom. I was in a large mixed ward with no means of attracting the attention of the night-staff other than shouting loudly and waking up about 30 other people. I decided to get to the bathroom on my own. I suppose that, being tired and on painkillers, I thought I was steadier than I really was. Anyway, the outcome was that I fell and screamed so loudly that I woke everyone up and was taken straight back to bed. The nurses were very unsympathetic and did not realize that I was very frightened. Twelve hours later, despite the fact that I had asked the nurses to check that the stump was OK and to reassure me that I had not damaged it, no one had done anything at all, even though blood had soaked through all the thick padding and bandages. As well as my having to deal with anxiety about the possibility that I had damaged the healing stump, the staff nurse decided that I did not need any painkillers until the evening session, and she refused to give me the ones I was prescribed for midday. I do not like taking drugs, and I desperately wanted to get better, but this lack of care and heartless attitude caused me the greatest upset in my entire stay in hospital. I think it was on this occasion that I first broke down in tears when my twin sister visited. I actually felt guilty about letting her down and allowing her to see how upset I really was. She took one look at me and ran out of the ward. I was very upset that the lack of nursing care and provision of pain relief on this occasion not only affected me but also had such a bad effect on a member of my family. All the other nursing staff were very kind and took time to talk to me.

I believe it is these two experiences that make me so nervous now of falling. I really hate icy weather, and have decided I will give skiing a miss! In fact, simply thinking about these two falls, despite the amount of time that has elapsed since then, still makes my stomach churn slightly – I feel physically sick if I dwell on these situations. Writing this account was difficult.

For me, the whole scenario of fear and emotions is inextricably linked to the actual feeling of pain, and I believe that these elements are remembered more vividly than the actual 'ouch' element.

The other problem associated with falling is that if one is wearing a limb, it usually 'pops off', and this means one ends up feeling humiliated and sitting in a public place with one's limb, as in Murphy's law, just out of reach. What is even more exasperating is that one minute one is not even thinking about it, and the next minute one's disability has in no uncertain terms slapped one in the face and brought back difficult memories. I shall never manage to walk across a nicely polished dance floor, a stage, a shining supermarket floor, or even wet stone paving slabs without some level of trepidation. I really have to concentrate on walking safely in these conditions.

I remember the actual accident, almost in short photosnaps of the event. I presume I was not conscious all the time, although I vividly remember someone telling a friend in a very loud voice not to look as it was a horrible sight. That really worried me, as no one could or would tell me what was happening. I remember looking at my leg and seeing the bone sticking through, although I did not know that my foot was twisted all the way round. Fortunately, my friend covered the leg with a jacket. I do remember seeing quite a large pool of blood and desperately trying to work out how much was actually there. I was fascinated by the fact that it was congealing from the outside of the pool inward.

The next memory perhaps sounds 'corny', and it is not something I have told people about before. I remember lying in total darkness. I was not afraid, just very relaxed – it was like lying on the edge of a shelf. I felt that it would be bad if I rolled backwards and that I had a choice – either to answer the voice that kept asking me my name, or just to give up and black out. In retrospect, I presume this feeling of lethargy was due to the dose of heroin I was given, as well as to the welcome amounts of gas and air.

I remember very little about the rest of the day of the accident itself, apart from someone cutting off my trousers, putting a drip in and getting me to sign something with my left hand. I remember waking up at some point later on and seeing my family there, then waking up again and seeing a large frame over the end of the bed. I have no recollection of being told about the amputation, although I do remember waking up later on my own and thinking that, in the movies, this is where I am supposed to look under the blankets and find out – this I duly did. I do not remember being shocked – it was as if I already somehow knew. Whilst I was in hospital there was so much going on that I did not really have much time to dwell on my situation. Things seemed to progress reasonably well, despite the need for a second operation; all I wanted to do was go home, and I was grateful when the day finally arrived. It was not until then that things really hit home and I realized how much I had to deal with. I was sitting in the car outside the house with all my family inside, delighted to have me back home, when I realized that I was never going to get my leg back – I was never going to get 'better' in the full sense of the word.

Support and encouragement

The level of support from my friends and, in particular, from my family was the most important element in my recuperation and in helping me to deal with the situation. Although I have always been the kind of person who gets on with a situation, I would never have made it without all their support. I am sure that at times I was unco-operative, uncommunicative and downright horrible to them, but they never complained. I spent quite a lot of time thinking about things, and I have never been one really to discuss my feelings. The other pressure I felt was that they had all given up so much in order to support me. The whole family travelled from London to the Orkney Isles to be 'there' for me; they kept me constantly cheerful. An early joke was when a nurse, about 5 days after the operation, asked me how tall I was. Quick as a flash, my sister replied that it depended which leg I stood on! Despite their support I did not want to upset my family, and I think that the pressure of trying not to let them know how upset I felt on occasion was the hardest thing of all.

The other factor was that after I came out of hospital I received no more official support to help me along. I did not know anyone else in the same position and I felt that it would be weak to ask for help. In fact, all the time I was in hospital it was only the nurses, with their general caring chatter, who provided any real support or care. Whether or not I would have accepted any offers to talk about how I was or was not coping I do not know. However, I am certain that, for people in the same position as me but without the support of a close family, such a situation must be very frightening. They must feel desperately lonely.

There's nothing phantom about the pain!

Within the first 2 weeks of the accident I was up and about, either in a wheel-chair or making my early attempts on crutches, which involved going to a gym-type area and pulling weights and so on. I enjoyed this and it took my mind off things, making me feel a little more as if I was back to a normal routine. The main problems I encountered at this stage were phantom pains (more of these later) and difficulty in trying to lower my leg to make the stump hang vertically. When I was first asked to do this I was surprised how painful it was (up until then I had had my leg supported and sticking out in front of me). Nobody had thought to warn me that it would hurt, and it took quite a bit of coaxing before I was prepared to try a second time. I suppose it was so painful because it was bruised and swollen and there was fluid running down into the area. Anyway, all my nerves were shouting: '*Stop! – What's happening?*' After a few days of trying to lower my leg for short periods of time the pain decreased. However, it was still much easier to rest with the stump resting on a pillow raised up slightly. One thing I should mention is that to this very day I hate the word 'stump'. There is something degrading and almost coarse or vulgar in its intonation. None of my family, early on, seemed to like to use the word – it was rather as if it was a taboo word. This was soon made light of since, for some reason, my stump was nicknamed 'Charlie' by my father, and the name has stuck to this day. The other thing about 'Charlie' is that I can look at it closely to rub it better when it aches, or to examine the scar tissue and sore areas. In fact, I view it at this level in almost a clinical and detached way. I still hate to see myself in a mirror or in photos without the limb on. It is as though that person is not me.

In those early days I was administered fairly strong painkillers on a regular basis, and they were very effective in allowing me to deal with the emotional issues. However, once the level of painkillers was reduced there seemed to be a constant background of pain. It was not a particularly severe pain – more of a dull ache – but it was a constant nagging pain that went on for hours. This still occurs, particularly if I have walked a long way, which for me is about 5 miles. Looking back I cannot tell which is worse, the shorter periods of severe pain or the longer periods of constant pain. The constant pain is very tiring and chips away at all one's resolve to be positive and to cope. Alongside the background pain there were often feelings of cramp.

I personally consider that phantom pain is poorly named since, for me, there is *nothing* phantom about it. In the early days it was very painful and felt like a mixture of cramp, pins and needles and a stabbing pain, as if someone was stabbing me with a large needle. What still frustrates me is that it occurs in the area that has been amputated. This means that not only do I have to cope with the leftover parts, but the part that has been removed *will not let me forget about it*. In the first few weeks the phantom pains occurred on a regular basis every few hours, lasting for perhaps 30 to 40 minutes. I actually felt a stabbing in my toes that were not there. The sensation is about 18 inches below the end of the stump. In my case the cramps seemed to be in exactly the spot where the bone was protruding through the skin at the scene of the accident.

I tried various methods to stop the pain. The standard painkillers would numb everything else, but did not touch the phantom pains. I remember desperately asking for some pain relief from one of the doctors who said that it was difficult, as there was nothing there to treat and it was almost one of those things that I would have to get on with. People said that the pains would go as soon as my brain realized that the leg was not there and so would eventually stop sending the messages. I tried dropping heavy books near to the end of the stump to jolt my unconscious into action, and I asked people to sit where the leg should have been. I would have tried any crackpot idea if I thought that it would help.

My phantom pains gradually grew less frequent, and nowadays it is rare for me to get the pains for any length of time. If I do experience them now it is often when I have been sitting for long periods, such as during a car journey or on a long flight. The first signs of aching start after about an hour and a half, and then gradually get worse. The best solution is to remove the limb, but this is not possible in public places unless one wants a lot of people staring and then fussing around one. What I do now is to tap the top of my knee (above the stump) continuously and forcefully. This seems to help until I can get up and walk around. Generally my phantom pains could best be described as a cramp-like feeling.

What is weird is that I can still feel my toes, and have even tried to scratch them in the past. In fact, as I am sitting writing this I can wriggle my big toe, although it feels as if it is halfway between where my foot should be and my stump. Phantom pains just seem to arrive, and I know from talking to other amputees at the limb-fitting centre that I am probably lucky and do not suffer from them too much. I have met a number of elderly amputees who live with constant phantom pain – many try a magnet at the bottom of the socket or laid in their bed by their stump. Some people say this works, while others get no relief and are obviously worn down by the constant nagging pain. Even if phantom pain is a psychological problem rather than a physical one, it would be helpful if the professionals knew more about it. Many people, including nursing staff and doctors, are fascinated by it. Indeed I guess I could be fascinated by it myself sometimes, but one ends up feeling like a medical quirk or curiosity, rather than a person who needs support and help.

In general terms, if I had to make a choice, I think I would rather suffer severe short-term pain rather than a lesser pain over a prolonged period. I think the body copes well with short periods of stress and has its own way of dealing with them. The psychological pressure of long-term pain must be unbearable.

Managing 'Charlie' – the stump

Once the stump had healed, I went for the first limb-fitting session. I imagined that I would be fitted with a lovely looking limb, put it on and walk away with it and be running around in 2 weeks and back rock-climbing again in 4 weeks. I was horrified to see the ugly looking limb that they initially fitted until the swelling went down. It was very unsightly with a large black rocker, although when I actually took it home they fitted it with a foot, but the whole contraption was held together with buckles and leather straps. It was very painful trying to squash a swollen stump with two wool socks into a leather-lined socket. Initially I could only wear it for 30 minutes to an hour before it started to ache and itch like mad. I only managed to walk with crutches for a few hundred yards for a week or two. However, as a result of perseverance and proper healing of the stump, after about 3 months I could get around reasonably well and started to regain some of the independence I had so badly missed. Just being able to go and do a little shopping on my own, or prepare a meal and carry it to the table meant real progress. I realized how much in life I had taken for granted. Have you ever tried carrying a cup of coffee into a separate room when you have no sense of balance? Most of it lands on the carpet!

Nowadays, a long day on my feet does still cause me to be very tired and the stump to ache and feel sore. If it is hot I frequently get blisters where the skin has rubbed raw. Even small blisters can be very painful. Even when the stump is sore I am loath to take the limb off and rest it, since this means that I am not so mobile and simple things like going to the bathroom, answering the door and making a drink become irksome tasks. I usually get blisters at the back of the stump where the pressure is great, or else along the scar tissue at the front of the stump. In hot weather, despite washing, wearing clean socks and applying plenty of highly absorbent talc, the stump gets very hot in its layers of socks. Fortunately, these days stump socks are similar to cotton sports socks, and not like the old thick wool ones. Once the stump gets hot it reacts like hands that have been in water too long – the skin gets soft, loses its resistance to abrasion and breaks down. In recent years I have used a silicon gel to prevent abrasion. In the past I bought Spenco Second Skin® which, although expensive, was excellent. The thinner silicone gel I now use is ideal, as it is washable and can be used repeatedly. I could not manage at all without it. If I ever run out, I get blisters within the first 6 hours of wearing the limb. In my case this may be due to the bad scarring at the front of the stump. People who have a neater stump as a result of a pre-planned operation may not suffer to the same degree.

A comfortable limb is a godsend. If professionals suggest a new limb, I always want to keep the old comfortable one in preference, even if it is a bit battered and the worse for wear. I suppose it is similar to choosing between wearing an old comfy pair of slippers and new shoes – there really is no choice to make.

Conclusions

The majority of the nursing care I received was very good. During the initial 2 weeks after the accident I was in a small hospital on the Orkney Isles. The friendliness of the staff, and the time they took to pop in and see me when passing

(while both on and off duty) was excellent. I suppose I was spoilt beca
I returned to a large busy hospital in outer London, I felt that I was bein
as just a patient, a number – a faceless person who had no feelings. I
medical care but that was all. The staff were very busy, but they did not
as an individual; I hated this period and longed to go home. The only difterence
between the two hospitals was in how they treated me as a person, and I can
assure you this was a very important aspect of my care. I know it must be easy
for staff to see one as just another amputee, but for people like me this is likely
to be the most important and devastating event in their lives.

Provision of adequate pain relief is essential in both physical and psychological care, and it is difficult to say which side of the coin is most important, as
they are so closely interlinked. Whilst professionals may be concerned that
some patients may wish to take more painkillers than necessary (whatever that
is), it is not really acceptable to allow people to feel pain if it can be managed
effectively. Who knows how bad the pain is – the patient or the nurses? As a
person who has experienced being denied painkillers when I needed them, I
know what it feels like. It made my whole experience of pain worse.

For me, pain has both physical and psychological effects, and perhaps the
psychological effects are underestimated and ignored by the professionals.
Whilst a dose of distalgesic could have helped my physical pain, it was only the
personal care of the professionals, family and friends that helped to heal the
painful longer term psychological scars.

Acknowledgements

Thanks to Mum, Dad, Dot and Bridget, who are still the best support I could
wish for!

Talking about pain

Marion V. Smith

A word is a bridge thrown between myself and another

(V.N. Volosinov, 1973)

Introduction

This chapter is about the importance of language and communication in the experience of pain. Because we use language (and in general use it effortlessly) most of the time and in all spheres of our lives, it is easy to overlook it and to be unaware of its power and complexity. This is particularly true when we come to talk about pain. When language is not overlooked, many would dismiss a study of its relationship to pain on the grounds that it is difficult – to the point of impossible – to describe pain. Yet when someone seeks help or advice for troublesome and worrying sensations, their first recourse is to language. There is no objective way of demonstrating that someone is in pain, or how much pain or what kind of pain they are experiencing. And although language is problematic in this area, in the last analysis it is sometimes all there is available. We respond to pain spontaneously and automatically, leaving no space for a considered reaction – and yet pain is a psychological phenomenon, and individual psychologies develop within languages and cultures. Pain language can provide meaningful categories into which an attempt is made to fit unordered and anomalous experience. If we can fit our sensations to a familiar experience or non-threatening disease pattern, then we gain the reassurance that there are appropriate treatments and a known trajectory back to health.

The word 'pain' can be used equally to refer to mental distress or suffering, and physically motivated pain of either trivial (e.g. being stung by nettles) or serious genesis. I shall discuss the relationship of language to both in the course of this chapter. I shall start with a short section on some features of language and their relevance to pain, before moving on to look at the importance of verbal expression. This will lead to a consideration of language and suffering as a broader concern of pain, before focusing on the phenomenon of pain itself. The experience of pain in western societies can become enmeshed in mind/body dualism, and after a brief consideration of the issues involved in this area, I shall move on to the role of culture in the experience of pain. Finally, I shall turn to the doctor–patient consultation and the use of pain descriptors such as *cramping, shooting* and *piercing*.

Language and pain

When asked why we have language, the usual immediate response is that it enables us to give each other information. People are often surprised – until they stop to think about it – to find that language is often not very good at conveying information, although we are reliant upon it to do so. Simple facts such as 'Today is Thursday' do not pose much of a problem, but take a slightly more complex example, such as 'I shop on Thursday'. Does this mean that I regularly go shopping on Thursdays, or that I will do so on the next Thursday, with no information as to when I will shop after that? Furthermore, am I saying that I will, whilst I am shopping, look for that item you particularly want? Or that I refuse to look for that item until Thursday? We can see already that so much of what precisely we are communicating depends on the context in which we say it. Because of this indeterminacy in language, there are multiple opportunities for misunderstandings and misleadings, accidental or otherwise. Aitchison (1996) reports a case where one small piece of crucial information was misunderstood, leading to the deaths of 583 people:

> 'We are now at take-off', said the pilot of a Boeing 747. He meant: 'We are now in the process of taking off.' The air-traffic controller assumed he meant: 'We are waiting at the take-off point.' In consequence . . . two aeroplanes collided on a runway in Tenerife.
>
> (Aitchison, 1996, p.16)

Aitchison (1996) is interested in what language is good at, as a way of approaching its early functions and origins. Her discussion has several points of interest for considering why it is so hard to talk about pain. Why do we say 'It hurts right in there' (with an eloquent gesture which will probably indicate how focused the pain is) rather than 'the pain is approximately 3 inches to the left of my navel and down a bit'? The answer is because: 'Language is bad at handling spatial information, whether for tying knots, following routes or learning about the circulation of the blood' (Aitchison, 1996, p.18).

It is so much easier and clearer to demonstrate manual skills or convey information diagrammatically. Aitchison continues by considering talk about sensations and emotions, both of which are again rarely represented well in language. This is a feature that has often been commented on by writers, including Virginia Woolf, who wrote:

> English, which can express the thoughts of Hamlet and the tragedy of Lear, has no words for the shiver and the headache . . . . The merest schoolgirl, when she falls in love, has Shakespeare or Keats to speak her mind for her; but let a sufferer try to describe a pain in his head to a doctor and language at once runs dry.
>
> (Woolf, 1967, p.194)

To Woolf, love at least has been captured and beautifully conveyed in language, but only by certain gifted practitioners of linguistic expression. The language of pain remains intractable, even to them.

The relationship between language and private experience is a particularly contentious area. When the experience cannot be shared, our reliance on the shared 'meanings' of words is complete. This is of course true of communication in general, but for many uses of everyday language there are both linguistic and non-linguistic opportunities to ascertain that meaning is shared or, if it is not shared, to establish understanding. As Aarsleff (1988, p.xxii) writes: 'language develops only socially as we keep testing the rightness of our words by adjusting them, so to speak, by trial upon others'. With pain words such as *aching, throbbing, crushing* and *lancinating*, or phrases like 'I feel fuzzy and wobbly in my head', opportunities to establish what precisely is shared when someone uses this kind of language do not arise under normal circumstances.

So far, we have looked at the shortcomings of language, some of which it appears vital to circumvent if we are to talk successfully about pain. Language is not very good at conveying information, particularly spatial information and information about sensations and emotion. So what is it good at?

According to Aitchison (1996), language is good at persuasion, lying and, most importantly for our discussion here, chatting. This perception was identified by the anthropologist Malinowski, who argued for the social importance of talking, even when there is nothing of note to be said. Long gossipy telephone calls, short polite exchanges with neighbours and light-hearted party or restaurant talk are all examples of occasions when we talk, often with immense enjoyment, seemingly without having anything to say. What was said is rarely what is memorable. This kind of talk, which serves to create and maintain our social relationships, is both commonplace and important. It is also crucial for how we talk with people in pain – chatting is difficult under these conditions, but it is the only way to keep an isolated person in connection with the social world.

The importance of the voice

The difficulties we have in communicating pain have been noted by Scarry (1985), who records that 'physical pain does not simply resist language but actively destroys it' (p.4). In her view, pain's 'resistance to language is not simply one of its incidental or accidental attributes but is essential to what it is' (p.5). This is intimately connected to the realization that pain is the only bodily state that has no object in the world. Hunger, love, fear, antipathy, etc. all have a focus beyond ourselves. Pain forces us back within our corporeal boundaries. It is not *for* anything; it has no place in the social world, which is constituted and maintained through talk. Scarry argues that the only way to counter this is to force pain into language, into the reality of the shared world. In medical terms, success in diagnosis or management often depends on the skill of the physician or nurse in coaxing pain into linguistic being and interpreting it.

Cassell (1985) reports that, as the symptom of pain is so important, doctors have developed a large descriptive vocabulary which can often point to the source with great accuracy. As lay people generally do not hold such a vocabulary (or only hold it passively), the onus is on the doctor to provide words with which the patient can compare the sensation. Descriptive terms such as *burning, dull, sharp* and *aching* are helpful, as are similes, such as 'Does it feel as if a balloon were being blown up in your finger?' (Cassell, 1985, p.61). The constancy (in waves, intermittent or continuous) and severity (irritating, unendurable or awful) of pain are also important factors. Information on private experience of this nature coupled with the history of onset, duration, recurrences and associated symptoms can be vital in tracking down the cause of discomfort. Scarry sees the development of the McGill Pain Questionnaire, an arrangement of words into 'coherent groups which, by making visible the consistency interior to any one set of words, work[s] to bestow visibility on the characteristics of pain' (Scarry, 1985, p.7), as an enabling device, assisting patients in the difficult task of pain description. However, the use of such a tool[1] is a procedure of such complexity that much more research is needed before such an instrument can be truly satisfactory. This is a point to which I will return towards the end of the chapter.

Communication is of vital importance throughout the entire medical encounter. There is more than the quality of pain at stake. In order to assist doctor–patient communication, various elements brought to the encounter have been selected as central by different researchers. For example, much work has been done to encourage doctors to alter their behaviour (e.g. Ley, 1979), but patients have also become the focus of attention in studies which have shown the benefits of encouraging them to take a more active role in the consultation (e.g. Roter, 1979; Mishler, 1984). Steps have also been taken towards finding ways of teaching medical students more effective and satisfactory techniques in history-taking. Among other factors, Maguire and Rutter (1976) found that medical students adopted a premature and restricted focus, were unsystematic and imprecise, asked 'closed' rather than 'open' questions, and were unresponsive to both verbal and non-verbal cues. Because of the difficulties intrinsic to the diagnostic interview, Katz and Shotter (1996) have experimented with the special practice of employing a third person in the interview to function as a 'cultural go-between' who mediates between the patient and the doctor. It is their role to pick up on subtle cues, in either verbal or body language, or both, as an unfolding synthesis, to discover the 'inner world' of the patient's experience that the doctor would otherwise miss.

Waddie (1996) writes of the challenge to nurses in dealing with patients' pain expressions. She discusses the language used to express pain, and the use of language as part of the pain experience, through the work of Wittgenstein. Pain experience and pain expression are inseparable, but lack of expression does not mean that there is no pain. Jarrett and Payne (1995) review a selection from the growing literature on nurse–patient communication, and find it critical of the quality and quantity of their talk, with the nurses being revealed as overly controlling and restricting the topics and course of conversation. However, as Jarrett and Payne point out, it takes two to talk, and the research has tended to concentrate on the nurses' contribution during isolated excerpts of

---

[1]The user is presented with short lists of words, with each group representing a particular aspect of sensation.

talk. Research must take into account the patients' contributions and the conversation as a whole. This is crucially true, but at the same time, in the medical encounter in particular, health professionals need to be aware of the balance of power in a conversation, and adapt themselves if the patient is lacking due to pain, fear, intimidating surroundings, etc. On the other side of the coin, Sofaer (1983) stresses the importance of good communication not only between nurses and patients, but also between nurses and doctors.

Other research has focused on how nurses talk in order to comfort patients who are in pain, or who are undergoing a painful procedure. Proctor *et al.* (1996) have examined the linguistic features of nurses' comfort talk, and report a distinctive register that is used only for patients. The talk is designed to achieve certain specific functions beyond 'simple' comforting. Through their talk, nurses believe that they can inspire patients with hope and courage, as well as encouraging them to 'hold on' through a particular episode. The talk can support, ensure the patient works with the nurse, give information about how a procedure is going and how near the patient is to the procedure being over, or, alternatively, provide distraction. The importance of such communication cannot be overvalued.

Advance preparation of the patient in terms of what is happening and why is also important. This can be at the relatively innocuous level of explaining the reason for taking a history, or at the more crucial level of giving preoperative information. Haywood (1975) writes of information as a prescription against pain and anxiety. Indeed, it has been found that information can reduce subsequent distress, aid recovery and shorten postoperative hospitalization by up to 2 days (Ley, 1976). It is particularly interesting that information on how much and what sort of pain to expect is also beneficial. It provides an opportunity for covert rehearsal, stimulates moderate fear and hence realistic expectations, increases the patient's feeling of control and, crucially for this chapter, provides names for experiences and sensations that would otherwise be unlabelled, and therefore more frightening and negative than they need to be (Ley, 1982). If people are given words for what they will undergo, then their sensations are more easily assigned to 'normal' and understood categories of experience which they see are perceived as familiar and unthreatening by doctors and nurses.

Language and suffering

In the case of those who suffer personal misfortune, the need for an explanation or the need to make sense exerts immense pressure. Pain experience is no exception – rather it is the more urgent to make sense of a situation of bodily suffering, partly because of its relationship to language, and partly because of the sufferer's loss of power. These two factors are connected. As Rawlinson (1986) notes, the 'lived body' is the domain of delimited access to and control over immediate social reality: 'In illness one discovers one's embodied self as an obstacle in one's own project of encountering and shaping the world' (Rawlinson, 1986, p.39).

An important part of the presence or extension of the self into the world is the voice (Scarry, 1985), and it is through talk that we have access to and control over the social worlds that we inhabit. However, physical pain and its concomitant emotional arousal are peculiarly resistant to language, stifling our projection of our reality into the social world. In experiencing pain, the individual is removed from the familiarity of habitual and likely events of daily life, knowledge of which and participation in which are shared by members of the social network. Replacing this, as part of the personal discomfort, is all the isolation and insecurity of an experience that has no object in the outer world, which delimits the self as a finite quantity, and which acts as an alienating factor not only in the relationship of the body to the self, but also in the relationship of the self to others. The lived realities that we shared in health can be shared no longer, and the relationship has to adjust to that. A corollary of this is the experience of not knowing what to talk about when visiting someone in hospital. The patient's voice is silenced – they have access to few experiences to which a healthy visitor can readily relate – and this stultifies the visitor's.

Rawlinson (1986) provides a typology of suffering consisting of four focal areas, all of which are important in the experience of pain. These provide a convenient summary thus far:

- in the body (the realm of embodied action);
- in the relationships that the sufferer has with others (the realm of intersubjective life);
- in the arena of the will – one's powers of self-possession, self-regulation and production as regards the external world;
- in the sphere of universal alteration (cf. Scarry, 1985, p.33; pain nullifies the claims of the world).

Powerlessness, alienation, loss of control, frustration and anomie are all aspects of suffering. Copp (1990) defines suffering as a state of anguish, and records that anticipation, fear and dire imaginings are intrinsic to the suffering associated with pain. Immediately, the value of communication is striking:

> Nurses can help prevent fear of the unknown. One cannot always be sure exactly what a patient's response to a medication will be or how one can relieve the pain – especially if fear not pain is the greater problem, but the ability to reduce one kind of suffering is within nursing's scope. Nurses can inform, educate, and help eliminate or minimize a person's fears and imaginings.
>
> (Copp, 1990, p.36)

The relationship between pain and anxiety is also of relevance here, opening another pathway through which communication can relieve suffering. Walsh (1993) studied pain and anxiety in an Accident and Emergency department, and recommends that nurses should alleviate worries about the injury or reason for attendance, and make sure that the patient knows what is going on with regard to tests or indeed delays. Walding (1991) reports that power-lessness increases anxiety, which in turn increases pain. Involving patients more in their own care could increase their sense of control, with beneficial effect. For example, Carter (1994, pp.76–80) describes the increasingly popular pain-relief method of patient-controlled analgesia for children, and reports that there is generally a high level of satisfaction with it. Yet another aspect of suffering involves generally held beliefs about 'appropriate' pain behaviour. The imaginings of a patient, or the meanings that a patient associates with their pain, may intensify their experience of pain beyond that which medical staff see as reasonable. The staff may then react as though the sufferer were an 'attention-seeker' or 'putting it on', and thereby increase suffering further. Beales (1986) explores the cognitive factors in pain experience, with special reference to the case of children who grow up with a chronic, painful illness such as arthritis. He points out that for older children: 'Differences in the way they perceive their condition can sometimes cause their suffering to be a good deal greater than that of a younger child' (Beales, 1986, p.410).

Suffering is inversely related to comfort. Morse et al. (1994) suggest (cor-rectly, in my view) that pain reduction is not equivalent to comfort, but rather that sensitive analysis is necessary to 'uncover the multidimensional complex-ity of comfort and how it is achieved' (Morse et al., 1994, p.189). They speak of comfort as 'a state of an integrated body' (p.190), and the divisive nature of suffering could certainly be characterized as a dis-integrated body. Their typo-logy of arenas for the attainment of comfort is also a typology of suffering, and the remedy or pathway to alleviation always involves talk (see Figure 3.1). Communication provides the link to the normalcy of the lost world of health, and the pathway to some small reattainment of it.

- the diseased body needs diagnosis and to be able to trust its carers;
- the disobedient body, no longer under control, needs help to find new areas of independence, competence and strength;
- the vulnerable body, consumed by anticipation, needs to be given security and support it can trust;
- the violated body, invaded and open to medical scrutiny, needs sensitive help to maintain some dignity;
- the enduring body, whose horizons are shrunk to inexorable discomfort, needs support;
- the resigned body, that has learnt to relinquish its former self, needs assistance to accept and rebuild;
- the deceiving body, through which illness has progressed silently to the point of a late discovery, needs reassurance with the appropriate treatment;
- the betraying body, that breaks down from hidden stress, needs watchful care, and assistance to recognize and resolve such problems;
- the betraying mind, that performs in unusual ways, needs support and encouragement.

Figure 3.1   Typology of suffering (from Morse et al., 1994)

So what is pain?

Pain is an extremely common experience, and yet it is one of the least understood symptoms in medicine (Bakal, 1979, p.139). Pain may occur without any apparent cause, it may be absent when physical damage is present, it can spread from the site of damage or occur in apparently unrelated sites, and it can trouble an area that no longer exists, as in phantom-limb pain. It is as much a psychological phenomenon as a somatic experience. Merskey (1973, p.251) emphasizes that pain is 'something that happens in the mind', despite the fact that it is related to events 'which are experienced as originating in the body'. Miller (1978, p.20) writes that pains do not occur in hands or heads or anywhere physical, but in the images of hands and heads. Under normal circumstances, 'the subjective image of these parts coincides with their physical existence'. Furthermore, the specificity of our body image is not usually in the foreground of our awareness. In normal health we rarely focus directly on our bodies. As Leder puts it, when 'functioning well this body is a transparency through which we engage the world' (Leder, 1990, p.82), but one 'is seized by a power holding sway . . . . In the face of pain, one's whole being is forcibly reoriented' (Leder, 1990, p.73). It is this quality that makes pain so difficult to get hold of – one's whole being plays a part in the pain, and to concentrate on the diseased or injured area misses the event.

The Subcommittee on Taxonomy for the International Association for the Study of Pain defines pain as 'an unpleasant sensory and emotional experience associated with actual or potential tissue damage, or described in terms of such damage' (Merskey and the International Association for the Study of Pain Subcommittee on Taxonomy, 1979, p.250).

They add in a note that this definition avoids tying pain to a stimulus – it is a *psychological state*, even though it often has a proximate physical cause. The theory that copes most completely with the rapidly growing experimental evidence is that of gate control. (For a detailed and technical explanation of gate control theory, see Wall, 1978; Yaksh, 1986; Melzack and Wall, 1988). As medical research continues, it is becoming increasingly evident that almost all of the brain plays a role in pain. Anxiety (as we have already seen), attention, suggestion and prior experience all have an effect, so seeing the source of an injury, or the lesion itself, hearing the sounds that accompany it and thinking about the consequences all contribute to pain. These processes interact with inputs either from the injured area, or from deafferented neurons that signal pain when injury has not occurred (Melzack and Wall, 1988).

Dualism and medicine

Two frequent criticisms of Western technological medicine are that, stemming from its Enlightenment traditions, it is pervaded by the assumption that the mind is separate from the body – and that it treats bodies as examples, rather than dealing with people. Armstrong (1983) writes that, in a medical examination, what is seen is not someone's body, but a representation of the twentieth-century anatomical atlas. Jewson (1976) traces the 'disappearance' of the *person* of the patient during the course of industrialization of Western societies (see also Mishler, 1986, chapter 5). Lupton reports (after Doyal, 1983, p.31) that, by the turn of the twentieth century:

> the views of the patient had lost their relevance and power in the medical encounter, and the responsibility for discovering and labelling illness had become the preserve of the medical practitioner. The disease had become more important than the person who harboured it.
>
> (Lupton, 1994, p.86)

More recently, the trend has been to take account of the social contexts of illness, and Armstrong (1984, p.739) contends that this has served to open to medical surveillance social and personal spaces that have hitherto been hidden. What it does not do, however, is attempt to reintegrate the body and the mind. Yet Leder (1990) does not wish to locate the separation of mind and body as emanating solely from the medical profession, and offers another perspective:

> This cleavage between body and self is not only initiated by the pain but may also serve as an adaptive response to it. As Bakan points out, when the affected part of the body becomes 'other' to the ego, one becomes more ready to take whatever means are necessary to rid oneself of it. A tooth may need to be pulled or a limb amputated; one is prepared for physical invasions and separations by an existential separation already effected. With pain that cannot be so removed, a process of distancing still provides consolation. To experience the painful body as merely an 'it,' that which is separate from the essential self, yields some relief and re-establishes one's integrity in the face of an overwhelming threat.
>
> (Leder, 1990, p.77)

Hence the separation of the mind and the body is under way before the consulting room has been reached. This is an interesting point, and there is no doubt that pain is divisive, but for some sufferers, at least, the distancing will be not a consolation but an estrangement to be grieved over.

The problem of mind/body dualism is clearly larger than medicine. It has been posited that in the Western world, this dualism is endemic, such that modern selfhood is intimately connected with the freedom of the mind from corporeality (Gordon, 1988). Williams (1996, p.706) argues for the notion of body-image, which he describes as an 'important third term linking body to mind and mind to body without serving to reduce one to the other.' However, simply as a term, it is hard to see it serving both mind and body equally when 'body' is part of the name. Language is powerful, and has itself contributed to the dualism. No one has a mechanistic image of the cognitive functions of the brain, but a common model for the functioning of the body in Western society is the metaphorical analogy of the body as machine (see, for example, Osherson and AmaraSingham, 1981). The body is constructed of various parts which may 'fail' and can sometimes be replaced. 'Fuel' is needed to power the body, and 'bitters', 'tonics' or vitamin pills are often thought of as necessary to this end. We are clockwork – 'I'm all wound up', 'What makes him tick?' – we are engines 'recharging our batteries' – or plumbing systems with 'bottled-up emotions' or 'overflowing feelings' (quoted in Lupton, 1994, p.59). The machine metaphor is also commonly used in hospitals as an explanatory model for patients. For example, 'Your heart isn't pumping so well'; 'You've had a nervous breakdown' or 'The current isn't flowing so well along your nerves' (Helman, 1984, p.16). Miller (1978, p.182) points out that it is not only patients who have found the metaphor helpful: 'whatever [these] devices were designed to do, they have incidentally provided conjectural models for explaining the human body'. Manning and Fabrega (1973) argue that it is this metaphor that is partly responsible for a growing sense of the self as separate from the body in Western society today. Whether or not this is true, many would be surprised to be reminded that these are figures of speech, rather than literalities.

Culture and pain

Bendelow and Williams (1995, p.140) argue that 'scientific medicine reduces the experience of pain to an elaborate broadcasting system of signals, rather than seeing it as moulded and shaped both by the individual and their particular socio-cultural context'.

This is an important aspect of bodies – although they are a natural environment, they are socially constituted and located (Turner, 1984). Grosz (1994, p.xi) speaks of their 'organic openness to completion': 'Part of their own "nature" is an organic or ontological "incompleteness" or lack of finality, an amenability to social completion, social ordering and organization.'

The particular relevance of this here is that, although we have neurological information about pain mechanisms, bodily experiences emerge as a cultural phenomenon. There is an active process in which the sufferer shapes the experience of illness or pain into an intelligible situation (Miller, 1978, p.45). Although the uniqueness of the individual's experience is undeniable, informing it are cultural aspects of situation, behaviour and belief. Various studies have classically been cited to demonstrate the connection between culture and pain behaviour. Zola (1966), for example, compared Irish and Italian Americans (with matched subsequent diagnoses) with regard to what was socially selected to be brought to medical attention. Amongst other findings, the Italian presentations featured pain, whilst the Irish tended to deny pain. Zborowski (1969) compared Italian, Jewish and 'Old' (Northern European) Americans for their reaction to the presence of pain. The 'Old' Americans tended to describe their pain without great emotion, and with an air of detachment. However, both Italians and Jews tended to be very emotional and to present their pain with a great deal of concern and emotion. Yet whereas the Italians soon disregarded their suffering once an analgesic had been administered, the Jews continued to worry about the underlying cause of the pain, and their inability to feel its possible progression while under medication. Zola (1966, p.630) comments that 'the very labelling and definition of a bodily state as a symptom or as a problem is, in itself, part of a social process'. Such studies as these, however, are lacking in the sensitivity needed to unpick the intensely complicated interplay of individual aspiration and experience, situation and culture (cf. DelVecchio Good *et al.*, 1992).

It is not possible to allocate pain behaviours to cultures and end up with an appropriate and useful analysis of individual experience. Nevertheless, culture is indubitably implicated in experience at all levels, from the pain to diagnosis and subsequent care. Kleinman (1986) has studied and compared the social origins of distress and disease in great detail in Chinese and Western society. He shows that what is perceived and communicated, in terms of bodily complaints in association with depressive illness, differs dramatically across cultures. His findings, among others, indicate 'forms of experience not available to members of our own society' (Kleinman, 1986, p.14). There is also an active process by which disease is shaped into a cultural entity, according to the explanatory framework of medical practitioners. As Turner (1984, chapter 9) points out, disease is not a fact but a product of a classificatory process – a new disease is not epistemologically like a new butterfly, but is linked to changes in institutionalized medicine and the nature of medical power (cf. Foucault (1973), who defines disease as a system of signs that can be read and translated in more than one way).

There is support, therefore, for the idea that aspects of illness behaviour and others' responses to illness are affected by cultural factors. In broad terms, cultural factors determine what is 'abnormal', they also help *shape* these diffuse emotional and physical changes into a pattern which is recognizable to both the sufferer, and those around him' (Helman, 1984, p.71).

However, the place of the individual should not be forgotten – social categories and medical categories meet, and are mediated by the specific instance of the individual.

> Current definitions of what is social and what is medical are simply too narrow and do not allow explanations of phenomena that are problematic to both social scientists and physicians. . .there is a need for an analytic framework that can accommodate relationships between body and self which is deeply rooted in biology and in the social and cultural forms in which phenomenological experience is cast.
>
> (Manning and Fabrega, 1973, p.252)

What is it that we take to the doctor?

Alongside the physiological and neurological mechanisms for pain detection and response, there is an intimate and dynamic relationship between this somatic side and individual mental states, consciousness and memory. Pain tolerance is variable depending on a range of factors, including expectation and the assignation of meaning. We have considered the personal nature of suffering, the loss of power over one's world and the consequent disruption of relationships and goals in the world. Set against the undeniably unique qualities of individual suffering may be relatively stable aspects – cultural patterns in the definition and presentation of symptoms, and the health beliefs that make individual experience into shared experience at the level of attributed significance and understanding or diagnosis. These cultural aspects bring frightening and diffuse personal changes into the social world where they can be fitted to meaningful configurations and, in most cases, rectifying behaviours.

At this most general level, language is important both to the sufferer who is seeking help and personal understanding, and to the healer whose task it is to diagnose and institute the appropriate restorative practices. For the sufferer, explanation is the crucial link between apparently random and uncontrolled experience and regularity and control – a name for a condition, a course of expected development and in most cases recession. As the person who provides treatment and reassurance (Tate, 1983), the medical practitioner steps between the sufferer and his or her body. This is a position of considerable power, and to use this power to advantage, to intervene successfully on the patient's behalf, the Western practitioner must be able to combine subjective and value-laden information with the objective signs that form the basis of scientific medicine (Cassell, 1985). Unfortunately, the modern technology of diagnosis and therapy leaves the patient out – their story becomes obtrusive or irrelevant, a voice to be bypassed in the search for the physical event. Yet doctors need to be able to take account of 'beliefs and fears, liver chemistries, family constellation, barium enema findings, hopes for the future, drug eccentricities, immediate needs, cardiac arrhythmias' (Cassell, 1985, p.2) and the like in their decision-making. The illness that a patient takes to a doctor is an interaction in Cassell's view between a biological disease entity and the person of the patient. The abstract and generalized pathophysiology is modified within a particular instance. However, psychosocial factors in illness are not as 'visible' as the physical factors on which medical training concentrates. Doctors need to understand the complexity of patients' presentations, and the only way to achieve this is through communication (Thompson, 1984). It is language which transforms the experience into the illness presented to the doctor.

In recent years there has been a move towards the study of doctor–patient communication (e.g. King, 1983; Pendleton and Hasler, 1983). Armstrong (1983) reports that the Goodenough Committee (1944) considered the patient to be a passive object from whom a history could be taken unproblematically, but the Todd Report produced some 20 years later was at pains to focus on the problems of vocabulary limitations, cultural attitudes and social prejudices. It is clear that using language carefully and sensitively holds great advantages for both doctor and patient and is of central importance in defining sensation and hence the allocation of significance to the experience. Within the context of the experience of pain, language has a further importance and centrality. There is no objective way of measuring how much or indeed whether pain is in fact being borne. The sufferer's knowledge confronts the carer's belief. Autonomic nervous system reponses (such as increased blood pressure or sweaty palms) are subject to learning and conditioning – our backgrounds and prior experiences contribute to how our bodies respond, so that there is considerable individual variation. Furthermore, the direction of response cannot be guaranteed. Pain is often associated with an increased rate of breathing, for example, but the rate can also decrease when pain originates from organs within the abdominal cavity (Bloch, 1985). As there are no physiological signs that uniquely indicate pain, language has provided, and probably will continue to provide, the best tool for the assessment and diagnosis of suffering. It is only through the pain vocabulary of a language that details of the nature and intensity of pain experience can be communicated:

> if the only external sign of the felt-experience of pain (for which there is no alteration in the blood count, no shadow on the X-ray, no pattern on the CAT scan) is the patient's verbal report (however itself inadequate), then to bypass the voice is to bypass the bodily event, to bypass the patient, to bypass the person in pain.
>
> (Scarry, 1985, p.6)

There is no doubt in the minds of many doctors that patients feel very strongly about the selection of words appropriate to their pain experience. For example, Melzack (1975, p.283) writes that, when given a word list 'patients are usually highly selective; they may reject word after word, until one comes up that is clearly "right"; they may smile, say "that's it!" with a sense of certainty, and continue the process of rejection and selection'.

Obviously, patients have a strong interest in being as clear and exact as possible where their future well-being is concerned. However, it remains to be shown that a symbolic token in a system of such tokens bears a constant relationship to a psychophysical symptom.

Studies of pain words

The question of similarity of usage of such terms as *throbbing, stinging* and *cramping* has motivated many experimental studies. Most have been conducted as medical research (for a review, see Smith, 1989), but many have relied on experimental pain (e.g. Gracely and Wolskee, 1983). Skevington (1995) reports that results from laboratory studies may be misleading because of the assumption that their subjects can feel sensation that is devoid of emotion. However, the most influential study of pain words was undertaken with the specific aim of developing a pain questionnaire for use with patients.[2] It is a categorization of (Canadian) English pain words on principles of sensory, affective and evaluative qualities. The inceptive study (Melzack and Torgerson, 1971) gathered and categorized pain words, and then had subjects judge

[2]This critique of the McGill Pain Questionnaire is taken from Smith (1989). See also Skevington (1995).

whether or not each word fitted within its assigned group. Each group consisted of from two to six words and represented a different quality, such as 'punctuate pressure' or 'brightness' (sensory groups), and 'punishment' or 'fear' (affective groups). However, words seldom have a straightforward relationship to each other, so this methodology is somewhat problematic. Pain adjectives can be categorized in many ways owing to their multidimensional nature. Melzack and Torgerson's arrangement could be perfectly acceptable without utilizing the most generally significant or salient dimensions for its organization, and their arrangement is unlikely to suit a different group of people. Subsequently, subject groups of students, doctors and patients placed the words of each group on intensity scales ranging from 1 to 5. The results showed very high levels of agreement for 16 of the 20 groups.

Because of the consistency of the intensity relationship between the majority of pain words (across subjects having different cultural, socio-economic and educational backgrounds), the McGill Pain Questionnaire (MPQ) was developed on the basis of this research. It consists of four main parts. The first part seeks to establish where pain is felt, and whether it is internal or external, and the third and fourth parts ask how the pain changes with time and how bad it is. The second part consists of the 20 groups of words, unlabelled (i.e. the trait that each group is intended to represent is not specified), and the instruction to choose one word from each appropriate group. As each group is meant to refer to one trait, by choosing a word within a group a patient is making a choice of intensity, as each word has been quantified to show how much pain it represents. The patient is not made aware of this.

The free categorization of pain words into groups has never been replicated by subjects (a different exercise from the 'validation task' of Melzack and Torgerson). So far as I am aware there has been one attempt at replication of the MPQ (Reading et al., 1982) before my own (Smith, 1989). Both replications show partial support for the MPQ groupings, but also show a number of important differences. Atkinson et al. (1982) point out that the assumption that language is employed in a systematic and precise manner is critical. Patients are only allowed to select one word from each group on the MPQ so the connections or common ground between the words in each group must be reliably assured, and the groupings should be the most significant. Scarry (1985) commends these groupings as their effect is to force pain characteristics into visibility. However, this cannot happen if particular groups make no sense to patients. This is a particular concern as the group characteristics (group headings such as 'temporal', 'incisive pressure', 'brightness', which are *not* given to patients) were selected by Melzack and Torgerson rather than elicited from sufferers. Furthermore, as patients may only select one word from each group, it is very likely that pain characteristics are not forced into visibility by the connections that are being made, but rather that they are hidden by the isolated and unrelated choices permitted.

The words in each group are ranked for intensity and numbered for position. The position numbers of all of the words that a patient selects are totalled to give the pain rating index based on the rank values of the words, or PRI(R). This index does not take into account either the different sizes of groups or the relative intensities of groups with regard to each other. Melzack (1975) has shown that this index correlates strongly with the PRI(S). This is a pain rating index based on the scale values found to be reliable for three different subject populations for 16 of 20 groups by Melzack and Torgerson (1971). However, the rank ordering for each group on the MPQ was taken from Melzack and Torgerson's experiment, and the latter did not compare different groups on the *same* intensity scale – they were rated on separate scales that were similarly numbered. Rather than the simple addition of position scores, it would be wise to establish the degree to which each item contributes to an overall score.[3] Any research utilizing these and other MPQ indices will yield results that are constrained by these difficulties.

There are other queries concerning the categorization of English pain adjectives as given on the MPQ. As Reading and Newton (1978) point out, the original groupings by Melzack and Torgerson along three dimensions (sensory, affective and evaluative) was a priori, and conformed to Melzack's three-factor account of pain. It was Merskey and Spear's (1967) earlier opinion that it is impossible to separate the 'components' of pain in its experience and so 'the idea of . . . distinguishable parts of [pain] experience . . . should probably be dropped' (Merskey and Spear, 1967, p.62). Fernandez and Turk (1994, p.213) have since reported that 'subjects are not inclined to distinguish between sensory versus affective aspects of pain' unless this is demanded of them – in a laboratory experiment (where the experience of pain is, of course, a different matter). Holroyd *et al.* (1996) tested the MPQ (along with other instruments) to see how clearly the three factors are distinguished. They found evidence that patients' descriptions of pain were influenced by the formal characteristics of the pain measurement instruments, and concluded that 'Inferences about distinct pain dimensions on the basis of patients' scores . . . appear problematic' (Holroyd *et al.*, 1996, p.264). As well as supporting a more multidimensional approach to pain, Crockett *et al.* (1977) point out the danger of attempting to characterize pain largely in terms of one general quality, such as intensity. This has also been noted by Bailey and Davidson (1976), who set out to determine whether intensity is indeed the most prominent dimension along which pain words vary. They used a selection of 39 adjectives only, but took ratings from two groups consisting of 93 and 90 subjects, respectively. They extracted six factors, of which the intensity factor accounted for only 15 per cent of the total variance of ratings. Factor 2 was sensory in nature, but no cogent pattern was discernible for the other factors.

As a representation of the semantic domain of (Canadian) English pain words, therefore, the McGill Pain Questionnaire and the methods used to construct it have some shortcomings from a linguistic point of view. This is not to deny its obvious utility for some purposes, however. Patients respond with relief to an orderly tool for communication, and 'it is still one of the better measures of subjective pain available to us' (Skevington, 1995, p.57). It is surely a sophisticated improvement on earlier pain chart methods (e.g. Keele, 1948) for the assessment of pain relief strategies.

[3]Furthermore, I remain to be convinced that words can be 'added up' in this way.

Pain descriptors in English model the experience on events that are logically unrelated to pain, such as *crushing, piercing, squeezing* and *gnawing*. These are metaphorical usages of the words, and they are typically characterized by energy, activity, deformation, violence and destruction. There is a strong sense of process, that something is actually happening (rather than simply residing), and this is not the case for pain vocabulary in all languages. However, we cannot compare pains, and so we cannot directly compare the use of pain words to ensure that we all use them in the same way as each other. The way round this is to look at pain words not as individual items (with set individual meanings – Melzack and Torgerson's mistake), but as an interrelated resource pool. In analysing the lexicon of a language, we are looking at distinctions and relationships that are treated as meaningful by a society. Within a language, therefore, the ideas expressed are not autonomous, each with a kind of individual essence, but are members of a system where each is defined by its relationships with the other members. Culler (1977) explicates this by pointing out that it is impossible to teach someone what 'brown' means unless one also teaches them 'red', 'grey' and 'black', etc. To discover the place of a word in our language – the work it does – we must investigate the system of relationships and distinctions that creates it.

It follows from this that it does not really make sense to speak of the meaning of individual words. Meanings change according to contexts of use, and what other possible words could have been used – the connotations of the choice of a particular word. When people are given the opportunity to sort pain words into similar groups themselves, it immediately becomes apparent that pain descriptors are multidimensional, and no one grouping is entirely satisfactory. Subjects attempting this task find it possible to arrange the words in different groupings, according to category headings they choose, but they could also rearrange them in alternative and equally satisfactory groups.[4] It is clear from this that selecting individual words from a list of pain words is not likely to yield much information about pain, unless the list provides a satisfactory context, and the relevance of that context is absolutely clear to the health professional and patient alike. An example from my own research revealed that *stabbing* could be in a group with *shooting* on the basis of movement, or in a group with *piercing* on the basis of sharpness (incision). On the MPQ, *stabbing* does not appear with *shooting* or *piercing*, but in a group with *pricking, boring, drilling* and *lancinating*, designating punctuate pressure. The group in which *piercing* appears is a sensory miscellaneous group, and *shooting* appears in a spatial group. *Boring* is another word that has a number of features that can be highlighted in context – sorted with *penetrating* it can mean sharp and moving inwards, with *dull* it can mean blunt or unfocused, and as one of my subjects (a sufferer of Crohn's disease) told me, she would choose *boring* to describe her pain because it went on and on and on.

Lists of words therefore need to be analysed in considerable linguistic depth before they can convey reliable information, and single words are unlikely to

[4]This is reported in Smith (1989) and in forthcoming work.

be helpful. Asking why a particular word is chosen may provide more information, but not everyone has the same reflective capacities for language,
particularly when they are in pain. It may be necessary to supply a context and
ask if it is right, or to attempt to pick out the feature the sufferer may be getting
at.

Conclusions

Creating a context for pain language without the help of a truly sensitive
instrument has to be done on a personal basis. A carer needs to know enough
about his or her patient to be able to put the patient's pain in the patient's own
context. Communication is always worthwhile. There is a danger in health care
today that, because we can do so much more for people than we could even a
relatively short time ago, we do not have to engage with them. However, being
able to do more does not mean that people suffer less. In some conditions, it
may mean that suffering is more long drawn out than it would have been in
former days.

Talking about pain, in a sympathetic and supportive atmosphere, has a
number of benefits. It allows the disoriented person a measure of reconnection
with their body; it allows self-expression when selfhood is under threat; it
helps to create a new context for this chapter of life when the old has fallen
away. Talking allows the beleaguered personality the chance to make his or her
experience real in the shared world, and this in itself can be a way of pushing
the pain away:

> When I feel really absolutely drained I always say something like the
> vampires have been at me because it's that feeling when you see our heroine
> bitten by the vampire and she goes all white and limp and feels like she can't move
> at all – you know like in these silly old films. Because . . . that helps me to feel
> better about it because it's silly and I think also shows in a general way how I am
> feeling.
>
> (Smith, 1989: taped interview with a Crohn's disease sufferer.)

Frank (1995) claims even more for talk than this. He believes that sufferers
need to recount their experiences, and that this has a healing effect. Telling the
story of their illness enables the reconstruction or new construction of their
position in their own life and its relationships, and engineers continuity in
their life experience.

Sometimes it is only through talk that an ill person can still participate in the
world.

References

Aarsleff, H. 1988: Introduction. In Von Humboldt, W., *On language* (translated by P.
Heath). Cambridge: Cambridge University Press, vii–lxv.

Aitchison, J. 1996: *The seeds of speech. Language origin and evolution.* Cambridge: Cambridge University Press.

Armstrong, D. 1983: *The political anatomy of the body: medical knowledge in Britain in the twentieth century.* Cambridge: Cambridge University Press.

Armstrong, D. 1984: The patient's view. *Social Science and Medicine* **18**, 737–44.

Atkinson, J.H., Kremer, E.F. and Ignelzi, R.J. 1982: Diffusion of pain language with affective disturbance confounds differential diagnosis. *Pain* **12**, 375–84.

Bailey, C.A. and Davidson, P.O. 1976: The language of pain: intensity. *Pain* **2**, 319–24.

Bakal, D.A. 1979: *Psychology and medicine. Psychological dimensions of health and sickness.* London: Tavistock Publications.

Beales, J.G. 1986: Cognitive development and the experience of pain. *Nursing* **11**, 408–10.

Bendelow, G. and Williams, S. 1995: Transcending the dualisms: towards a sociology of pain. *Sociology of Health and Illness* **17**, 139–65.

Bloch, G. 1985: *Body and self. Elements of human biology, behavior, and health.* Los Altos, CA: William Kaufmann, Inc.

Carter, B. 1994: *Child and infant pain.* London: Chapman & Hall.

Cassell, E.J. 1985: *Talking with patients.* Cambridge, MA: MIT Press.

Copp, L.A. 1990: The spectrum of suffering. *American Journal of Nursing* **90**, 35–9.

Crocket, D.J., Prkachin, K.M. and Craig, K.D. 1977: Factors of the language of pain in patient and volunteer groups. *Pain* **4**, 175–82.

Culler, J. 1977: *Ferdinand de Saussure.* Harmondsworth: Penguin.

DelVecchio Good, M.-J., Brodwin, P., Good, B. and Kleinman, A. 1992: *Pain as human experience: an anthropological perspective.* Berkeley, CA: University of California Press.

Doyal, L. 1983: *The political economy of health.* London: Pluto Press.

Fernandez, E. and Turk, D.C. 1994: Demand characteristics underlying differential ratings of sensory versus affective components of pain. *Journal of Behavioral Medicine* **17**, 375–90.

Foucault, M. 1973: *The birth of the clinic: an archaeology of medical perception.* London: Tavistock.

Frank, A.W. 1995: *The wounded storyteller: body, illness, and ethics.* Chicago: Chicago University Press.

Gordon, D.R. 1988: Tenacious assumptions in western medicine. In Loch, M. and Gordon, D. (eds), *Biomedicine examined.* Dordrecht: Kluwer, 19–56.

Gracely, R.H. and Wolskee, P.J. 1983: Semantic functional measurement of pain: integrating perception and language. *Pain* **15**, 389–98.

Grosz, E. 1994: *Volatile bodies. Toward a corporeal feminism.* Bloomington, Indianapolis, IN: Indiana University Press.

Haywood, J. 1975: *Information, a prescription against pain.* London: Royal College of Nursing Publications.

Helman, C. 1984: *Culture, health and illness.* Bristol: John Wright and Sons.

Holroyd, K.A., Talbot, F., Holm, J.E., Pingel, J.D., Lake, A.E. and Saper, J.R. 1996: Assessing the dimensions of pain: a multitrait-multimethod evaluation of seven measures. *Pain* **67**, 259–65.

Jarrett, N. and Payne, S. 1995: A selective review of the literature on nurse–patient communication: has the patient's contribution been neglected? *Journal of Advanced Nursing* **22**, 72–8.

Jewson, N.D. 1976: The disappearance of the sick man from medical cosmology. *Sociology* **10**, 225–44.

Katz, A.M. and Shotter, J. 1996: Hearing the patient's voice: toward a social poetics in diagnostic interviews. *Social Science and Medicine* **43**, 919–31.

Keele, K.D. 1948: The pain chart. *Lancet* **2**, 6–8.

King, J. 1983: Health beliefs in consultation. In Pendleton, D. and Hasler, J. (eds), *Doctor–patient communication*. London: Academic Press, 109–25.

Kleinman, A. 1986: *Social origins of distress and disease*. New Haven, CT: Yale University Press.

Leder D. (1990). *The absent body*. Chicago: University of Chicago Press.

Ley, P. 1976: Toward better doctor–patient communications. In Bennett, A.E. (ed.), *Communication between doctors and patients*. London: Oxford University Press for the Nuffield Provincial Hospitals Trust, 75–98.

Ley, P. 1979: Improving clinical communication: effects of altering doctor behaviour. In Oborne, D.J. Gruneberg, M.M. and Eiser, J.R. (eds), *Research in psychology and medicine. Vol. 2*. London: Academic Press, 221–9.

Ley, P. 1982: Giving information to patients. In Eiser, J.R (ed.), *Social psychology and behavioural science*. Chichester: John Wiley and Sons, 339–73.

Lupton, D. 1994: *Medicine as culture*. London: Sage.

Maguire, P. and Rutter, D.R. 1976: Teaching medical students to communicate. In Bennett, A.E. (ed.), *Communication between doctors and patients*. London: Oxford University Press for the Nuffield Provincial Hospitals Trust, 45–74.

Manning, P.K. and Fabrega, H. 1973: The experience of self and body: health and illness in the Chiapas Highlands. In Psathas, G. (ed.), *Phenomenological sociology: issues and applications*. London: John Wiley and Sons, 251–301.

Melzack, R. 1975: The McGill Pain Questionnaire: major properties and scoring methods. *Pain* **1**, 277–99.

Melzack, R. and Torgerson, W.S. 1971: On the language of pain. *Anesthesiology* **34**, 50–9.

Melzack, R. and Wall, P. 1988: *The challenge of pain*, 2nd edn. Harmondsworth: Penguin.

Merskey, H. 1973: The perception and measurement of pain. *Journal of Psychosomatic Research* **17**, 251–5.

Merskey, H. and Spear, F.G. 1967: The concept of pain. *Journal of Psychosomatic Research* **11**, 59–67.

Merskey, H. and The International Association for the Study of Pain Subcommittee on Taxonomy 1979: Pain terms: a list with definitions and notes on usage. *Pain* **6**, 249–52.

Miller, J. 1978: *The body in question*. London: Jonathan Cape Ltd.

Mishler, E.G. 1984: *The discourse of medicine: dialectics of medical interviews*. Norwood, NJ: Ablex.

Mishler, E.G. 1986: *Research interviewing. Context and narrative*. Cambridge, MA: Harvard University Press.

Morse, J.M., Bottorff, J.L. and Hutchinson, S. 1994: The phenomenology of comfort. *Journal of Advanced Nursing* **20**, 189–195.

Osherson, S. and AmaraSingham, L. 1981: The machine metaphor in medicine. In Mishler, E.G., AmaraSingham, L.R., Hauser, S.T., Liem, R., Osherson, S.D. and Waxler, N.E. *Social contexts of health, illness, and patient care*. Cambridge. Cambridge University Press, 218–49.

Pendleton, D. and Hasler, J. (eds) 1983: *Doctor–patient communication*. London: Academic Press.

Proctor, A., Morse, J.M. and Khonsari, E.S. 1996: Sounds of comfort in the trauma center – how nurses talk to patients in pain. *Social Science and Medicine* **42**, 1669–80.

Rawlinson, M.C. 1986: The sense of suffering. *Journal of Medicine and Philosophy* **11**, 39–62.

Reading, A.E. and Newton, J.R. 1978: A card sort method of pain assessment. *Journal of Psychosomatic Research* **22**, 503–12.

Reading, A.E., Everitt, B.S. and Sledmere, C.M. 1982: The McGill Pain Questionnaire: a replication of its construction. *British Journal of Clinical Psychology* **21**, 339–49.

Roter, D. 1979: Altering patient behaviour in interaction with providers. In Oborne, D.J., Gruneberg, M.M. and Eiser, J.R. (eds), *Research in psychology and medicine Vol.2.* London: Academic Press, 230–7.

Scarry, E. 1985: *The body in pain.* New York: Oxford University Press.

Skevington, S. 1995: *Psychology of pain.* Chichester: John Wiley and Sons.

Smith, M.V. 1989: *Language and pain.* Unpublished PhD thesis, University of Cambridge.

Sofaer, B. 1983: Pain relief – the importance of communication. *Nursing Times* **79**, 32–5.

Tate, P. 1983: Doctor's style. In Pendleton, D. and Hasler, J. (eds) *Doctor–patient communication.* London: Academic Press, 75–85.

Thompson, J. 1984: Communicating with patients. In Fitzpatrick, R., Hinton, J., Newman, S., Scambler, G. and Thompson, J. *The experience of illness,* London: Tavistock, 87–108.

Turner, B.S. 1984: *The body and society: explorations in social theory.* Oxford: Basil Blackwell.

Volosinov, V.N. 1973: *Marxism and the philosophy of language.* London: Seminar Press.

Waddie, N.A. 1996: Language and pain expression. *Journal of Advanced Nursing* **23**, 868–72.

Walding, M. 1991: Pain, anxiety and powerlessness. *Journal of Advanced Nursing* **16**, 388–97.

Wall, P.D. 1978: The gate control theory of pain mechanisms: re-examination and a re-statement. *Brain* **101**, 1–18.

Walsh, M. 1993: Pain and anxiety in A & E attenders. *Nursing Standard* **7**, 40–2.

Williams, S.J. 1996: Medical sociology, chronic illness and the body: a rejoinder to Michael Kelly and David Field. *Sociology of Health and Illness* **18**, 699–709.

Woolf, V. 1967: On being ill. In *Collected essays. Vol.4.* New York: Harcourt, Brace & World Inc., 193–203.

Yaksh, T.L. 1986: *Spinal afferent processing.* Plenum: New York.

Zborowski, M. 1969: *People in pain.* San Francisco: Jossey-Bass Inc.

Zola, I.K. 1966: Culture and symptoms – an analysis of patients' presenting complaints. *American Sociological Review* **31**, 615–30.

Effective pain management: is empathy relevant?

4

Judith H. Watt-Watson

Introduction

Effective pain management continues to be a challenge. Inadequate pain relief has been documented repeatedly for over 20 years, from Marks and Sachar's (1973) seminal work to the present (Watt-Watson et al., 1997). Patients in acute care settings continue to experience moderate to severe pain despite prevalent pain literature, education and treatment options. Furthermore, patient self-reports of pain and professional caregiver ratings differ (Teske et al., 1983; Iafrati, 1986; Camp and O'Sullivan, 1987; Seers, 1987; Grossman et al., 1991; Paice et al., 1991; Zalon, 1993). In addition, prescribed analgesia is often not given despite patients' reports of moderate to severe pain (Marks and Sachar, 1973; Donovan et al., 1987; Close, 1990; Paice et al., 1991; Watt-Watson and Graydon, 1995; Watt-Watson et al., 1997). Compounding these issues are patients' reluctance to disclose that they are hurting (Carr, 1990; Owen et al., 1990; Lavies et al., 1992; Watt-Watson et al., 1997) and their satisfaction with their care despite moderate to severe pain (Miaskowski et al., 1994; Ward and Gordon, 1994, 1996). Despite these inconsistencies, the nurse–patient inter-action in the process of pain management has been only minimally docu-mented. Consequently, the degree to which nurses attend to cues from patients in pain, and empathically respond to them, is not known.

The assessment of another's pain is not easy as pain is subjective and responses to pain are highly variable (Melzack and Wall, 1965, 1996). Fre-quently, no objective tests or physical evidence exist to indicate or validate a person's pain, unlike other symptoms such as fever or diabetic ketoacidosis. Therefore, caregivers need to understand as much as possible about the patients' pain experience in order to help them manage it. We need to ask patients about their pain and value their self-report, that is, believe what they say. The wish to know and understand what other people are experiencing in order to help them defines empathy (Gallop et al., 1990a). Empathic care, which focuses on the individual's unique experience, may be critical to changing current ineffective pain management practices.

For many years, empathy has been discussed in most nursing literature as the basis of a therapeutic relationship, but the concept has remained elusive. In the last decade, however, major developments in the conceptualization of empathy have been published (Wheeler, 1988; Gallop *et al.*, 1990a; Williams, 1990). In addition, measures have been developed by nurses to measure empathy in settings other than psychotherapy (La Monica, 1981; Gallop *et al.*, 1990b). However, the contribution of empathy to patient outcomes, such as pain relief, has been minimally discussed. If effective pain management requires an understanding of another's pain, then the relevance of empathy needs to be considered in this context.

An examination of empathy needs to address several questions. What has been documented about the interpersonal process between caregivers and patients in managing pain? How is empathy defined, and what tools are available to measure it? What evidence is available about the relationship between empathy and patient outcomes, including patients' pain? Discussion of these questions is important for determining the relevancy of empathy for effective pain management.

Pain management and interpersonal process

The subjectivity of pain

Pain is a subjective phenomenon that varies with each individual and each painful experience. The International Association for the Study of Pain (IASP) has defined pain as 'an unpleasant sensory and emotional experience associated with actual or potential tissue damage, or described in terms of such damage' (Merskey and Bogduk, 1994, p.210). The explanatory note with this definition emphasizes the subjectivity of the pain experience, that pain is more than a noxious stimulus, and that patients' self-reports of pain should be accepted even when tissue damage is not clearly evident.

Unrelieved acute pain can result in pulmonary, circulatory, and gastro-intestinal complications (Craig, 1981; Benedetti *et al.*, 1984; Kehlet, 1986; Kollef, 1990). Atelectasis after cardiovascular surgery has been found to be greater in patients with higher pain intensity (Puntillo and Weiss, 1994). Moreover, early postoperative pain for thoracotomy patients was the only factor that significantly predicted pain 18 months later (Katz *et al.*, 1996). However, well-managed postoperative pain can result in fewer complications, earlier mobilization and shorter hospital stays (Finley *et al.*, 1984; Wasylak *et al.*, 1990; Tuman *et al.*, 1991). Most important of all is research evidence which suggests that early treatment of acute pain, where possible before it begins, may prevent ensuing long-term pain (Bach *et al.*, 1988; Dworkin, 1996; Kalso, 1996). Therefore, it is problematic that patients in a variety of settings continue to report moderate to severe acute pain.

Perceptions of and responses to pain vary considerably, and this variability is explained by Melzack and Wall's (1965, 1996) gate control theory (GCT), ding to which a person's thoughts and emotions can influence inhibitory rotransmitters in the descending nervous system to modulate pain transmission in the dorsal horn by opening or closing the 'gate'. Painful stimuli enter an already active nervous system that is a substrate of the individual's past experience, culture, anticipation and emotions. As a result, the amount and quality of pain are determined by individual factors, resulting in major implications for effective pain management. The continuing prevalence of pain suggests that these unique responses either have not been well recognized in management strategies, or have been discounted as not being pertinent to management decisions.

Interaction between nurses and patients in pain

Pain assessment is an interactive process between patients and caregivers. Patients' input is crucial for determining the extent and impact of their pain and optimal treatment options. Yet minimal analysis has been reported about the interpersonal process that occurs between nurses' pain assessment and patients' responses. The analyses that are available indicate that there are problems with this interaction. Watt-Watson *et al.* (1997) report that the majority of their coronary bypass patient sample did not remember being asked a specific pain question such as a 0 to 10 rating, although the majority of their nurses stated that they usually used a pain rating scale; most of these patients were experiencing moderate to severe pain. An important ongoing question is why patients with pain in acute care settings are not only prescribed inadequate analgesia but also receive less than half of these doses (Donovan *et al.*, 1987; Paice *et al.*, 1991; Maxam-Moore *et al.*, 1994; Watt-Watson *et al.*, 1997).

Paired caregiver–patient research has been focused mainly on discrepancies in pain intensity ratings (Graffam, 1981; Walkenstein, 1982; Teske *et al.*, 1983; Hodgkins *et al.*, 1985; Iafrati, 1986; Seers, 1987; Sutherland *et al.*, 1988; Holmes and Eburn, 1989; Van der Does, 1989; Choiniere *et al.*, 1990; Grossman *et al.*, 1991; Paice *et al.*, 1991; Zalon, 1993; Cleeland *et al.*, 1994). Discrepancies have also existed between nurses' documentation and patients' pain descriptions (Camp and O'Sullivan, 1987). Nurses have underestimated the severity of patients' pain (Seers, 1987; Zalon, 1993), specifically for patients with moderate to severe pain ratings (Grossman *et al.*, 1991; Watt-Watson *et al.*, 1997). Choiniere *et al.* (1990) compared patient and nurse assessments of pain intensity during therapeutic procedures for severe burn injuries. Nurses' ratings were found to be correct for 49 per cent of patients at rest and 30 per cent of patients during procedures; no analgesia was given to almost 25 per cent of these patients. Teske *et al.* (1983) found a low correlation between nurses' judgements of pain based on non-verbal behaviour and self-reports of pain from both acute ($r = 0.32$, $P < 0.05$) and chronic ($r = 0.28$, $P < 0.06$) pain patients.

Caregivers' assessments may be based not on patient input, but on misbeliefs which preclude effective pain relief (Watt-Watson, 1992). Donovan *et al.*, (1987) found no significant relationship between severity of pain and (a) the nurse having discussed the pain with the patient, (b) the identification of pain as a problem on the care plan or (c) the presence of a progress note about pain. The majority of the patients in this sample and one third of Paice *et al.*'s (1991) sample indicated that nurses did not discuss patients' pain with them. Therefore, nurses' assessment and/or interpretation of patients' pain cues are frequently not accurate, especially with regard to severe pain. This problem is compounded when patient self-reports are not valued.

Few investigations have been conducted of nurses' responses to patients in pain. An examination of nurses' responses to patients' expressions of distress indicated that 62 per cent of these episodes were related to pain (Graffam, 1970). In almost 50 per cent of the patient-initiated complaints, nurses were at the bedside for another reason, and for only 2 per cent of the time were patients first approached by nurses. In over 50 per cent of the distress incidents, nurse interaction concluded within 1 minute, and only 13 per cent of nurses explored the cause of the distress with the patient. Blocking behaviours, such as not following patient cues, changing the subject, and leaving the room after the patient had made an emotional statement, were observed. Nurses' predominant responses included informing (33 per cent), suggesting relief (17 per cent), giving comfort (15 per cent) or directing patients (14 per cent). Comments that did not focus on patient needs (17 per cent) included scolding, contradicting, ridiculing, controlling, and making no comments or making multiple comments. There was minimal inquiry into the patient's pain experience, and most interactions were initiated by the patient.

In summary, little research has been published that describes the interpersonal process involved in managing pain, including nurses' responses to patients with pain. Caregivers and patients are not similar in their pain ratings, particularly where pain is moderate to severe. Moreover, caregivers' assumptions about pain, without patient validation, may contribute to ineffective pain management. For example, Graffam's (1970) examination of interaction issues identified difficulties in both recognizing distress and responding to it.

Conceptualization of empathy

No consensus has existed on how empathy should be defined or measured. The variety of definitions has often been related to the various instruments used to measure empathy. Empathy has frequently been reduced to a communication skill or a personality characteristic without there being any discussion of the empathic interaction and/or the factors influencing it. This reductionistic approach has precluded the very essence of empathy – that of the experience of the self, the other, and the interaction between the two.

Conceptual confusion

Nurses have utilized various conceptualizations and measures of empathy developed in the psychoanalytical and counselling fields. The nursing literature therefore reflects the diversity and confusion evident in these fields.

Early conceptualizations tended to compartmentalize empathy into components, such as behaviours (Barrett-Lennard, 1962; Truax and Carkhuff, 1967) and characteristics or emotions (Hogan, 1969; Mehrabian and Epstein, 1972), and in particular differentiating between an affective or cognitive focus. In the recent nursing models (Wheeler, 1988; Gallop *et al.*, 1990a; Williams, 1990), emotional and cognitive components are integrated.

The conceptual fit of empathy for nursing practice has been challenged, partly because of the body of confusing and equivocal literature surrounding the meaning and components of empathy (Pike, 1990; Morse *et al.*, 1992a). Morse *et al.*'s (1992a) premise, that empathic approaches are not realistic in acute care, confuses empathy with psychological counselling. Empathy does not require the '30 minutes or longer listening to one patient' (Morse *et al.*, 1992a, p.278) that they suggest. Empathy is a sensing of any person's experience, whether simple or complex, and is not restricted to a time frame. Rather, empathy has a timeless quality and can occur in a brief interaction of minutes or over a period of years (Wheeler, 1988; Gallop *et al.*, 1990a).

An examination of definitions of empathy in the nursing literature has pointed to confusion and/or disagreement surrounding two major issues (Watt-Watson *et al.*, 1997). The first debate relates to the appropriate objective–subjective balance of the therapeutic relationship, and is often polarized into sympathy versus empathy. The degree of acceptable involvement with others ranges from maintaining one's identity and emotional distance to losing oneself and merging with the client's experience. Distinctions between empathy and sympathy have not always been clearly understood or discussed (Ehmann, 1971; MacKay *et al.*, 1990; Morse *et al.*, 1992a). Kalisch (1973) emphasized that an empathic caregiver was always aware of his or her own separateness from the other, and that a nurse who sympathetically loses her own identity may need help herself.

Secondly, some definitions move beyond understanding feelings and meanings to include empathy as an intervention or learned skill as well. The latter define empathy then on two levels, as a way of being with another person and as a measurable and teachable communication skill (Watt-Watson *et al.*, 1997). An important question to examine is whether communicating empathic understanding to another is a component of empathy or an outcome of an empathic exchange. Validation of the accuracy of one's understanding was highlighted by Rogers (1975) and identified by Forsyth (1980) as a criterion whenever empathy exists. Does this validation need to be taught, and does it require techniques? Morse *et al.* (1992b) argue that empathy has been reduced to a mechanistic patter, or to standardized learned approaches, which caregivers use to decrease their emotional responses to clients. Their premise may be true where the use of rote communication strategies are mistaken for being empathic. However, their argument does not include a discussion of the three major nursing conceptualizations of empathy (Wheeler, 1988; Gallop *et al.*, 1990a; Williams, 1990). Gallop *et al.*'s (1989) definition of therapeutic empathy as the wish to know or understand the subjective experience of another suggests that empathy is not ritualistic, but forms the basis of all therapeutic interventions.

Major nursing models of empathy

In the last decade, nurses have published three major conceptualizations of empathy which do not fragment empathy into a personality trait, a learned skill or a contextual factor. Wheeler (1988) conceptualized empathy as an energy field pattern emerging from the continuous interaction between people and their environment. Nurses were described as resonating instruments who share and reflect patients' needs and emotions through the empathic process. She described this model as an initial effort to explore the nature of empathy by using a nursing science approach instead of borrowing concepts from psychological models.

Williams (1990) described empathy as a multidimensional phenomenon and as a unitary construct with emotional, cognitive, communicative and relational components. She addressed the empathy–sympathy issue by suggesting that inadequate analysis and reality testing results in either over-identification and experiencing the empathized emotion as one's own, or intellectualization and distancing. This model focused only on the empathizer, and not on the interaction with the other. Neither of these models was operationalized to measure empathy, unlike the model of Gallop *et al.* (1990a).

Gallop *et al.* (1990a) conceptualized empathy as a three-phased, cyclical process rather than a multidimensional phenomenon (Table 4.1), each phase being mediated by patient, context and staff variables that determine whether the process continues or stops.

In the initial inducement phase, the process continues when caregivers become engaged with and attend to the person who is expressing some need. The caregivers' willingness to be involved can be affected by mediators such as their affective sensitivity to cues, mood or cultural beliefs, and by patient characteristics such as gender. In the next matching phase, the engaged caregiver postulates what the patient may be experiencing and, if correct, continues to the next phase. The process ends if the caregiver overidentifies and is too distressed to help the other, or if he or she is perplexed and unable to understand what is actually happening. The mediators of this phase involve mainly the caregivers, the theoretical belief system, such as highly valuing empathy, may determine his or her motivation to participate. The final participating–helping phase has four possible outcomes:

- do nothing despite experiencing matching because of knowledge of the situational context or role expectations;
- offer non-specific emotional support;
- engage in instrumental problem-solving, such as information or advice; and
- demonstrate understanding of the patient's experience, such as the cause of the feeling.

The mediators influencing this phase relate mainly to:

- the caregiver, such as role, state, stereotypical beliefs, gender, habit, communication skills, and knowledge of empathic process and of the event;

- the situational context, such as ward policies; and
- the patient's state and willingness to communicate distress.

Gallop *et al.* (1990a) have addressed some of the conceptual difficulties of previous models, such as distinguishing mediators of empathy from the process itself. This model does not fragment empathy into context, empathizer or recipient, but examines the interrelationship of all three throughout the cycle of the empathic process. Gladstein (1983) emphasized that therapists may have

Table 4.1 Three phases of empathy

Phase	Mediators[a]	Possible outcomes of each phase
Inducement phase (an event is observed)	Prior role	1. Overwhelmed
	Role of observer Affective sensitivity Experiential congruence Context Expressivity of observed culture and gender	2. Disinterested 3. *Engaged*
Matching phase (an observer is engaged)	Ability to fantasize	1. Overidentification
	Ability to generate hypothetical situations	2. Perplexed state 3. Defensive state
	Perspective taking Sensitivity to cues Knowledge about event Vulnerability domains Self/other differentiation Motivational distortion	4. *Wish to help*
Participatory–helping phase (an empathic helper results)	Situational context	1. Do nothing
	Role of observer	2. Non-specific emotional support
	State of observer Stereotyping Gender Habit Expressivity of observed	3. Problem-solving
	State of observed Knowledge about empathic process Knowledge about event Communications skills Repeat the empathic process	4. *Demonstrate understanding*

[a] Examples of mediators; others are possible.

Source: Gallop, R., Lancee, W. and Garfinkel, P. 1990: The empathic process and its mediators: a heuristic model. *Journal of Nervous and Mental Disease* **178**, 649–54. Reproduced with permission of Williams and Wilkins.

the capacity to feel empathic, but may not act on this because of other factors. This dilemma has serious implications for clinical practice, and Gallop *et al.*'s (1990a) delineation of mediators as separate from the empathic process permits a closer examination of this issue.

Mediators of empathy in the context of pain management

Mediators that may determine whether pain management practices empathically reflect patient needs include the following:

- nurses' knowledge-beliefs about pain, their age, nursing experience, and birthplace;
- patients' gender, age, culture and beliefs about expressing pain; and
- situational context variables, such as ward policies, beliefs, and habituated practices.

There is empirical support for the view that some of these variables influence empathy.

Nurse mediators

Knowledge about empathy, communication skills and the current event involving the patient may influence outcomes (Gallop *et al.* 1990a). Little research has been conducted on pain knowledge and beliefs as a mediator of empathy; Watt-Watson *et al.* (1997) found that nurses' knowledge and beliefs about pain were problematic, regardless of whether their empathy levels were high or low. What has been established is that nurses have not valued patients' self-reports (Ferrell *et al.*, 1991; Brunier *et al.*, 1995), have mistrusted and disagreed with patients' pain intensity ratings, have used assessment tools minimally (Watt-Watson, 1987), and have used their own beliefs as a basis for care (Dalton, 1989). Nurses have expected patients to experience moderate to severe pain and have not seen this as unacceptable (Cohen, 1980; Weis *et al.*, 1983; Watt-Watson, 1987; Kuhn *et al.*, 1990; Lavies *et al.*, 1992). Nurses' communication with patients has tended to be brief and to focus mainly on giving advice or solutions, rather than on understanding the individual's experience (Graffam, 1970; Gallop *et al.*, 1990b). The gaps in nurses' knowledge and misbeliefs about pain assessment and management have not been recognized in their self-evaluation, particularly with regard to their reluctance to give opioids (Brunier *et al.*, 1995; Clarke *et al.*, 1996).

Nurses' characteristics, such as age, nursing experience, education level, inservice education and cultural background, may also influence the empathic process. Nurses who are younger and/or less experienced have generally been more empathic (Forsyth, 1979; Mynatt, 1985; Pennington and Pierce, 1985; Gallop *et al.*, 1990b; Reid-Ponte, 1992; Watt-Watson *et al.*, 1997). Nursing education level has been positively related to empathy (Forsyth, 1979; Kunst-Wilson *et al.*, 1981; Layton and Wykle, 1990). Nurses' empathic levels have improved after empathy-focused educational programmes (Kalisch, 1971; La Monica *et al.*, 1976; Layton, 1979; Olson and Iwasiw, 1987). The influence of nurses' birthplace on empathy is not known. Nurses' cultural background has been associated with differences in their pain knowledge levels (Brunier *et al.*, 1995; McCaffery and Ferrell, 1995) and in their inferences of patients' suffering (Davitz and Pendleton, 1969; Davitz *et al.*, 1976).

Patient mediators

Patient characteristics have been reported to influence nurses' responses. For example, nurses' empathic behaviours have been found to vary with the patient's diagnostic category, minimal levels of empathic responses being evident with borderline personality patients (Gallop *et al.*, 1990b). Nurses responded empathically only 25 per cent of the time with burn patients (Hughes *et al.*, 1990). Different levels of nurses' verbal empathy have depended on the types of client affective communication, as nurses most frequently identified patient feelings related to pain rather than to anger or depression (Olson and Iwasiw, 1989).

No research was found that examined the relationship between nurses' empathy and patients' age, gender, birthplace or pain beliefs, such as willingness to communicate pain. However, patient characteristics have influenced caregivers' perceptions of patients' pain and need for intervention. Female patients have received fewer analgesics after surgery than male patients (Faherty and Grier, 1984; Calderone, 1990; McDonald, 1994), older adult patients have received fewer analgesics than younger adult patients (Melzack *et al.*, 1987; Winefield *et al.*, 1990; Duggleby and Lander, 1994), and patients from ethnic minority groups have received less opioid analgesia postoperatively than have Caucasian patients (McDonald, 1994). Patients' own beliefs about pain may influence their seeking and accepting help (Ward *et al.*, 1993). Patients do not necessarily tell a caregiver when they are in pain (Carr, 1990; Owen *et al.*, 1990; Lavies *et al.*, 1992) – yet nurses have inferred more pain when patients verbalized their discomfort or asked for relief (Baer *et al.*, 1970; Oberst, 1978).

Context mediators

The influence of the nursing work environment on empathy is not clear. Sparling and Jones (1977) found that nurses working in a psychiatric setting were significantly more empathic than those working in other settings. However, Forsyth's (1979) and Brunt's (1985) work did not support this finding. Moreover, no significant differences were found between empathy ratings for nurses working in five psychiatric settings (Gallop *et al.*, 1990b) and nurses working in four cardiovascular surgical settings (Watt-Watson *et al.*, 1997). No research was found that described the relationship between nurses' empathy and the ward context in relation to philosophies or policies. However, nurses with greater pain knowledge and expertise experienced conflict with both

nursing and medical colleagues when they attempted to improve pain management for their patients (Ferrell *et al.*, 1993).

In summary, the complexity of the conceptualization of empathy has been
problematic and has been reflected in the variety of instruments that have been
borrowed from other disciplines and used in nursing research. Gallop *et al.*'s
(1990a) conceptualization of empathy is a major development. It has been
operationalized in a measure that examines the process of empathy separately
from its mediators.

Measures of empathy

The confusion in the conceptualization of empathy is reflected in the variety of
measures that have evolved, mainly from the counselling and psychotherapy
literature. The first empathy measures with reliability and validity were developed by Truax (1961), Barrett-Lennard (1962), Truax and Carkhuff (1967),
Hogan (1969), and Mehrabian and Epstein (1972). It is difficult to make comparisons between these measures as researchers varied in their focus on the
patient and/or therapist, in their use of self-report or judged ratings, and in
their choice of real, simulated or standard stimulus situations. Measures also
differ in their conceptualization of empathy as a behaviour, personality characteristic or process, as outlined in Table 4.2.

Most nurse researchers originally examined empathy by using instruments
from other disciplines. Early measures developed by nurses (Brunclik *et al.*,
1967; Kalisch, 1973; Clay, 1984) had no demonstrated reliability and validity
and were not used by other researchers. La Monica *et al.* (1987) developed an
empathy scale, known as the Empathy Construct Rating Scale (ECRS), to
measure the effects of nurse empathic training on client outcomes. This 84-item
measure asks about one's feelings or actions toward another on a 6-point Likert
scale. Internal consistency, but minimal convergent and discriminative validity, have been reported for this scale (La Monica, 1981; Shamian *et al.*, 1986), and
no published data have been found for a later version, known as the La Monica
Empathy Profile.

Gallop (1989), influenced by Barrett-Lennard (1962), developed a measure
of empathy as a multiphase time-sequenced process. Her measure, known
as the Staff Patient Interaction Response Scale (SPIRS) (Gallop *et al.*,
1990b), has reliability and validity, and includes a stimulus-set protocol and
scoring method. On each of the four parallel pages of this questionnaire are a
patient vignette and five patient statements to which caregivers write their best
response. Gallop *et al.*'s (1990b) scoring manual outlines 11 categories
of potential responses that reflect three ordered levels of care in the process of being empathic. Many of the predicted outcomes in the conceptualization of empathy, as described by Gallop *et al.* (1990a), are operationalized in
these categories. Within three levels of *no care, solution* and *affective involvement*,
each response category has been assigned a weight of −1, 0, 1 or 2, depending
on whether responses are (a) belittling or contradictory (−1), (b) platitudes (0),

Table 4.2 Major measures of empathy used in nursing research

Measure	Empathy definition	Description	Psychometric properties	Use in nursing research
Empathy as a behaviour				
Empathic Understanding Scale (EU) (Carkhuff, 1969, 1971)	Ability to recognize, sense and understand others' expressed feelings and to accurately communicate understanding to other	From Truax (1961) and Truax and Carkhuff's (1967) Accurate Empathy Scale. 5-point rating of therapists' verbal responses with minimally facilitative level being the midpoint of 3 (therapist and person express same affect and meaning). Judges rate interviews or audiotapes	Narrow range of scores. *Reliability*: inter-rater differences at high levels. Little test-retest evidence. Few raters for many segments with few therapists. *Validity*: lacks discrimination from other ratings, e.g. warmth	Used in Hills and Knowles, 1983; Kalisch, 1971b; La Monica, 1976; Layton, 1979; Mansfield, 1973; Mynatt, 1985; Pennington and Pierce, 1985; Sparling and Jones, 1977; Williams, 1979. Scores low. Content of response unknown
Relationship Inventory (RI) Empathy Subscale (Barrett-Lennard, 1962)	A multi-level complex process with three phases of relational response, each differing in locus and content: I, empathic recognition; II, expressed empathy of therapist; III, received empathy of patient. Experiencing process and content of others' awareness	16 items within 64-item RI, rated on 6-point scale of agreement with no neutral position. Rating of self by therapist (myself-to-other [MO]) and by patients (other-to-self [OS])	*Reliability*: split-half and test-retest. *Validity*: factor analysis for construct; little agreement between MO-OS ratings and conclude that there are different sources of assessment; not developed for hospital populations	Used in Brown, 1990; Forsyth, 1979; Gagan, 1983; Hardin and Halaris, 1983; Kalisch, 1971b; Layton, 1979; Layton and Wykie, 1990; Stetler, 1977. Suitability for hospital setting questioned
Empathy Construct Rating Scale (ECRS) (La Monica, 1981)	Accurate perception of the client's world by therapist, communication that understands the client, and client's perception that the therapist understands	84 items rated on 6-point Likert scale. Raters are clients, peers or therapist. Paper and pencil self-report. Revised unpublished measure – La Monica Empathy Profile (LEP) – 30 forced choice items to minimize social desirability not controlled for in ECRS	*Reliability*: split-half. *Validity*: little discriminative ability. No published data for LEP	Used in La Monica, 1981, 1987; Reid-Ponte, 1992; Rogers, 1986; Shamian et al., 1986. First nurse-designed measure with published psychometric data

Empathy as a personality characteristic

Questionnaire Measure of Emotional Empathy (QMEE) (Mehrabian and Epstein, 1972)	A personality attribute; a vicarious emotional response where one has a heightened responsiveness to another's emotional experience and is more likely to engage in helping behaviour	33 statements ask therapist to rate self on responses to situations involving feelings; agree–disagree on 4-point scale	*Reliability:* split-half *Validity:* minimal construct validity regarding broad definition and discriminative ability	Used in Gallop (1989) for construct validity
Empathy Scale (Hogan, 1969)	Act of reconstructing for oneself another's mental state; capacity to adopt a broad moral viewpoint	39 true-false questions ask about four components of social self-confidence, even-temperedness, sensitivity, and non-conformity	*Reliability:* test-retest *Validity:* factor-analysis confirmed three constructs; relevance of several items questionable	Used in Brunt, 1985; Forysth, 1979; MacDonald, 1977. Trait measure

Empathy as a process

Staff Patient Interaction Response Scale (Gallop, 1989; Gallop et al., 1990b)	Wish to know or understand the experience of another; a process dependent on attention of nurses to meanings and interpretations patients give to events in their lives; a 3-phased, time-sequenced process with mediators and potential outcomes at each phase	Four equivalent pages, each with a patient description and 5 patient statements to which the nurse writes verbal responses. Order of 5 statements randomized per page. Responses are rated using 11 scoring categories of responses grouped within 3 levels of care: I, no care; II, solution; III, affective involvement	*Reliability:* inter-rater reliability and test-retest *Validity:* construct with QMEE	Used in Burcher, 1992; Eastabrook, 1993; Gallop, 1989; Gallop et al., 1990b; Lancee et al., 1995; Olson, 1993, 1995. Nurse-designed measure based on Gallop's conceptual model of empathy. Includes nurses, patient and context mediators. Scoring manual standardized interpretation

Table 4.3   Examples of levels of nurses' empathic responses to SPIRS vignettes

Charles is a patient in his mid-thirties. He was admitted to hospital 2 days ago for severe chest pain. Charles says: 'I don't want to burden my family with my problem'

Nurses' levels of empathic responses

Level 1 – No care
- Your family needs to know
- Your well-being is the most important concern of your family
- You'll be alright

Level 2 – Solution
- Why do you feel this way?
- What do you mean?
- I can talk to them if that would help

Level 3 – Affective involvement
- You seem concerned about how your family will cope
- Is your family worried about what is happening to you?

(c) seeking solutions (1) or (d) reflecting affective involvement (2). An example of the three levels of nurses' empathic responses to a patient statement is given for one patient vignette in Table 4.3.

In conclusion, Hornblow (1980) has suggested that empathy be defined in a broad way rather than by focusing on selected characteristics or components. Furthermore, Gagan (1983) concluded that a measure is needed to examine the empathic process within the nurse–patient relationship. Unlike other measures, the SPIRS differentiates between the process of empathy and the mediators influencing it. The question of why caregivers may not act on their empathic feelings has serious clinical implications, and the SPIRS appears to be the only tool available to examine this issue.

Relationship between empathy and therapeutic outcomes

Patients' mood

Considerable evidence in the counselling and psychotherapy literature suggests that empathy is essential to therapeutic outcomes (Gladstein, 1983). The minimal research examining the relationship between nurses' empathy and patient outcomes has demonstrated positive changes in patients' mood or self-concept. The self-concept of institutionalized elders improved with empathic nurses (Williams, 1979), and cancer patients experienced less anxiety and hostility when they were cared for by nurses receiving empathy training (La Monica *et al.*, 1987). Brown (1990), in a qualitative interview approach, found a positive relationship between nurses' empathy and patients' satisfaction with their care. These patients identified nurses' 'being there' and 'taking time to sit and listen' as most important in their relationship. Reid-Ponte (1988) and Olson (1993) disagreed about the impact of empathy on distress levels, but their results were confounded by the fact that both patient samples had low baseline distress scores. Lancee *et al.* (1995) found that psychiatric patients reacted with less anger to nurse actors who used an interpersonal style which combined affective and solution responses.

Patients' pain management

Only one study has examined nurses' empathy and their pain management practices. Watt-Watson *et al.* (1997) compared nurses' empathic responses and their pain management as reflected by their patients' pain intensity and the analgesic doses given after coronary bypass graft surgery. Patients received less than half of the analgesia prescribed, despite their moderate to severe pain. Patients with more empathic nurses did not report less pain or receive more analgesia than patients with less empathic nurses. It was problematic that the more empathic nurses did not have much greater pain knowledge than the less empathic nurses. Although the nurses expressed confidence in their knowledge and management of pain, they were not seen by their patients as resources concerning their pain. It is important to note that these nurses had graduated on average 10 years earlier from a diploma programme with little or no recent in-service education on pain. These data point to the need to explore further the role of knowledge as a mediator of empathy in the pain context. Nurses may be empathic but have inadequate knowledge with which to help the patient.

Conclusions

The recent proliferation of both pain education programmes and research reports in journals and textbooks has not significantly changed the continuing frequency of poor pain relief. Moreover, research that examines caregiver–patient interactions in managing pain is minimal, and indicates that patient self-reports are frequently not valued. In addition, inadequate analgesic prescription and administration continue for patients in acute care despite their moderate to severe pain. Consequently, new models for directing practice and research are needed in order to solve this dilemma.

Effective pain assessment and management require that caregivers try to understand patients' unique experiences of pain, in order to help them to choose appropriate interventions. However, there has been minimal exploration of why some caregivers are more attentive to patients' cues of pain and their need for optimal pain management than others. The role of empathy in improving pain management practices is only now beginning to be considered, and the paucity of reliable and valid measures of empathy has probably contributed to this gap. Previously, the confusion within and diversity of the concept and related measurement of empathy have yielded equivocal findings about its usefulness.

Major developments in measurement (Gallop *et al.*, 1990a,b) permit an examination of the process of empathy as well as its potential mediators. Relationships between caregiver, patient and context mediators of empathy need to be included in future pain research. For example, caregivers may have an understanding of the patient's experience, but may not help because of knowledge gaps, ward culture or patient characteristics. Initial data suggest that empathy has a positive influence on patients' mood and is influenced by caregivers' knowledge and beliefs, e.g. about pain. Further research is needed before the relevance of empathy to effective pain management can be established.

Acknowledgement

I would like to thank Dr Ruth Gallop and Dr Paul Garfinkel for their invaluable contribution to my understanding of empathy.

References

Bach, S. Noreng, M. and Tjellden, N. 1988: Phantom limb pain in amputees during the first 12 months following limb amputation, after preoperative lumbar epidural blockade. *Pain* 33, 297–301.

Baer, E., Davitz, L., and Lieb, R. 1970: Inferences of physical pain: in relation to verbal and nonverbal communication. *Nursing Research* 19, 388–92.

Barrett-Lennard, G.T. 1962: Dimensions of therapist response as causal factors in therapeutic change. *Psychological Monographs* 76, 1–36.

Benedetti, C., Bonica, J. and Belluci, G. 1984: Pathophysiology and therapy of postoperative pain: a review. In Benedetti, C., Chapman, C.R. and Moricca, G. (eds.), *Recent advances in the management of pain*. New York: Raven Press, 373–407.

Brown, K. 1990: *The nurse, empathy and patient satisfaction*. Unpublished doctoral thesis, University of Utah, Salt Lake City.

Brunclik, H., Thurston, J. and Feldhusen, J. 1967: The empathy inventory. *Nursing Outlook* 15, 42–5.

Brunier, G., Carson, G. and Harrison, D. 1995: What do nurses know and believe about patients in pain? Results of a hospital survey. *Journal of Pain and Symptom Management* 10, 436–45.

Brunt, J. 1985: An exploration of the relationship between nurses' empathy and technology. *Nursing Administration Quarterly* 9, 69–78.

Burcher E. 1992: *The investigation of public health nurses' inquiry into the subjective experience of new mothers prior to giving advice*. Unpublished masters thesis, University of Toronto, Toronto.

Calderone, K. 1990: The influence of gender on the frequency of pain and sedative medication administered to postoperative patients. *Sex Roles* 23, 713–25.

Camp, D. and O'Sullivan, P. 1987: Comparison of medical, surgical and oncology patients' descriptions of pain and nurses' documentations of pain assessments. *Journal of Advanced Nursing* 12, 593–8.

Carkhuff, R. 1969: *Helping and human relations.* New York: Holt, Rinehart and Winston Inc.

Carkhuff, R. 1971: *The development of human resources: education, psychology and social change.* New York: Holt, Rinehart & Winston.

Carr, E. 1990: Postoperative pain: patients' expectations and experiences. *Journal of Advanced Nursing* 15, 89–100.

Choiniere, M., Melzack, R., Girard, N., Rondeau, J. and Paquin, M. 1990: Comparisons between patients' and nurses' assessments of pain and medication efficacy in severe burn injuries. *Pain* 40, 143–52.

Clarke, E., French, B., Bilodeau, M., Capasso, V., Edwards, A. and Empoliti, J. 1996: Pain management knowledge, attitudes and clinical practice: the impact of nurses' characteristics and education. *Journal of Pain and Symptom Management* 11, 18–31.

Clay, M. 1984: Development of an empathic interaction skills schedule in a nursing context. *Journal of Advanced Nursing* 9, 343–50.

Cleeland, C., Gonin, R., Hatfield, A. *et al.* 1994: Pain and its treatment in outpatients with metastatic cancer. *New England Journal of Medicine* 330, 592–6.

Close, S. 1990: An exploratory analysis of nurses' provision of postoperative analgesic drugs. *Journal of Advanced Nursing* 15, 42–9.

Cohen, F. 1980: Postsurgical pain relief: patients' status and nurses' medication choices. *Pain* 9, 265–74.

Craig, D. 1981: Postoperative recovery of pulmonary function. *Anaesthesia and Analgesia* 60, 46–52.

Dalton, J. 1989: Nurses' perceptions of their pain assessment skills, pain management practices, and attitudes toward pain. *Oncology Nursing Forum* 16, 225–31.

Davitz, L. and Pendleton, S. 1969: Nurses' inferences of suffering. *Nursing Research* 18, 100–7.

Davitz, L., Sameshima, Y. and Davitz, J. 1976: Suffering as viewed in six different cultures. *American Journal of Nursing* 76, 1296–7.

Donovan, M., Dillon, P. and McGuire, L. 1987: Incidence and characteristics of pain in a sample of medical-surgical inpatients. *Pain* 30, 69–78.

Duggleby, W. and Lander, J. 1994: Cognitive status and postoperative pain: older adults. *Journal of Pain and Symptom Management* 9, 19–27.

Dworkin, R. 1996: *Acute herpes zoster and postherpetic neuralgia.* Paper presented at the meeting of the Eighth World Congress on Pain, Vancouver, British Columbia, 18 August 1996.

Eastabrook, S. 1993: *Factors influencing adherence in persons with schizophrenia attending depot medication clinics.* Unpublished doctoral thesis, University of Toronto.

Ehmann, V. 1971: Empathy: its origin, characteristics and process. *Perspectives in Psychiatric Care* 9, 72–80.

Faherty, B. and Grier, M. 1984: Analgesic medication for elderly people post-surgery. *Nursing Research* 33, 369–72.

Ferrell, B., McCaffery, M. and Grant, M. 1991: Clinical-decision making and pain. *Cancer Nursing* 14, 289–97.

Ferrell, B., Rhiner, M. and Ferrell, B. 1993: Development and implementation of a pain education program. *Cancer* 72, 3426–32.

Finley, R., Keeri-Szanto, M. and Boyd, D. 1984: New analgesic agents and techniques shorten postoperative hospital stay. *Pain* 2, S397.

Forsyth, G. 1979: Exploration of empathy in nurse-client interaction. *Advances in Nursing Science* 1, 53–61.

Forsyth, G. 1980: Analysis of the concept of empathy: illustration of one approach. *Advances in Nursing Science* 2, 33–42.

Gagan, J. 1983: Methodological notes on empathy. *Advances in Nursing Science* 5, 65–72.

Gallop, R. 1989: *The influence of diagnostic labelling on the expressed empathy of nursing staff.* Unpublished doctoral thesis, University of Toronto, Toronto.

Gallop, R., Lancee, W. and Garfinkel, P. 1989: How nursing staff responded to the label 'borderline personality disorder'. *Hospital and Community Psychiatry* 40, 815–19.

Gallop, R., Lancee, W. and Garfinkel, P. 1990a: The empathic process and its mediators: a heuristic model. *Journal of Nervous and Mental Disease* 178, 649–54.

Gallop, R., Lancee, W. and Garfinkel, P. 1990b: The expressed empathy of psychiatric nursing staff. *Canadian Journal of Nursing Research* 22, 7–18.

Gladstein, G. 1983: Understanding empathy: integrating counseling, developmental and social psychology perspectives. *Journal of Counseling Psychology* 30, 467–82.

Graffam, S. 1970: Nurse response to the patient in distress – development of an instrument. *Nursing Research* 19, 331–6.

Graffam, S. 1981: Congruence of nurse-patient expectations regarding nursing intervention in pain. *Nursing Leadership* 4, 12–15.

Grossman, S., Sheidler, V., Swedeen, K., Mucenski, J. and Piantadosi, S. 1991: Correlation of patient and caregiver ratings of cancer pain. *Journal of Pain and Symptom Management* 6, 53–7.

Hardin, S. and Halaris, A. 1983: Nonverbal communication of patients and high and low empathy nurses. *Journal of Psychosocial Nursing and Mental Health Services* 21, 14–20.

Hills, M. and Knowles, M. 1983: Nurses' levels of empathy and respect in simulated interactions with patients. *International Journal of Nursing Studies* 20, 83–7.

Hodgkins, M., Albert, D. and Daltroy, L. 1985: Comparing patients' and their physicians' assessments of pain. *Pain* 23, 273–7.

Hogan, R. 1969: Development of an empathy scale. *Journal of Consulting and Clinical Psychology* 33, 307–16.

Holmes, S. and Eburn, E. 1989: Patients' and nurses' perceptions of symptom distress in cancer. *Journal of Advanced Nursing* 14, 840–46.

Hornblow, A. 1980: The study of empathy. *New Zealand Psychologist* 9, 19–28.

Hughes, J., Carver, E. and MacKay, R. 1990: The professional's use of empathy and client care outcomes. In MacKay, R., Hughes, J. and Carver, E. (eds.), *Empathy in the helping relationship.* New York: Springer Publishing Company, 107–19.

Iafrati, N. 1986: Pain on the burn unit: patient vs. nurse perceptions. *Journal of Burn Care and Rehabilitation* 7, 413–16.

Kalisch, B. 1971: An experiment in the development of empathy in nursing students. *Nursing Research* 20, 203–11.

Kalish, B. 1973: What is empathy? *American Journal of Nursing* 73, 1548–52.

Kalso, E. 1996: *Prevention of chronicity.* Paper presented at the meeting of the Eighth World Congress on Pain, Vancouver, British Columbia, 19 August 1996.

Katz, J., Jackson, M., Kavanagh, B. and Sandler, A. 1996: Long-term post-thoracotomy pain is predicted by acute post-operative pain. In *Abstracts of the Eighth World Congress on Pain,* 20 August 1996. Seattle: IASP Press, 260.

Kehlet, H. 1986: Pain relief and modification of the stress response. In Cousins, M. and Phillips, G. (eds.), *Acute pain management.* New York: Churchill Livingstone, 4–6.

Kollef, M. 1990: Trapped-lung syndrome after cardiac surgery: a potentially preventable complication of pleural injury. *Heart and Lung* 19, 671–5.

Kuhn, S., Cooke, K., Collins, M., Jones, J. and Mucklow, J. 1990: Perceptions of pain relief after surgery. *British Medical Journal* 300, 1687–90.

Kunst-Wilson, W., Carpenter, L., Poser, A., Vennohr, I. and Kushner, K. 1981: Empathic perceptions of nursing students: self-reported and actual ability. *Research in Nursing and Health* **4**, 283–93.

La Monica, E. 1981: Construct validity of an empathy instrument. *Research in Nursing and Health* **4**, 389–400.

La Monica, E., Carew, D., Winder, A., Haase, A. and Blanchard, K. 1976: Empathy training as the major thrust of a staff development program. *Nursing Research* **25**, 447–51.

La Monica, E., Wolf, R., Madea, A. and Oberst, M. 1987: Empathy and nursing care outcomes. *Scholarly Inquiry for Nursing Practice: An Institutional Journal* **1**, 197–219.

Lancee, W., Gallop, R., McCay, E. and Toner, B. 1995: The relationship between nurses' limit-setting styles and anger in psychiatric inpatients. *Psychiatric Services* **46**, 609–13.

Lavies, N., Hart, L., Rounsefell, B. and Runciman, W. 1992: Identification of patient, medical and nursing attitudes to postoperative opioid analgesia: stage 1 of a longitudinal study of postoperative analgesia. *Pain* **48**, 313–19.

Layton, J. 1979: The use of modelling to teach empathy to nursing students. *Research in Nursing and Health* **2**, 163–76.

Layton, J. and Wykle, M. 1990: A validity study of four empathy instruments. *Research in Nursing and Health* **13**, 319–25.

McCaffery, M. and Ferrell, B. 1995: Nurses' knowledge about cancer pain: a survey of 5 countries. *Journal of Pain and Symptom Management* **10**, 356–69.

McDonald, D. 1994: Gender and ethnic stereotyping and narcotic analgesic administration. *Research in Nursing and Health* **17**, 45–9.

MacKay, R., Hughes, J. and Carver, E. 1990: *Empathy in the helping relationship.* New York: Springer Publishing Company.

Mansfield, E. 1973: Empathy: concept and identified psychiatric nursing behaviour. *Nursing Research* **22**, 525–30.

Marks, R. and Sachar, E. 1973: Undertreatment of medical inpatients with narcotic analgesics. *Annals of Internal Medicine* **78**, 173–81.

Maxam-Moore, V., Wilkie, D. and Woods, S. 1994: Analgesics for cardiac surgery patients in critical care: describing current practice. *American Journal of Critical Care* **3**, 31–9.

Mehrabian, A. and Epstein, N. 1972: A measure of emotional empathy. *Journal of Personality* **40**, 525–43.

Melzack, R. and Wall, P. 1965: Pain mechanisms: a new theory. *Science* **150**, 971–9.

Melzack, R. and Wall, P. 1996: *The challenge of pain.* Toronto: Penguin Books.

Melzack, R., Abbott, F., Zackon, W., Mulder, D. and Davis, M. 1987: Pain on a surgical ward: a survey of the duration and intensity of pain and the effectiveness of medication. *Pain* **29**, 67–72.

Merskey, H. and Bogduk, N. 1994: *Classification of chronic pain: descriptions of chronic pain syndromes and definitions of pain terms,* 2nd edn. Seattle: IASP Press.

Miaskowski, C., Nichols, R., Brody, R. and Synold, T. 1994: Assessment of patient satisfaction utilizing the American Pain Society's quality assurance standards on acute and cancer-related pain. *Journal of Pain and Symptom Management* **9**, 5–11.

Morse, J., Anderson, G., Bottorff, J. *et al.* 1992a: Exploring empathy: a conceptual fit for nursing practice? *Image* **24**, 273–80.

Morse, J., Bottorff, J., Anderson, G., O'Brien, B. and Solberg, S. 1992b: Beyond empathy: expanding expressions of caring. *Journal of Advanced Nursing* **17**, 809–21.

Mynatt, S. 1985: Empathy in faculty and students in different types of nursing preparation programs. *Western Journal of Nursing Research* **7**, 333–48.

Oberst, M. 1978: Nurses' inferences of suffering: the effects of nurse-patient similarity, and verbalizations of distress. In Nelson, M.J. (ed.). *Clinical perspectives in nursing research*. New York: Teachers College Press, 38–60.

Olson, J. 1993: *Relationships between nurse-expressed empathy, patient-perceived empathy and patient distress*. Unpublished doctoral thesis, Wayne State University, Michigan.

Olson, J. 1995: Relationships between nurse-expressed empathy, patient-perceived empathy and patient distress. *Image* 27, 317–22.

Olson, J. and Iwasiw, C. 1987: Effects of a training model on active listening skills of post-RN students. *Journal of Nursing Education* 26, 104–7.

Olson, J. and Iwasiw, C. 1989: Nurses' verbal empathy in four types of client situations. *Canadian Journal of Nursing Research* 21: 39–51.

Owen, H., McMillan, V. and Rogowski, D. 1990: Postoperative pain therapy: a survey of patient's expectations and their experiences. *Pain* 41, 303–7.

Paice, J., Mahon, S. and Faut-Callahan, M. 1991: Factors associated with adequate pain control in hospitalized postsurgical patients diagnosed with cancer. *Cancer Nursing* 14, 298–305.

Pennington, R. and Pierce, W. 1985: Observations of empathy of nursing-home staff: a predictive study. *International Journal of Aging and Human Development* 21, 281–290.

Pike, A. 1990: On the nature and place of empathy in clinical nursing practice. *Journal of Professional Nursing* 6, 235–40.

Puntillo, K. and Weiss, S. 1994: Pain: its mediators and associated morbidity in critically ill cardiovascular surgical patients. *Nursing Research* 43, 31–6.

Reid-Ponte, P. 1988: *The relationships among empathy and the use of Orlando's deliberative process by the primary nurse and the distress of the adult cancer patient*. Unpublished doctoral thesis, Boston University.

Reid-Ponte, P. 1992: Distress in cancer patients and primary nurses' empathic skills. *Cancer Nursing* 15, 283–92.

Rogers, C. 1975: Empathic: an unappreciated way of being. *The Counseling Psychologist* 5, 2–9.

Rogers, I. 1986: The effects of undergraduate nursing education on empathy. *Western Journal of Nursing Research* 8, 329–42.

Seers, K. 1987: Perceptions of pain. *Nursing Times* 2, 37–42.

Shamian, J., Leprohon, J. and Zamanck, A. 1986: *Clients' and nurses' perceptions of empathy levels of personnel in an emergency department*. Poster session presented at the International Nursing Research Conference, Edmonton, Alberta, June 1986.

Sparling, S. and Jones, S. 1977: Setting: a contextual variable associated with empathy. *Journal of Psychiatric Nursing and Mental Health Services* 15, 9–12.

Stetler, C. 1977: Relationship of perceived empathy to nurses' communication. *Nursing Research* 26, 432–8.

Sutherland, J., Wesley, R., Cole, P., Nesvacil, L., Daly, M. and Gepner, G. 1988: Differences and similarities between patient and physician perceptions of patient pain. *Family Medicine* 20, 343–6.

Teske, K., Daut, R. and Cleeland, C. 1983: Relationships between nurses' observations and patients' self-reports of pain. *Pain* 16, 289–96.

Truax, C. 1961: A scale for measurement of accurate empathy. *Psychiatric Institute Bulletin* 1, 12.

Truax, C. and Carkhuff, R. 1967: *Toward effective counselling and psychotherapy*. Chicago: Aldine Publishing Co.

Tuman, K., McCarthy, R., March, R., DeLaria, G., Patel, R. and Ivankovich, A. 1991:

Effects of epidural anaesthesia and analgesia on coagulation and outcome after major vascular surgery. *Anesthesia Analgesia* **73**, 696–704.

Van der Does, A.J. 1989: Patients' and nurses' ratings of pain and anxiety during burn wound care. *Pain* **39**, 95–101.

Walkenstein, M. 1982: Comparison of burned patients' perception of pain with nurses' perception of patients' pain. *Journal of Burn Care Rehabilitation* **3**, 233–6.

Ward, S. and Gordon, D. 1994: Application of the American Pain Society quality assurance standards. *Pain* **56**, 266–306.

Ward, S. and Gordon, D. 1996: Patient satisfaction and pain severity as outcomes in pain management: a longitudinal view of one setting's experience. *Journal of Pain Symptom Management* **11**, 242–51.

Ward, S., Goldberg, N., Miller-McCauley, V. *et al.* 1993: Patient-related barriers to management of cancer pain. *Pain* **52**, 319–24.

Wasylak, T., Abbott, F., English, M. and Jeans, M. 1990: Reduction of postoperative morbidity following patient-controlled morphine. *Canadian Journal of Anaesthesia* **37**, 726–31.

Watt-Watson, J. 1987: Nurses' knowledge of pain issues: a survey. *Journal of Pain and Symptom Management* **2**, 207–11.

Watt-Watson, J. 1992. Misbeliefs. In Watt-Watson, J. and Donovan, M. (eds), *Pain management: nursing perspective*. St Louis, MO: Mosby Year Book, 36–58.

Watt-Watson, J. and Graydon, J. 1995: Impact of surgery on head and neck cancer patients and their caregivers. *Nursing Clinics of North America* **30**, 659–671.

Watt-Watson, J., Garfinkel, P., Gallop, R., Stevens, B. and Streiner, D. 1997: *The relationship between nurses' empathic responses and pain management in acute care*. Unpublished doctoral thesis, University of Toronto.

Weis, O., Sriwantanakul, K., Alloza, J., Weintraub, M. and Lasagna, L. 1983: Attitudes of patients, housestaff and nurses toward postoperative analgesic care. *Anaesthesia Analgesia* **62**, 70–74.

Wheeler, K. 1988: A nursing science approach to understanding empathy. *Archives of Psychological Nursing* **2**, 95–102.

Williams, C. 1979: Empathic communication and its effect on client outcome. *Issues in Mental Health Nursing* **2**, 15–26.

Williams, C. 1990: Biopsychosocial elements of empathy: a multidimensional model. *Issues in Mental Health Nursing* **11**, 155–74.

Winefield, H., Katsikitis, M., Hart, L. and Rounsefell, B. 1990: Postoperative pain experiences: relevant patient and staff attitudes. *Journal of Psychosomatic Research* **34**, 543–52.

Zalon, M. 1993: Nurses' assessment of postoperative patients' pain. *Pain* **54**, 329–34.

Cultural dimensions of pain

Bryn D. Davis

Introduction

If one patient responds to postoperative pain with obvious verbal and non-verbal expressions of pain and requests for relief, and yet another patient in the same situation lies quietly and seems to be in much less pain, why is this?

Another patient suffering from chronic pain relates this to the fact that they have been in some way guilty of some sin, or regret some action in the past. Yet another believes that the pain is a challenge from God, as part of life's experience and through which there is a greater likelihood of entering heaven. The first is very depressed, full of regret and finds it difficult to cope, whereas the second fights on, trying to make the most of life. What factors are operating to bring about these different ways of expressing or giving meaning to pain?

The basic insights about the mechanism and experience of pain that allow these differences to occur, and enable this kind of chapter to be written, are embodied in the gate control theory of pain that was promulgated by Melzack and Wall in 1965, and which has been the basis of much further research and development since then. A major advantage of this model for the pain mechanism and experience is the potential for influence from the cerebral cortex – and with that for psychological, sociological and cultural influences – on the pain experience.

For example, we have individual behaviours that are affected by social processes, which include sensations, emotions, motivations and expectations. We have interpersonal relationships where we share beliefs about pain and its management, relationships such as those with our family, friends or health care professionals, from which we receive social motivation such as support, approval and resources. We also belong to various groups and have inter-group relationships from which we gain social representations of pain, group beliefs, group experiences, personal and social categorizations, and social identification. Finally, we are influenced by higher order factors (dealing with society and culture) such as health culture, ideology, politics, quality of life, and economic aspects (see Figure 5.1).

Skevington (1995), in a comprehensive review and discussion of the psychological and social aspects of the pain experience, offers a detailed model of social and cultural influences covering these four levels, which she explores in some depth and for which she draws on a wide range of literature. Many of the points covered by this model will be the focus of discussion in the various sections of this chapter, and will form the basis of the nursing implications which are explored in the concluding section.

It is perhaps important to clarify at this stage that pain is seen as being 'all in the mind', in that what we experience as pain is the result of stimuli reaching various parts of the brain and being interpreted as, and experienced in the conscious mind as, pain. The stimuli – that is, the impulses that travel from the periphery to the central nervous system, wherever they might start and

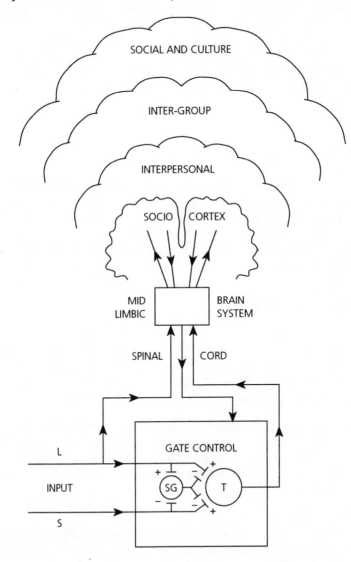

Figure 5.1 Socio-cultural extension of the gate control model of pain (after Melzack and Wall, 1996, and Skevington, 1995). L, large diameter fibres; S, small diameter fibres; SG, substantia gelatinosa; T, transmission cells; +, excitation; –, inhibition

through whatever routes they travel – are not the pain. Pain is an experience by the conscious mind, and sometimes it is very difficult, if not impossible, to identify any particular set of nervous impulses that might have brought about that experience. However, in most instances of a pain experience there are clear indications of particular nervous impulses from a source that could cause pain.

The focus of this chapter, then, is on the social and cultural factors that can influence the experience of and response to pain. In the first section, the concept of culture will be explored in order to gain some insight as to how it might affect the way that we interpret and interact with the world in which we live. In the second section we shall explore in general terms the influences of culture on our perceptions and behaviour regarding health and illness. Then, in the next section, we can look specifically and in some detail at the relationship between culture and pain. In conclusion, we can then consider the implications for nursing of these cultural influences on pain.

Culture

Before we can start to consider the influence that culture might have on pain experience and behaviour, it is important that we clarify what is meant by the term. In an attempt to arrive at an interpretation that is suitable for the present purposes, a review of some approaches will be undertaken and a definition reached which will form the basis of the following discussions concerning health, illness and pain.

Approaches to culture

Keesing (1981, cited in Helman, 1994) has offered the following definition from the field of social anthropology: 'systems of shared ideas, systems of concepts and rules and meanings that underlie and are expressed in the ways that humans live' (p.68). Helman himself offers:

> a set of guidelines (both explicit and implicit) which individuals inherit as members of a particular society, and which tell them how to view the world, how to experience it emotionally and how to behave in it in relation to other people, to supernatural forces or gods, and to the natural environment.
>
> (Helman, 1994, p.2)

Leininger identifies culture as 'values, beliefs, norms and life-ways of a particular group that guide their thinking, decisions and actions in patterned ways' (Leininger, 1991, p.47).

As a shared set of guidelines or understandings, culture does not exactly specify particular behaviours, but the individuals in social groups then develop agreed behaviours with varying ranges of tolerance about them with respect to social phenomena – such as health and illness. Every culture has subgroups that follow major identifying understandings about the world, supernatural forces or gods and the environment, but which have relatively minor differences regarding some of these understandings. These subgroups can focus around religious beliefs, geographical areas with regional character-istics such as language dialects, or be related to particular ways of life such as farming or certain industries. These subgroups can be fiercely loyal to their particular way of life, religion or language variant, even though they do acknowledge and share the overall cultural understandings.

Some cultures are less tolerant than others in the degree to which such deviations can occur, e.g. with only one religion and one way of practising that religion being allowed. Tribal or sectarian conflicts over such issues can lead to warfare or pogroms against the subgroup that is seen to be too different, or taking too much.

Another term that is used in this context of culture is 'ethnic'. Smooha has defined 'ethnic' as relating to a descent group with a common culture who 'perceive themselves as a distinct ethnic group ("we" and "they" feelings) who sense a common fate, interact more among themselves than with outsiders and think and behave similarly' (Smooha, 1985, p.267).

An ethnic group may be a separate culture with distinct geographical boundaries, or it may be a subgroup within a larger cultural group, embracing the majority of the larger group cultural understandings, but retaining some understandings and behaviours associated with the subgroup which gives it a slightly different identity to the rest of the larger cultural group (Lipton and Marbach, 1984).

'Race' is a term that is sometimes used to discriminate between people, usually with regard to physical or biological characteristics rather than psy-chological, sociological or behavioural ones. Certain of the latter may be imputed by some to be corollaries of the physical or biological characteristics (Dobson, 1991). It is a term that is frequently used in a derogatory sense, but one that does not really have much scientific validity. It is a concept that is frequently used as a basis for inter-group conflict and aggression, with neg-ative stereotypical behavioural characteristics being attributed to one group. Such stereotypical attitudes are known as prejudice, and can influence behav-iour in quite subtle ways. Simplistic models of culture can be merely prejudice, with members of particular subgroups or ethnic groups being classified and categorized according to stereotypes rather than as individuals. Professionals who are attempting to include culture as one aspect of care in any health care situation must beware of this danger.

Transcultural nursing has been developing as an approach to care over the last two or three decades, and there are now quite a few textbooks offering models of care involving culture as a major determinant. Leininger (1991), for example, has published regularly, and her sunrise model, which illustrates all of the possible influences on a person's perception of and response to health problems, is well known. Other writers in the field include Orque et al. (1983)

from the USA. Dobson (1991) reflects the situation in the UK, and also contains a useful review of other models.

These books are useful for gaining insights into the general dynamics of different cultures, often based on the experiences of the authors with various cultural groups. However, the information is frequently anecdotal, or based on interviews with small samples. The information should be seen as a guide to gaining relevant information through individual interviews with patients to find out just how much of the general information applies to that particular person and his or her health care problem.

Conclusions

Within the subgroups and the larger group there are always individual variations in the shared understandings, guidelines and behaviours, within a range of tolerance that is acceptable to the particular culture or society. As these understandings are shared and transmitted, there is much opportunity for the development of individual nuances, particularly within families. Certainly for anyone working within large cultural groupings, e.g. in the delivery of health care, sensitivity to the subtleties of understandings and behaviours in the various subgroups and between individuals is vital. This point will be developed further below, particularly in the section on nursing management.

One of the major aspects of life that might be influenced by the within-group and between-group influences is that of health. If we refer to Figure 5.1 again we can see the variety of levels from which influence might percolate to affect the individual's views of and reactions to health problems. In the next section, some of the ways in which culture can influence perceptions, values and behaviours with regard to health and illness will be explored.

Culture and health

Within this section we shall address those aspects of culture that relate to perceptions and practices concerning health and illness. Different societies have varying histories, experiences and problems concerning health issues for which they develop solutions to suit their general belief and value systems. They may have the same problems as other societies, but find or develop different solutions. They will evolve different values and different concepts and meanings of illness and health, and life and death (Twaddle and Hessler, 1977). Nevertheless, within each society definitions of health problems and responses will be developed, organized and even codified. Moreover, within each culture we will find that medicine – the treatment or management of ill health – is itself a separate subculture within the dominant culture. There will be a separate, arcane language and rituals to be learned and practised by the practitioner, whatever he or she may be called. The specialization of language and ritual or practice of health care often makes this an alien subculture.

Cultural perceptions of health and illness

There are generally four sources of ill health acknowledged in most societies:

1. factors within the individual;
2. factors in the natural world;
3. factors in the social world;
4. factors in the supernatural world or worlds (e.g. witchcraft).

Explanations of ill health in non-industrial societies commonly involve combinations of (3) and (4), (Helman, 1994). This can often take the form of accusations of witchcraft or magic, resulting from a breakdown in interpersonal relationships.

Other explanations can involve spiritual and religious factors whereby, under the influence of religious or spiritual trances, individuals or groups can undergo what in other circumstances would be regarded as very painful experiences. Melzack and Wall (1996) described some examples of these when they first introduced their gate control theory of pain to the wider readership. They describe individuals being suspended from hooks, walking on hot coals or undergoing invasive surgical procedures without any usual anaesthetic. Indeed, it was an awareness of experiences such as this that informed the development and intuitive acceptance of the new theory.

Blaxter (1983, cited in Skevington, 1995) proposed three main concepts of what is meant by 'healthy' from responses to a large-scale survey of attitudes. These were:

- a sense of positive fitness, energy and strength, with an efficient and athletic body;
- the ability to perform roles normally, having a hardy personality;
- being unstressed, unworried, coping, and being in tune with the world as perceived within the particular culture.

Often the ways in which the entities of disease, illness and sickness are conceptualized in different cultures can be helpful in understanding an individual's particular problems. Helman (1994) has offered a comprehensive discussion of the concepts of disease, illness and sickness. The following definitions summarize his arguments:

- disease usually has some biological, physical dimension, based on some biomedical model and some understanding of the mechanisms which keep the body going;
- illness is usually conceptualized as a psychological or abstract phenomenon. It has social, moral, psychological and physical aspects. It can affect social functioning and can overlap with;
- sickness, which is the way in which the disease or illness affects the ability of the individual to meet his or her social role responsibilities.

Kleinman (1988) offers the idea of 'explanatory models', and argues that disease is the practitioner's problem, and that illness has meaning for the sufferer – the experience of symptoms. It could be added that sickness affects the group or society to which an individual belongs.

Culture can also influence the language in which ill health might be reported, as well as the non-verbal behaviour that might express it.

- Some cultures tend to expect a more emotional tone to the reporting of symptoms of ill health, whilst others demand a less emotional presentation.
- Some cultures expect it to be presented in the third person, as if the symptoms belong to someone else or to a doll or figurine.
- There are often gender issues here as well, with women in particular being expected to perform or behave in particular ways.
- In some situations the illness itself may be referred to as a person or entity that is invading the body or mind of the sufferer.
- The illness may also be presented by the family, all reporting on behalf of the sufferer who may not be allowed to report, or who may call upon his or her family members to confirm the story being told.
- The symptoms are frequently reported as a story, a description of a process or of relationships, and of a breakdown in relationships which is linked to the particular symptoms.

In many cultures there are at least two languages relating to health and illness, namely the 'official' medical or practitioner language, and the lay or folk language. These different languages may reflect different understandings of the nature, causation and treatment of health problems. Folk views of illness frequently have symbolic meanings of a psychological, social or even moral nature. Often emotional or social stress may be converted into physical symptoms, and in many societies certain diseases are seen as symptoms not, say, of infection but of immoral or self-indulgent behaviour, e.g. lung cancer or AIDS.

Attempts have been made to classify some of these, such as that by Helman (1994), who suggests three models, namely a plumbing model (all pipes, tubes and pumps), a machine model (using fuel and energy) and a mechanical model (with different working parts leading to mechanical breakdown and damage to the system). Many ideas about the treatment or management of ill health and disease employed in folk medicine utilize models such as these, and the language used by the patient and also by the practitioner may relate to such explanations.

Some of the explanations can become quite elaborate, have a history of many centuries of development, and form the basis of very sophisticated medical systems. Chinese medicine is a good example, with acupuncture being a familiar treatment method. Herbal medicine similarly has a great heritage, and spans the Eastern and Western worlds. In the UK there are now some well-established courses preparing practitioners in Chinese medicine and acupuncture, and in herbal medicine at master's and bachelor's degree levels. As a university adviser to such courses, the present author has direct experience of the sophistication and firm grounding of the theory and practice of these approaches to health and illness.

Chinese medicine has its foundations in another very different culture, but has found ways of linking in with our Western medicine to offer complementary approaches to care. Herbal medicine, deriving from an approach to health and illness that is much more closely related to nature than to the laboratory, can be seen as a subcultural approach within our Western model, but also as relating to other models from other cultures. It makes an interesting bridge between cultures and peoples.

There are many alternative approaches to treatment of ill health, which are often based on folk models of health, and practised within or alongside orthodox medicine. Many of these involve physical contact and time spent discussing the nature of the health care problem with the patient or client. These interpersonal approaches reflect some of the ways in which external factors and processes can influence individual understandings of and responses to illness, as described in Figure 5.1. There are very many of these, some of them being very similar. Nanke and Canter (1993) refer to 33 types in their attempt to categorize and classify them. Many of them are used in the management of pain, of course, and we shall consider these in the next section.

Conclusions

Thus there seem to be some diversities and some universalities in the way in which people conceive of illness, disease and sickness. However, different cultures and subgroups within cultures have different ways of expressing these and of practising health care. Language seems to play a very important part, and can even make the practitioners part of an alien culture (or they may make themselves intentionally such for reasons of power and control).

In the next section, in what might be seen as the main part of this chapter, we shall consider how culture can influence the experience and/or the expression of pain, and following that, we shall examine the implications for the management of pain in people from different cultures.

Culture and pain

There have been many studies of the experience and management of pain in different cultures. This introductory section will start with a general review of key aspects of the work, followed by a main section in which the research will be considered more critically and from an historical slant. Finally, conclusions will be drawn with regard to the main implications of the research for the nursing management of pain.

In their various versions of *The Challenge of Pain* (the latest published in 1996), Melzack and Wall have reported a range of evidence indicating the ways in which people from different cultures cope with or tolerate pain. They refer to studies of hook-swinging in Indian villages (Kosambi, 1967), where young men hang from long poles above carts, suspended by hooks through their abdominal wall as they are carried from village to village as part of a religious ceremony. This is also reported by Helman (1994) as being a practice of the Cheyenne in the Great Plains of the USA. He also refers to the work of Pugh (1991), who describes the social and cultural influences on the pain experience and the way it is described in North India, where pain is seen as a mixture of meanings relating to social, spiritual and emotional issues reflecting the integrated body–mind system of culture, as well as being a physical event. Emotional distress may also be described in terms of physical pain.

Melzack has shown films, which have been seen by the present author, of people in African villages undergoing the operation of trepanning, whereby a section of the cranium is removed after the scalp has been cut and turned back to reveal the bone, the patient assisting in the procedure and chatting to the 'hakim' during it. One example showed a young man crouching at the side of a track in the bush, holding a large wooden bowl to catch the blood running from his scalp as it was cut, and discussing the procedure with the man performing the operation, and being watched by fellow villagers. All of the individuals involved seemed to be treating the situation in a most calm and matter-of-fact way, whilst Western viewers of the film were stunned.

Examples of the use of folk medicine in the treatment of pain are referred to by Melzack and Wall (1996), including the application of pain to treat pain, with 'cupping', scarification and cautery (all of which are examples of counter-irritation) and acupuncture being common methods. However, the evidence for these tends to consist of historical reports or observational studies, rather than properly controlled experimental designs. The gate control theory of pain is the only modern theory that offers a mechanism which could explain some of these phenomena.

From some of these studies, often those of an anthropological nature, models have evolved which can help the practitioner. An example is that of Helman (1994), who argues that (1) not all sociocultural groups may respond to pain in exactly the same way, (2) perceptions and responses to pain in the self and in others are influenced by the cultural and social background, and (3) communication of pain is influenced by social and cultural factors. This approach was very much influenced by the work of Zborowski (1952), who suggested as a result of his studies that the expectations and acceptance of pain are cultural.

However, Helman (1994) does differentiate between private and public pain. He argues that the way in which pain is described by patients depends on a number of factors, including language facility, familiarity with medical terms, individual experiences of pain, and lay beliefs about the structure and functions of the body. He suggests that public pain implies a social relationship, and expectations regarding the expression of pain influence that expression (in terms of the nature of the response to the pain behaviour and the relative costs and benefits to the expression of pain).

Helman supports the argument of Engel (1950) and Lewis (1981) that, even in childhood, experiences of pain are very important in general psychological development, and may become associated with being 'bad' or feeling guilty and punishing oneself, as well as with gaining attention. Zborowski (1952) also reported that he believed that the cultural values of parents and other family members help to develop attitudes to and expectations of pain. Most of these views and proposals are contained within the psychosocial model offered by Skevington (1995), and are summarized in the introduction to the chapter.

Research evidence

There has been quite a long history of attempts to study the relationship between culture and the experience and expression of pain. One of the earliest was that of Le Barre (1947) who identified non-verbal behavioural differences and, in 1950, Engel was arguing for the importance of pain in psychological development. Pain in this context was seen as a warning of the dangers of the environment. It can also be associated with punishment and being 'bad' in childhood, and thus lead to adult interpretations of pain as being a challenge or a punishment, or seeking atonement through their suffering. This was also reported by Zborowski (1952), with parents manifesting different approaches to pain or environmental dangers that might lead to pain being experienced by their children.

From a review of a variety of studies Melzack and Wall (1996) offer three levels of pain threshold:

- the sensation threshold, for which there seems to be no evidence of cultural difference (Sternbach and Tursky, 1965);
- the pain perception threshold (that is, the sensation changes from non-pain to pain), e.g. the difference reported by Hardy et al. (1952) between perception of heat by people of Mediterranean origin and northern Europeans, and also of the tolerance of Nepalese porters (Clark and Clark, 1980), who required higher levels of electric shock before they reported them as painful, compared to their Western employers; and
- the pain tolerance threshold (that is, the point at which an increasingly painful stimulus can no longer be tolerated), where people from different cultures tolerate different levels of pain (Zborowski, 1952; Lambert et al., 1960; Woodrow et al., 1972; Clark and Clark, 1980).

From the 1960s the research seemed to focus on studies of the expression of pain in various cultures, e.g. the studies of Zola (1966) and Woodrow et al. (1972), as well as the earlier work of Zborowski (1952). In particular, Fabrega and Tyma (1976) demonstrated linguistic and semantic differences between groups where the same word had different meanings or different words were used to generate the same meaning. Patients tend to construe their own meaning with reference to chronic pain. Robinson (1990) identified three themes of meaning from patients with such illnesses, namely tragic, sad and heroic. Much of this is due to uncertainty – uncertainty about the cause of the pain, about the outcome of treatment and about the future consequences or expectancy.

These meanings can be culturally determined as well. Two interesting studies have demonstrated that pain might have different meanings in different cultural groups or subgroups. Skultans (1976) showed that Welsh Spiritualists shared their pain and thus, through making their pain 'public', helped the pain. Similarly, McGuire (1988) later showed that Episcopalian communities used their pain to come closer to God. The present author, working in Muslim countries, has found that Shi'ite Muslims also see pain as a way of getting closer to God, whereas the Sunni Muslims would prefer to seek pain relief. Some of these meanings can be developed in childhood, where ideas of pain as a punishment or as resulting from bad behaviour have been found in young children (Perrin and Gerrity, 1981; Gaffney and Dunne, 1987). Savedra *et al.* (1982) have also identified three categories of thinking about the causes of pain that reflected the Piagetian phases of cognitive development, which were also similar to those derived by Brewster (1982). In this model, phase one involved pain as punishment or the result of external hits or falls. The second phase involved the idea of disease and surgery and something of the mechanism of pain perception. The third, older phase involved an understanding of the psychological aspects, and a more thorough understanding of the physio-logical process was possible, together with the possibility of predicting likely outcomes of events. Earlier workers had postulated that the parents influence this developmental process. For example, Zborowski (1952) reported that Jew-ish and Italian Americans responded quickly if their children expressed pain, and made them fear pain, whereas Old Americans encouraged their children to expect and cope with pain, and not to come running to them with every little hurt.

Several studies spanning the period from the 1960s to the 1990s have looked at the influence of pain on integration into the main group. The more inte-grated a person is, the more he or she will follow the main cultural pattern. However, if the individual is not so well integrated into his or her main cultural group, then a more personal way of expressing pain will be demonstrated. For example, Buss and Portnoy (1967) showed that the degree of identification with a cultural group could influence the tolerance of pain, on the basis of a study of Jewish women who, from a sense of loyalty to their cultural group, tolerated higher levels of pain than other groups. Bates *et al.* (1993) found that ethnic group identity and feelings of being in control (or not) had a powerful influence, particularly in the case of Italians.

Although some of the results of the studies presented here might seem fairly persuasive, there have been criticisms of many of them. In particular, meth-odological critiques have been offered by Weisenberg (1977), Wolff and Lang-ley (1977) and Wolff (1985). The main criticisms concern the nature of the data collected, often by self-report and without adequate controls, and using small samples. Different methods of inducing and measuring pain have been used, which have led to differences in results. Moreover, in some studies there has been a tendency to amalgamate people from different cultures into larger cultural groups. For example, Zborowski (1952) amalgamated Japanese, people from the Philippines and Asians into a single cultural group. Lipton and Marbach (1984), along with a critique of Zborowski's work, found in their own study that there was a high level of homogeneity between cultural groups, with more differences between subgroups. However, they reported that descrip-tions and levels of intensity of pain did show cultural differences.

In the previous section, alternative models of health and illness and also approaches to treatment were discussed, and in particular a range of these were identified as being related to the management of pain. A recent review of the effectiveness of these approaches considered 49 studies published over a period of more than two decades (Sindhu, 1996). Looking at only randomized controlled trials of such non-pharmacological approaches to the management of pain, following a meta-analysis, the author was unable to demonstrate an overall significant effect. This was influenced by the wide variety of interventions. However, an attempt was made to analyse subgroups of a more homogeneous nature, but again no significant effect was demonstrated. The only interventions that did approach the level of significance were relaxation and patient teaching.

In a meta-analysis of the use of similar interventions with children, Broome et al. (1989) did find some significant effects, but they commented that again there were methodological limitations to this research. The authors mentioned small sample sizes, invalid indices of pain (quiet vs. noisy behaviour), little testing of the validity of the medium (Did relaxation really occur? Was information that was given actually received and understood?), and also the wide range of slightly different interventions, often consisting of mixtures of interventions, rather than single ones.

Conclusions

In summary, there would seem to have been some evidence produced demonstrating that the meaning of pain, and the language and expression of pain, can be influenced by cultural or subcultural affiliations. There is some indication that the degree of personal identification with a particular culture is important in determining whether or not an individual is influenced by that cultural stereotype. There is also evidence that some of these meanings and forms of expression are learned in childhood, during the developmental process and through parental influence.

Nevertheless, there is also evidence that there is much heterogeneity within cultural groups, and some of the studies suffered from methodological limitations which prevent them from offering findings that can be generalized to a whole culture. Skevington (1995) has suggested that there is a need for at least three levels of knowledge or understanding about social influences on pain. The first level is that of socially based individual differences, which has been quite thoroughly researched. The second level is that of interpersonal and group dynamics – how people are influenced socially. Relatively little is known with regard to pain. Finally, Skevington suggests that research into the effects of inter-group relationships on pain must be included (Skevington, 1995, p.80).

It would seem that we are thrown back on the understanding that pain is in the mind of the person suffering it, and that any cultural influences can only be derived from that person him- or herself. The imposition of any cultural stereotypical interpretations or expectations on any assessment of an individual in pain is not valid, and certainly there is no research to justify it. The implications for the nursing management of pain will be the focus of the next and final section of the chapter.

Culture and the nursing management of pain

In the various sections of this chapter so far we have covered many aspects of culture in relation to both health and the management of pain. From a consideration of what is meant by culture, we have explored the influence of culture on perceptions and understandings of health and illness, and we have looked specifically at the problem of pain. In this final section, the nursing implications of the points raised and the evidence offered above will be discussed.

This section is not concerned with the details of drugs or other specific treatments for pain, or even with particular alternative or complementary therapies. Nor is it concerned with any particular methods for the assessment of pain, acute or chronic. However, it is concerned with the assessment of patients in pain, and with the consideration of their individual needs, whatever their culture. It is concerned with the management of pain, taking into account any particular individual needs that might reflect a different point of view about pain from the one with which we are usually familiar.

In many ways this is supposed to be the basis of the approach to nursing care in the Western world as part of the nursing process, and as espoused by many of the models of nursing presented and forming the basis of practice over the last two decades. A consideration of models of transcultural nursing as reviewed briefly in the above section on culture and health emphasizes the importance of the nurse–patient relationship. This is going to be the main implication of this chapter for nursing practice, and of course it underpins all nursing models, in particular that of Leininger (1988, 1991), who discusses culture care as being the basis of all nursing. Thus 'culture care presentation' involves the practitioner in assisting, supporting or enabling the client from a particular culture to preserve or maintain health, or to recover from illness, and to face death (as cited in Dobson, 1991). Consideration of the role of the nurse in dealing with cultural aspects of health care in general and the management of pain in particular will be dealt with in more detail in the following final section of this chapter.

Nursing issues

Whatever model of nursing might be operating, when we look at the cultural mix in the general population in the UK, and in the profession of nursing, there are many therapeutic relationships with patients that might reflect differing cultural points of view. We may have indigenous orthodox health care staff caring for one or more ethnic subgroups in a particular health care setting. Alternatively, we may have a member of the health care staff from one ethnic subgroup caring for patients from another ethnic subgroup, as well as patients from the indigenous group. Here we can see the beginnings of the complicated cultural relationships that might exist in the caring situation, never mind the within-group variations that we may find, or the varying levels of identification that individuals might show with particular cultures (Davis, 1986).

As some of the research mentioned above demonstrates, there is often much homogeneity between cultural groups – or 'universalities', to use Leininger's word for it (Leininger, 1991). Although there may be cultural differences in the expression of pain or in the meaning of pain, the way in which a particular individual might respond depends on a variety of factors, as well as on any cultural label. Often cultural labels are applied by others rather than by the individual. Zola (1983) and Kleinman et al. (1992), among others, warn against the dangers of using stereotyped expectations as a basis for determining the needs of patients in pain. However, they do highlight the importance of being culturally aware of the possibility of variations in expression, response or meaning.

However, there is evidence that nurses tend to be influenced by a patient's culture. Research reported by Davitz and Pendleton (1969) and Davitz and Davitz (1985) indicated that nurses were influenced not only culturally but also by such factors as age and social class. Recent calls to individualize patient care and to plan care on the basis of individual assessments of patient need would seem to be the solution to a culturally aware but non-stereotyped approach to pain management.

The presentation of the patient, as either expressive and emotional or quiet and reserved when in pain, is not sufficient evidence on which to base a plan or to recommend medication. We must remember that pain is in the patient's mind – that it exists to the extent that he or she says it does, and that the approach to management has to include the meaning that the patient attaches to the pain as well as its intensity or bearability. Leininger has defined culturally congruent care as being 'tailor-made to fit with individual, group or institutional values, beliefs and life-ways, in order to provide or support meaningful, beneficial and satisfying health care or well-being services' (Leininger, 1991, p.49). As discussed in the section on culture and health, she argues along with others that health is culturally defined, and she emphasizes that although there may be differences between groups, there are also great universalities. Medicine itself can be an alien culture, with its special language and concepts and models, whether based on biomedical sciences or other, perhaps supernatural, concepts.

Leininger also argues for the validity of what she calls 'folk-ways' or lay models of health and treatment, and Helman too has recognized the value of such models in dealing with the client's or patient's understanding of the health care problem (pain) (Helman, 1994). He found that many practitioners themselves, particularly GPs, held lay beliefs or understandings which influenced the way in which they dealt with their patients. Models of care that include the patient in decision-making about the diagnosis or the assessment of the health care problem (in this case pain) are much more likely to be culturally sensitive. The nurse who is making the assessment must not be too wedded to the (Western) scientific biomedical model, but needs to be able to appreciate the patient's perhaps lay description of the problem. It is important to ask questions in the assessment that enable the nurse to explore those aspects of the social and cultural aspects of the patient's experience of his or her pain, so that the ensuing cultural awareness will lead to the development of an individual but cultural care plan and the meeting of the patient's needs.

Conclusions

How can this occur? And what are the requirements to ensure that this happens? What is not required is a list of different cultures or religions which identifies particular characteristics of patient response to particular situations, which nurses can learn or refer to when they plan care. This is the way to standardized, routinized care that will not meet individual patients' needs. All of the points made in this section indicate the vital importance of receiving from the patient, client or sufferer in whatever context, a thorough history that includes an exploration of the individual's perceptions and understandings of the nature of the problem.

Many alternative or complementary approaches to health that are becoming increasingly important in Western medicine do rely on extensive history-taking and the development of a physical, psychological and social assessment to explore all of the ramifications of the issue that has brought the individual into the care of the practitioner. Some of these approaches to health care are based on or derive from models from other cultures. Frequently, the time spent in this activity is seen as important in determining the uptake of treatment and the outcome.

As indicated above, we are concerned with the assessment of pain, but in a way that puts the patient in the driving seat. Whether the form of assessment measurement involved is one of the more objective types, such as a Visual Analogue Scale, or one that uses more subjective verbal descriptions, it must be the patient who makes the assessment. If necessary, family members can be involved as well, to help to make clear the nature of the patient's understanding and experience of the pain. Translation may be necessary, too.

However some knowledge of the general aspects of health beliefs of a particular culture can inform the nurse in her approach to the patient's individual experience and assessment of it. If she is dealing frequently with people from a particular culture, it is obviously helpful to discuss health care issues with leaders and influential people from that culture. If other nurses from that culture are available then they too should be consulted if they are not themselves involved in the care. In this way the nurse will be able to ask pertinent questions and to discuss aspects of the patient's care in an informed and sensitive way.

The real solution to this issue would seem to be that of education and skills training for nurses in cultural aspects of health care. This should be at both pre-registration and post-registration levels. Lectures and workshops on cultural aspects of care, as argued by Leininger (1991), and others such as Dobson (1991), and Brink (1990) should form an important part of nurse preparation. They could usefully form part of communication and interpersonal modules for example (Davis, 1986, 1990). Communication and interpersonal skill have been identified for some time as important aspects of nursing, yet there is still a need for continued emphasis of the importance of this. The essence of nursing care is the individual patient and her or his needs. The only way to establish these and, from them, to develop a care plan is to get to know the patient through a structured conversation, including reference to relatives if necessary.

The term culture, as well as having the meanings considered in the sections above, also has the meanings of artistic expression, sophistication, intelligence, knowledge and, above all, of sensitivity. From an awareness of general transcultural issues and detailed personal information, the pain as experienced, interpreted, felt and expressed by the individual patient will then be managed in a professional and cultured way.

References

Bates, M.S., Edwards W.T. and Anderson K.O. 1993: Ethnocultural influences on variation in chronic pain perception. *Pain* 52, 101–12.

Blaxter, M. 1983: The causes of disease; women talking. *Social Science and Medicine* 17, 59–69.

Brewster, A.B. 1982: Chronically ill hospitalised children's concepts of their illness. *Pediatrics* 69, 355–62.

Brink, P.J. 1990: *Transcultural nursing, a book of readings*. Prospect Heights, Illinois: Waveland Press Inc.

Broome, M.E., Lillis, P.P. and Smith, M.C. 1989: Pain interventions with children: a meta-analysis of research. *Nursing Research* 38, 154–8.

Buss, A.H. and Portnoy, N.W. 1967: Pain tolerance and group identification. *Journal of Personality and Social Psychology*, 1, 106–8.

Clark, W.C. and Clark, S.B. 1980: Pain responses in Nepalese porters. *Science* 209, 410–12.

Davis, B.D. 1986: Culture in psychiatric nursing: implications for training. In Cox, J.L. (ed.), *Transcultural psychiatry*. Beckenham: Croom Helm, 218–33.

Davis, B.D. 1990: Empathy in transcultural nursing practice. In Mackay, R.M., Hughes, J.M. and Carver, J. (eds), *Empathy in the helping relationship*. New York: Springer, 153–6.

Davitz, L.L. and Pendleton, S.H. 1969: Nurses' inferences of suffering. *Nursing Research* 18, 100–7.

Davitz, L.L. and Davitz, J.R. 1985: Culture and nurses' inferences of suffering. In Copp, L.A. (ed.), *Recent advances in nursing (perspectives on pain)*. Edinburgh: Churchill Livingstone, 17–28.

Dobson, S.M. 1991: *Transcultural nursing*. London: Scutari Press.

Engel, G. 1950: 'Psychogenic' pain and the pain-prone patient. *American Journal of Medicine* 26, 899–909.

Fabrega, H. and Tyma, S. 1976: Culture, language and the shaping of illness: an illustration based on pain. *Journal of Psychosomatic Research* 20, 323–37.

Gaffney, A. and Dunne, E.A. 1987: Children's understanding of the causality of pain. *Pain* **29**, 91–104.

Hardy, J.D., Wolff, H.G. and Goodell, H. 1952: *Pain sensations and reactions*. Baltimore, MD: Williams and Wilkins.

Helman, C.G. 1994: *Culture, health and illness*, 3rd edn. Oxford: Butterworth Heinemann.

Keesing, R.M. 1981: *Cultural anthropology: a contemporary perspective*. New York: Holt, Rinehart and Winston.

Kleinman, A.R. 1988: *The illness narratives: suffering, healing and the human condition*. New York: Basic Books.

Kleinman, A., Brodwin, P.E., Good, B.J. and DelVecchio-Good, M.J. 1992: Pain as human experience: an introduction. In Good, Brodwin, P.E., Good, B.J. and Kleinman, A. (eds), *Pain as human experience: an anthropological perspective*. Berkeley, CA: University of California Press, 1–28.

Kosambi, D.D. 1967: Living prehistory in India. *Scientific American* **216**, 105–14.

Lambert, W.E., Libman, E. and Poser, E.G. (1960) Effect of increased salience of membership group on pain tolerance. *Journal of Personality* **28**, 350–7.

Le Barre, W. 1947: The cultural basis of emotions and gestures. *Journal of Personality* **16**, 49–68.

Leininger, M.M. 1988: Leininger's theory of nursing. Culture care diversity and universality. *Nursing Science Quarterly* **1**, 152–60.

Leininger, M.M. (ed.) 1991: *Culture care diversity and universality: a theory of nursing*. New York: National League for Nursing Press.

Lewis, G. 1981: Cultural influences on illness behaviour: a medical anthropological approach. In Eisenberg L. and Kleinman A. (eds), *The relevance of social science for medicine*. Dordrecht, Reidel, 151–62.

Lipton, J.A. and Marbach, J.J. 1984: Ethnicity and the pain experience. *Social Science and Medicine* **19**, 1279–98.

McGuire, M.B. 1988: *Ritual healing in suburban America*. New Brunswick: Rutgers University Press.

Melzack, R. and Wall, P.D. 1965: Pain mechanisms: a new theory. *Science* **150**, 971–9.

Melzack, R. and Wall, P.D. 1996: *The challenge of pain*. Harmondsworth: Penguin.

Nanke, L. and Canter, D. 1993: The multivariate structure of treatment practices in complementary medicine. In Lewith, G.T. and Aldridge, D. (eds), *Clinical research methodology for complementary therapies*. London: Hodder and Stoughton, 189–203.

Orque, M.S.D., Bloch B. and Monrroy, L.S.A. 1983: *Ethnic nursing care. A multicultural approach*. St Louis, MO: C.V. Mosby.

Perrin, E.C. and Gerrity, P.S. 1982: There's a demon in your belly: children's understanding of illness. *Pediatrics* **67**, 841–9.

Pugh, J.F. 1991: The semantics of pain in Indian culture and medicine. *Culture, Medicine and Psychiatry* **15**, 19–43.

Robinson, R. 1990: Personal narratives, social careers and medical courses: analysing life trajectories in autobiographies of people with multiple sclerosis. *Social Science and Medicine* **30**, 1173–86.

Savedra, M.C., Gibbons, P., Tesler, M.D., Ward, J. and Wegner, C. 1982: How do children describe pain? A tentative assessment. *Pain* **14**, 95–104.

Sindhu, F. 1996: Are non-pharmacological nursing interventions for the management of pain effective? – a meta-analysis. *Journal of Advanced Nursing* **24**, 1152–9.

Skevington, S.M. 1995: *Psychology of pain*. Chichester: John Wiley.

Skultans, V. 1976: Empathy and healing: aspects of Spiritualist ritual. In Loudon, J.B. (ed.), *Social anthropology and medicine.* London: Academic Press, 190–222.

Smooha, S. 1985: Ethnic groups. In Kuper, A. and Kuper, J. (eds), *The social science encyclopaedia.* London: Routledge and Kegan Paul, 267–9.

Sternbach, R.A. and Tursky, B. 1965: Ethnic differences among housewives in psycho-physiological and skin responses to electric shock. *Psychophysiology* 1, 217–18.

Twaddle, A.C. and Hessler, R.M. 1977: *A sociology of health.* St Louis, MO: C.V. Mosby.

Weisenberg, M. 1977: Pain and pain control. *Psychological Bulletin* 84, 1008–44.

Wolff, B.B. 1985: Ethnocultural factors influencing pain and illness behaviour. *Clinical Journal of Pain* 1, 23–30.

Wolff, B.B. and Langley, S. 1977: Cultural factors and the response to pain. In Landy, D. (ed.), *Culture, disease and healing: studies in medical anthropology.* New York: Macmillan, 313–19.

Woodrow, R.M., Friedman, G.D., Siegelaub, A.B. and Collen, M.F. 1972: Pain tolerance: differences according to age, sex and race. *Psychosomatic Medicine* 34, 548–56.

Zborowski, M. 1952: Cultural components in responses to pain. *Journal of Social Issues* 8, 16–30.

Zola, I.K. 1966: Culture and symptoms – an analysis of patients presenting complaints. *American Sociological Review* 31, 615–30.

Zola, I.K. 1983: *Some medical inquiries: recollections, reflections and reconsiderations.* Philadelphia, PA: Temple University Press.

Researching pain: paradigms and revolutions

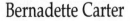

Bernadette Carter

> Scientists have seldom stopped to ask what it is that characterizes what they do. Being pragmatic people, they have simply got on and done it. Philosophers, on the other hand, have spent a great deal of time worrying about how we should define science and how we might distinguish it from religion (if indeed we can). Both groups have, in the end, been concerned with the same central issue, namely the certainty of our knowledge about the world, but their perspectives have been very different.
>
> (Dunbar, 1995, p.157)

Introduction

The dichotomy suggested by Dunbar (1995) concerning the differences between scientists and philosophers is intrinsically the same as the one that existed between research and philosophy. In the past the terms research and science/scientific method have often been used, albeit unwisely, interchangeably. Dunbar (1995) states that scientists have just got on with the job of 'doing' science, without really stopping to think about it from a philosophical perspective. It could be argued that modern science (that is, science during the past 400 years) arose out of activity rather than (philosophical) thinking.[1] This vision of what science *is*, and thus what research *is*, has had inevitable consequences for the direction of research in all fields of activity, including pain.

This chapter arose out of my own interest in pain research and philosophy and a desire to explore the relationship between how we *think* about pain and research. The ways in which we think about pain and research interact and affect each other. When exploring this interaction, some type of structure or framework for analysing this thinking is necessary. This is where the notion of

[1]However, it needs to be acknowledged that initially there was not such a clear division between philosophy and science (see Francis Bacon's work from the fifteenth century). Philosophy itself is seen to give rise to religion, science and sociology. It is only relatively recently that science has become divorced from its philosophical roots.

paradigms needs to be introduced. A paradigm is a representation of a world view or a 'cognitive road map' (Kuhn, 1962). Paradigms provide useful frameworks for expressing our thinking, and I shall explore them in more detail later in this chapter. As with any writing that claims to have some philosophical 'pretensions', I have not found *the* or indeed *any* answer(s). This is a personal perspective – a reflection of my interpretation of events, the presentation of linkages that I see exist. However, scrutiny of the interplay between the development of pain research and research philosophies or paradigms merits attention. This interplay has affected the way in which pain research has developed, and provides clues to the directions for future research.

In undertaking this examination, I have chosen to use Kuhn's (1962, 1970) notion of scientific revolutions as the framework for presenting the ways in which old thinking is overthrown by new thinking. Kuhn views science progressing in an open-ended way which was summarized by Chalmers (1982) as follows: *pre-science → normal science → crisis-revolution → new normal science → new crisis*. Broadly, a period of *normal science* is characterized by scientists working within the ruling paradigm, during which time they test and probe it, finding new evidence that supports it. This is a period of growth of knowledge and understanding within the boundaries of the science. It is characterized by a process of questioning the 'boundary conditions' of the paradigm, but with an underlying certainty of its 'rightness'. The *crisis-revolution* stage is the period when the certainty of the paradigm governing *normal science* is increasingly questioned until the frameworks for thinking are so undermined that it becomes evident that *normal science* thinking is simply inadequate and that new explanations/theories are needed. As new or revolutionary thinking occurs, there is a move away from the old normal science to a new normal science. This process is cyclical, with new revolutions occurring and followed by periods of paradigm exploration (Kuhn, 1970; Chalmers, 1982; Dunbar, 1995). An example of a paradigm shift would be the revolutionary change in thinking from the theory that the earth was flat to the new 'round-earth' thinking.

Within this chapter I shall note some of the conflict and dissent that can occur when researchers from different disciplines meet. Where well-established multidisciplinary pain research teams exist, such conflict may not occur. However, in less favoured areas, different approaches to pain research can cause feelings of discomfort. This chapter aims to highlight why these tensions exist.

Are we all talking about the same thing?

Researching pain is not easy. Pain is multidimensional. It can equally be seen as something tangible, existing in the real world, for which evidence can be established, or as something less tangible, which exists solely within the individual's experience of it. In fact, pain is generally perceived as being somewhere between these extremes. Common sense suggests that it is both tangible and intangible. Part of the problem in researching pain lies in trying to define exactly what it is one is trying to research. Pain definitions provide good working frameworks for practice, but may not provide a specific focus for research. Indeed, trying to research pain within a broadly based definition, such as that proffered by the International Association for the Study of Pain (1944) (see Figure 6.1), may inevitably result in the researcher attempting to research the whole world, as so many factors are implicated in pain. Conversely, by narrowing down the definition to something that is intrinsically researchable the researcher then faces the difficulty of knowing that some of the richness, complexity and reflexivity is lost. A pedantic argument perhaps, but it is possible to argue that adopting a differing definition of pain fundamentally changes that which is actually being researched. Pain is *always* more than the sum of its parts. It is this very point that provides such an immense challenge to research.

The language of pain, or perhaps the associated tortuous semantic debates, can result in the researcher finding it very difficult to frame the research question. Pain, suffering and distress – as terms – can become confusingly interchangeable. There is an obvious linguistic distinction between pain and suffering, but they are often so closely linked as an *experience* that separating them decontextualizes the suffering from perhaps a somatic cause. This changes the experience and is generally not the way in which pain is experienced. However, the debate as to whether the research question is focused on pain or suffering is still often one that provides an interesting discourse.

An unpleasant sensory and emotional experience with actual or potential tissue damage, or described in terms of such damage.

Note: Pain is always subjective. Each individual learns the application of the word through experiences related to injury in early life. Biologists recognize that those stimuli which cause pain are liable to cause tissue damage. Accordingly, pain is that experience which we associate with actual or potential tissue damage. It is unquestionably a sensation in a part or parts of the body, but it is also always unpleasant and therefore an emotional experience. Experiences which resemble pain but are not unpleasant, e.g. pricking, should not be called pain. Unpleasant abnormal experiences (dysaesthesias) may also be pain but are not necessarily so because, subjectively, they may not have the usual sensory qualities of pain.

Many people report pain in the absence of tissue damage or any likely pathophysiological cause; usually this happens for psychological reasons. There is usually no way to distinguish their experience from that of tissue damage if we take the subjective report. If they regard their experience as pain and if they report it in the same ways as pain caused by tissue damage, it should be accepted as pain. This definition avoids tying pain to the stimulus. Activity induced in the nociceptor and nociceptive pathways by a noxious stimulus is not pain, which is always a psychological state, even though we may well appreciate that pain most often has a proximate physical cause.

Figure 6.1   Definition of pain (from Merskey and Bogduk, 1994)

Defining pain is important, even though language itself is almost always inadequate. A current consensus definition of pain, albeit an expert consensus definition, is that which reflects the reigning paradigm. This pain paradigm may be the best way of articulating current beliefs, values and world views, but it almost always misses out individual definitions (even when the individuality of pain is acknowledged). It is important to note that, whilst definitions of pain (arising from the dominant paradigm) have changed over the past several thousand years, pain *itself* has not changed. Changing paradigms do not change the issue being discussed. They merely change or reflect current perspectives and thinking.

Pain may be elusive but research is vital. The contribution that pain research has made and will make is significant. The history of pain research, certainly within the world of Western allopathic thinking, is relatively short. For too long pain was seen as something which had to be borne – a punishment or penance, or a natural and inevitable consequence of disease and/or treatment of that disease. The impact that pain has on the person, beyond 'obvious' physical consequences, is now much better appreciated. The person who experiences pain is now seen to have an important role to play in developing our understanding of the experience of pain.

Research paradigms and the quest for knowledge: a brief history

Some would argue that the type of research question asked provides the trigger for the paradigm within which the research is undertaken. Others would contest this by saying that the paradigm itself is the most important starting point for research, as it essentially informs and underpins the framing of the question (see Figure 6.2). Regardless of the stance which is adopted, it is obvious that the paradigm and the research question(s) are closely linked. The chosen research paradigm may strongly reflect the pain paradigm and/or may reflect the individual researcher's view of the world. Thus again they are actually strongly interlinked.

The current paradigm embodies the belief in the multidimensionality of pain and accepts that pain can be somatic in origin, as well as having no diagnosable somatic origin. This paradigm is worlds away from the historical, scientific belief of the previous 400 years or so, that pain was purely physical. There was little real acknowledgement of the complex interplay of social,

Paradigm exerts effects on ⬦ Framing of research question(s)	Framing of research question(s) exerts effects on ⬦ Choice of paradigm

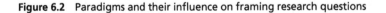

Figure 6.2 Paradigms and their influence on framing research questions

cultural, spiritual and cognitive factors. The mind/body duality paradigm of pain was broadly reflective of the scientific, reductionist mode of thinking that was first evident during the Age of Enlightenment, and which gained favour and currency as scientists became increasingly interested and were able to delve into the mechanistic functioning of the body. Descartes, for example, modelled pain on a mechanistic theory. The search for reductionist explanations for pain broadly reflected the quest for understanding, control and power over the natural world. Reductionism meant that pain research focused on the desire to find simple solutions and answers to the challenge of pain. Despite increased knowledge and improved instrumentation and techniques, no simple solutions were forthcoming. However, this did little to slow the search for reductionist explanations such as single pain pathways and a pain centre. Even when other models for pain were proposed, the dominance of pain as a physical entity persisted. It took the accumulation of a large body of contradictory evidence finally to demonstrate that this paradigm was untenably flawed. At this point, what Kuhn would term a *crisis-revolution* occurred and scientific revolution was inevitable. New thinking about pain and new approaches to research were made possible as the era of *new normal science* emerged and exploration of the boundaries of the new science developed.

Gate control theory, revolutions and paradigm shifts

Perhaps the most recent key scientific revolution in terms of the quest to understand pain came with gate control theory in 1965. Melzack and Wall's work had an immensely significant impact on pain thinking. The revolution that they stimulated resulted from so-called *normal science* reaching a crisis point. However, Melzack and Wall both acknowledge the work that had gone before:

> It was our unexpected good fortune that the theory came at a time when the field was ripe for change. In the 1960s, a wave of new facts and ideas (that had evolved gradually) was beginning to crest, and the gate-control theory rode in on the wave of the times.
>
> (Melzack and Wall, 1988, preface)

The elegance of gate control theory provided the fuel for a radical change in thinking, and a new pain paradigm emerged and was adopted, albeit not instantaneously, by practitioners. The perspective from which practitioners (researchers, scientists, clinicians and therapists) were to perceive pain was to change for ever. What had been seen as revolutionary was incorporated into the definition proposed by the International Association for the Study of Pain (IASP) in 1979[2] – a ringing endorsement of the theory and acknowledgement of its acceptance as new normal scientific thinking.

[2]This was re-examined, but remained unchanged, in 1994 by the Task Force on Taxonomy (see Merskey and Bogduk, 1994).

It is with this legacy that current practitioners and researchers must question their beliefs and understanding about the nature of pain. This current paradigm, which adopts a much more holistic stance, is radically different to that which went before. The new pain paradigm to a large degree governs approaches to research, the framing of research questions and those questions which are posed. One of the implications of the new paradigm lies in the diversity of professionals involved in research.

Differing paradigms: conflict and collaboration

Some 20 years into the *new normal science*, the normality of this thinking can mislead current researchers and practitioners into believing that this is the way that it has always been. Indeed, recounting relatively recent pain history to students who have been brought up on gate control theory is interesting. They invariably cannot 'wrap their heads around' the tenets of the previous paradigm. It is a credit to the strength and depth of the theory, and the huge amount of other research evidence, that the paradigm is so widely accepted. The appreciation of the complexity and plasticity of pain has legitimated the involvement of researchers from backgrounds as diverse as, for example, anthropology, psychology, biochemistry and genetics.

Each of these disparate disciplines is based within its own paradigm, its own way of thinking about the world, research, practice, and so on. Each discipline offers unique insights into the problem of pain, and the complexity of pain necessitates this diversity of approach. Each discipline has its own historical approach to enquiry, its own traditions, rules and perspectives on how it sees its own discipline, other disciplines and the world. These different world views result in an amazingly rich offering to the issue of pain, even though there will inevitably be some dissonance between them. In many instances these disciplinary world views are poles apart – yet they are united by a common interest in pain. Pain research requires all disciplines to be intrigued by the research strategies and findings of other disciplines. Clues from one speciality or discipline may lead to the advancement of knowledge in another discipline or the trigger to consider the problem in a different way. Pain may not be unique as a case for this stimulating interplay of so many disciplines, but it is certainly a prime example.

However, there can be tensions between the disciplines as a result of their differing paradigmatic perspectives in relation to the way in which they see the world. The education, training and experiences of a neuroanatomist, for example, are widely different to those of an anthropologist. Research methodologies that are almost 'sacred cows' in one discipline may not be considered to be 'good' methods in another discipline. This has perhaps been most evident in the tensions[3] that exist between qualitative and quantitative research. Qualitative research, for example, may be seen as an assault on the traditions of

[3]These tensions are not inevitable, but have been the focus of much debate (see Hammersley, 1992).

quantitative research (Denzin and Lincoln, 1994). The notions of 'good research' may be founded on radically different criteria. Fundamentals – such as objectivity, detachment, absence of bias, and statistical significance – may be highly prized and seen as *the* way to approach research. Alternatively, polar opposites – such as subjectivity, reciprocity, involvement and acceptance of bias – may be seen as being *the* appropriate way of tackling research. As professionals become more involved with the research methods and philosophies of other disciplines those barriers are gradually being eroded. However, they still exist. They are real and can still act as considerable obstacles to good pain research dialogue. The old arguments as to whether one method is better than another – the search to find the *true* research approach – are now less vociferous.

Pain research provides excellent examples of collaborative (cross-disciplinary) research that stretches across traditional research paradigm boundaries. There is appreciation that different research paradigms are essential if pain is to be explored comprehensively. The available range of research paradigms allows the most appropriate philosophical approach and research tools to be utilized for specific pain research problems. The multi-dimensionality of pain makes it essential for many perspectives to be adopted. Research methodologies appropriate for utilization of a randomized controlled trial, often described as the gold standard of research, are of virtually no use for research attempting to explore the lived experiences of people with pain. However obvious this may appear to be, it has not always stopped the arguments (good natured or otherwise) that continue amongst the disciplines.

Exploring research paradigms

Research paradigms can provide definition for researchers in terms of what it is they are about and what are the boundaries of legitimate research.[4] Guba and Lincoln (1994) see paradigms as being important in terms of understanding approaches to research. They provide the following definition of the nature of a paradigm:

> A paradigm may be viewed as a set of *basic beliefs* (or metaphysics) that deals with ultimates or first principles. It represents a *worldview* that defines, for its holder, the nature of the 'world', the individual's place in it, and the range of possible relationships to that world and its parts, as, for example, cosmologies and theologies do.
> (Guba and Lincoln, 1994, p.107, original authors' emphasis)

---

[4]It should be acknowledged that some writers do not see focusing on paradigms as being particularly useful. Firestone (1990), for example, suggests that 'paradigms are more analagous to cultures than philosophical systems' (Firestone, 1990, p.108), since their boundaries are not always clear and because diffusion and intermingling of differing approaches can be creative and fruitful.

Guba (1990) suggests that different paradigms can be characterized by a framework that takes account of three basic questions: the ontological question, the epistemological question and the methodological question. Guba and Lincoln (1994) propose the following:

- *The ontological question* – What is the form and nature of reality and, therefore, what is there that can be known about? . . .;
- *The epistemological question* – What is the nature of the relationship between the knower or the would-be knower and what can be known? . . .;
- *The methodological question* – How can the inquirer (would-be knower) go about finding out whatever he or she believes can be known? (Guba and Lincoln, 1994, p.108, emphasis in original).

These questions underpin all types of research (even though they may not be actively considered prior to starting the study). These three key questions can generally be used to analyse any type of paradigm. However, paradigms are tricky – all paradigms are of human construction and thus they are subject to human error.

Guba (1989) proposes four paradigms: positivism, postpositivism, critical theory and constructivism. Appreciation of these differing (some might say, competing) paradigms allows an understanding of what types of beliefs, values, properties and characteristics are involved in the way in which different researchers approach their studies. Considering how deeply entrenched some of these fundamental beliefs are, it is not surprising that disciplines can be suspicious of 'alien' philosophies, laying claim to the 'sanctity' of their own world view.

Positivism and postpositivism

The strongest tradition in research and, thus generally the one with the highest perceived status, lies with the positivists, whose scientific, conventional, reductionist and deterministic stance is generally well understood by other disciplines as well as, to differing degrees, by the public. Experimental controlled studies that utilize manipulative, chiefly quantitative, methodologies reflect a belief that truth is out there and reality can be apprehended. Researchers adopt a detached and objectivist approach to their study (dualist/objectivist epistemology). The aim of the positivist is to verify a priori hypotheses. This type of research has resulted in studies which have contributed to the development of knowledge in areas such as the pharmacology of pain, the neuroanatomy of pain, and pain biochemistry.

However, with the complexity of pain being accepted and the obvious need for pain research to embrace non-experimental, less completely controlled research environments, the postpositivist paradigm arose from a dissatisfaction with the constraints of positivism. Some writers, such as Guba and Lincoln (1994), suggest that it 'represents a kind of "damage control" rather than a reformulation of basic principles' (Guba and Lincoln, 1994, p.116).

Postpositivism accepts that it is impossible to apprehend reality perfectly (our human-ness prevents this), but that by the use of a number of critical data collection techniques the researcher can get close to the truth of the situation – that is, close to reality. The aim of postpositivism is to falsify a priori hypotheses. The methodological approaches include quantitative and some qualitative techniques, and the studies are undertaken in more naturalistic settings than the rigidly controlled positivist settings.

These two approaches have provided excellent studies that have developed the knowledge base of specific areas of pain. However, those characteristics which gave these paradigms strength were not suited to transformative research, in which a fundamental aim of research is actually to change the status quo.

Critical theory and constructivism

Critical theory is a broad term which covers a range of approaches to research; it developed to address the need for transformative research. Guba (1990, p.24) notes that 'Inquiry becomes a *political act*' (original author's emphasis). Proponents of critical theory adopt a critical realist ontology and acknowledge that values mediate the findings of the study. There is an overt political dimension to this paradigm. For example, this type of research has allowed the voice of the people experiencing pain to be heard. The people participating (both the researchers and those being researched) are active within the research process and are changed by it. Methodologies within the critical theorist paradigm are based on those which require dialogue between the researcher and the participants. This dialogue needs to be in the form of a debate or discourse that results in change – that is, it is transformative. It aims to promote 'emancipation and empowerment' (Smith, 1990, p.183). Kincheloe and McLaren (1994) propose that critical theory produces 'undeniably dangerous knowledge' (p.138) which can, for example, threaten the status quo of institutions.

Whilst the previous three research paradigms would seem to offer approaches that cover all types of research, they cannot deal with researchers who hold a relativist ontology. The research paradigm that embraces such an ontology is contructivism. In this approach to research there is the intention of true equality between the researcher and the researchee, and there is an acceptance that the resulting constructions are reflective of multiple mental constructions which are experientially based. Thus they are dependent on/reflective of those who participated in the study. Methodologically, constructivism aims to capture holistically realities that are developed between and among the participants and the researcher. It is described as being hermeneutic (interpretative) and dialectic. Any research conducted using a constructivist philosophy acknowledges that research can never be value free. Schwandt (1994) states of constructivism that 'Truth is a matter of the best informed and most sophisticated construction on which there is consensus at a given time' (p.128).

The fifth paradigm

Much of the new movement in research has grown out of the belief that the power balance between the researcher and the subject in conventional research needs to be addressed so that there is an equality or true partnership, a real collaboration in all aspects of the study. These types of values and beliefs, expressed by Reason and Rowan (1981), are seen to be new paradigm research or, as Heron (1996) proposes, co-operative enquiry or participating enquiry (Heron and Reason, 1997). This type of research adopts both quantitative and qualitative approaches, but is fundamentally participative research in which participants are co-subjects and co-researchers. Heron (1996) believes that co-operative inquiry 'rests on a related, but distinct, fifth inquiry paradigm, that of participative reality' (p.10). In this fifth paradigm the ontology is based on a mind-shaped reality, and the epistemology is subjective–objective with an active relationship between the knower and the known. It has an intrinsically political element to it which acknowledges that 'human flourishing is intrinsically worthwhile (Heron, 1996, p.11). It further acknowledges the primary value of 'practical knowing' (Heron and Reason, 1997).

This discussion of the five paradigms of research is not a diversion from pain research. The fact that new perspectives/paradigms on research methods have been developing over a period broadly similar to the history of twentieth-century pain research mirrors the fact that society is becoming aware of the complexity of issues and the need to explore these in innovative ways. Society as a whole has become more interested in being involved, being active consumers, having active information, being accepted, and working *with* rather than being worked *on*. This more equal holistic consideration of issues is reflected in the generation of the development of research paradigms. Some paradigms (for example, co-operative participative enquiry) will have greater resonance for some disciplines than for others. However, it is prescriptive to suggest that disciplines could and should be pigeon-holed into specific paradigms. Hammersley (1996) emphasizes that an open mind is important when considering fundamental choices about research. He states:

> What is required, then, in my view, is a methodologically aware eclecticism in which the full range of options is kept in mind, in terms of methods and philosophical assumptions. The practical character of research decisions should be recognised, but this must not lead us to ignore the methodological problems and debates that are involved.
> (Hammersley, 1996, p.174)

Growth or conflict?

It is therefore important that pain researchers appreciate the possibilities open to them for approaches to research, and that they make informed decisions about these choices. There are unique opportunities for both growth and conflict as a result of these often differing world views. The opportunity for growth is obvious when considering the rich melting-pot of ideas that can occur with such diversity in thinking, background, aims and responsibilities. The potential for conflict is evident in exactly those factors which are seen as opportunities. The need for the disciplines to work collaboratively and cooperatively and without hindering other disciplines is vital if we are to explore the possibilities, strengths and weaknesses of our current understanding about pain. There have been and will continue to be clashes between the various disciplines, and analytical criticism of each other's methods, approaches, and analytical tools. This can foster truly innovative research that will encourage exciting new ways of thinking about pain. This can only be of benefit to the end user of the research – the person in pain. Each discipline and perspective has much to offer, although there is no single paradigm that can provide *the* answers – all must be respected and embraced if they are to contribute effectively to pain research and the quest for knowledge.

Research: dormant domains and research for the future

All areas of pain research are under-addressed and need to be the focus of attention, and whilst this may be true it does not actually help to move things forward. As with any research area there is a need to target resources so that money, skill, expertise, time and other resources can be channelled appropriately. The need for some consensus about research directions must be addressed if the outcomes of research are to have a beneficial outcome. Some areas have received relatively high levels of attention compared to others, perhaps reflecting access to resources, a perceived need or a potentially positive outcome. If a need or problem is not acknowledged, then the research is simply not done. Thus many areas are hidden from view and are research dormant. My own specific areas of research interest lie in child and infant pain – an area that has received very little research attention until relatively recently. The culture that supported such a dearth of research resulted from a number of inappropriate beliefs (often referred to in the literature as myths) (Carter, 1994). This thinking included the belief that children and infants were incapable of experiencing pain. Thus whilst these beliefs were dominant little research was undertaken. Basically, there was no stimulus to research. This may be an oversimplification, but it is a reasonable reflection. Lack of research results in practice which is not evidence-based – the result can be chaos. However, once pain research focusing on children was undertaken, new evidence was generated and a new way of thinking emerged. It is now commonly accepted that children and infants do experience pain. This is now part of everyday thinking. The same is true of other areas of pain research, such as the patient's experience of pain (Sofaer, 1998).

Domains of research

Three key domains of research can be identified. These domains are, to a degree, artificial, as some of the issues overarch these domains and there is, as already discussed, great interplay between all aspects of pain. The three domains can be categorized as bioscience, political and psychosocial. Whilst the value of categorizing pain may be questioned, the vastness of the subject area suggests that some form of flexible categorization can be helpful in structuring thinking. The categorization I offer draws on Copp's (1990) domains of pain research (although Copp chose not to categorize the areas). Each of these three major domains contains sub-domains (see Figure 6.3). Categorization attracts debate, and whilst these domains and subdomains have not been made arbitrarily, they will inevitably provoke discussion. For example, each of the sub-domains could easily be subjected to further division as they, in themselves, are vast areas. This categorization is proffered as a starting point for discussion and thinking about potential areas of pain research.

Overarching issues		
<ul><li>Assessment of pain</li><li>Measurement of pain</li><li>Allopathic management</li><li>Complementary management</li></ul>		
Bioscience domain	**Political domain**	**Psychosocial domain**
<ul><li>Prenatal influences</li><li>Physiological research and theories</li><li>Age-related effects</li><li>Pharmacological influences</li><li>Treatment interventions</li><li>Pathology of pain</li><li>Conditions associated with pain</li></ul>	<ul><li>Quality, standards and bench-marking</li><li>Documentation</li><li>Research agendas and programmes</li><li>Ethics, consent and advocacy</li><li>Partnership, power and vulnerability</li><li>Pain as a moral emergency</li><li>Public impressions/role of the media</li></ul>	<ul><li>Perception, cognition and experience of pain</li><li>Communication and expression of pain</li><li>Linguistics of pain</li><li>Religion, culture and gender</li><li>Effects on family life</li><li>Coping styles</li><li>Effects of context, situation and meaning</li><li>Philosophical issues</li><li>Listening, empathy and intuition</li><li>Education and training issues</li><li>Detached concern</li><li>Professional perceptions</li><li>Lay/client perceptions</li></ul>

Figure 6.3 Domains of pain (developed from ideas in Copp, 1990)

Research for the future?

The need to develop evidence-based practice (the current watchword, at least in the UK) requires research efforts to be directed towards collaborative and interdisciplinary rather than cross-disciplinary working. A cross-disciplinary approach reflects practitioners and researchers working within their own disciplinary paradigm and its own boundaries. Interesting research can and does take place, but truly innovative research that breaks down the disciplinary boundaries is more resonant of an interdisciplinary approach. Interdisciplinary working reflects a much greater commitment to real respect and understanding of the beliefs, values and philosophies of the 'other' disciplines. As true interdisciplinary working develops, new approaches to thinking about pain will evolve and a new understanding of pain is likely to be proposed. This will require commitment. Revolutions in thinking require new ways of considering concepts and issues, and this will be made possible by interdisciplinary working. Disciplines will be able to challenge one another's assumptions and beliefs, and a clearer appreciation of pain will emerge. A new pain paradigm will not necessarily explain everything, but it will provide a more sophisticated understanding of an incredibly complex phenomenon. By investigating together, interdisciplinary research will ensure that pain is examined and explored from many perspectives – pain research will be the richer for this diversity of consideration. Pirsig (1974) states:

> Some things you miss because they're so tiny you overlook them. But some things you don't see because they're so *huge*. We were both looking at the same thing, talking about the same thing, thinking about the same thing, except he was looking, seeing, talking and thinking, from a completely different *dimension*.
>
> (Pirsig, 1974, p.62, original author's emphasis)

Recognizing that other ways of looking, seeing, talking and thinking about pain exist is important. What is even more important is that there is an active research dialogue and that the debate is continued.

References

Carter, B. 1994: *Child and infant pain: principles of nursing care and management.* London: Chapman & Hall.

Chalmers, A.F. 1982: *What is this thing called science?* 2nd edn. Milton Keynes: Open University Press.

Copp, L.A. 1990: The patient in pain: USA nursing research. In Bergman, R. (ed.), *Nursing research for nursing practice: an international perspective.* London: Chapman & Hall, 124–44.

Denzin, N.K. and Lincoln, Y.S. 1994: *Handbook for qualitative research.* Thousand Oaks, CA: Sage Publications.

Dunbar, R. 1995: *The trouble with science.* London: Faber and Faber.

Firestone, W.A. (1990) Accomodation: toward a paradigm-praxis dialectic. In Guba, E.G. (ed.) *The paradigm dialog.* Newbury Park, CA: Sage Publications, 105–124.

Guba, E.G. (ed.) 1990: *The paradigm dialog.* Newbury Park, CA: Sage Publications.

Guba, E.G. and Lincoln, Y.S. 1994: Competing paradigms in qualitative research. In Denzin, N.K. and Lincoln, Y.S. (eds) *Handbook for qualitative research.* Thousand Oaks, CA: Sage Publications, 105–17.

Hammersley, M. 1992: The paradigm wars: reports from the front. *British Journal of Sociology of Education* 13, 131–43.

Hammersley, M. 1996: The relationship between qualitative and quantitative research: paradigm loyalty versus methodological eclecticism. In Richardson, J.T.E. (ed.), *Handbook of qualitative research methods for psychology and the social sciences.* Leicester: BPS Books, 159–74.

Heron, J. 1996: *Co-operative inquiry. Research into the human condition.* London: Sage Publications.

Heron, J. and Reason, P. 1997: A participatory inquiry paradigm. *Qualitative Inquiry* 3, 274–9.

Kincheloe, J.L. and McLaren, P.L. 1994: Rethinking critical theory and qualitative research. In Denzin, N.K. and Lincoln, Y.S. (eds) *Handbook for qualitative research.* Thousand Oaks, CA: Sage Publications, 138–57.

Kuhn, T.S. 1962: The structure of scientific revolutions. *International Encyclopedia of Unified Science Foundations of the Unity of Science. Volumes 1 and 2.* Chicago: University of Chicago Press.

Kuhn, T.S. 1970: *The structure of scientific revolutions,* 2nd edn. Chicago: University of Chicago Press.

Melzack, R. and Wall, P. 1988: *The challenge of pain,* 2nd edn. Harmondsworth: Penguin.

Merskey, H. and Bogduk, N. 1994: *Classification of chronic pain,* 2nd edn. Seattle: IASP Task Force on Taxonomy, IASP Press.

Pirsig, R.M. 1974: *Zen and the art of motorcycle maintenance.* London: Vintage.

Reason, P. and Rowan, J. (eds) 1981: *Human inquiry: a sourcebook of new paradigm research.* Chichester: Wiley.

Schwandt, T.A. 1994: Constructivist, interpretivist approaches to human inquiry. In Denzin, N.K. and Lincoln, Y.S. (eds), *Handbook for qualitative research.* Thousand Oaks, CA: Sage Publications, 118–37.

Smith, J.K. 1990: Alternative research paradigms and the problem of criteria. In Guba, E.G. (ed.), *The paradigm dialog.* Newbury Park, CA: Sage Publications, 167–87.

Sofaer, B. 1998: *Pain: principles, practice and patients,* 3rd edn. Cheltenham: Stanley Thornes.

Psychotherapy, fetal memory and pain

Chris Sparks

Introduction

Much of this chapter will revolve around Hugh's story. This is the story of a man, now in his late sixties, who until recently suffered a variety of emotional, physical and, one might say, some spiritual pains as well. The writer's aim in telling Hugh's story is to illustrate some fundamental aspects of how and why pain is experienced which could be of great importance to the caring professions. Hugh's story is a true story about one man. As such it is unique, but the principles that it illustrates are universal. I will draw on a mix of anecdote and theory, although experience is generally to the fore. The writer will allow the reader to theorize.

Principles of psychotherapy

In order to appreciate Hugh's story and the journey he made through therapy, it is important to understand the basic principles which underpin psychotherapy. First, the principle of 'splitting' which is a basic self-defence mechanism, occurs when an experience is unbearable and a person must split it off in order to survive. Neurologically, this is like pulling the plug on it; it becomes disconnected from the person's consciousness. However, the memory circuits which 'hold' the events continue to reverberate in the brain. This can be likened to a CD playing with the volume turned down to zero, but Janov highlights the fact that the situation is not as simple as that (Janov, 1970, 1971, 1975, 1980, 1991). A split-off or dissociated experience is one that has not been fully processed, and thus the pain of that experience has not been expressed. For example, if you hit your thumb with a hammer it hurts like hell; you may need to shout and you probably swear. Shouting and expletives help to carry away the energy of the pain. However, if you do not shout or swear but quietly count to ten, then the pain will probably last much longer. If the pain is unexpressed, then the energy remains within it to fuel various kinds of neurotic behaviour. Neurotic behaviour is sometimes referred to as 'acting-out'. In therapeutic work acting-out achieves little; it can release some of the emotional pressure, but this simply builds up until the next acting out.

A therapist, however, will 'look with' the client for ways of acting-in – that is to say, finding ways of connecting to the painful memory. Here language is instructive. We say 'I remember', but what happens when we fully remember? When remembering a painful event we can often also feel something of the emotion connected with it. In therapy, a person is encouraged to feel fully any physical sensation so as to experience the original pain and to express any accompanying emotion. If the emotion was fully expressed when the event first occurred it will not be present when the event is recalled. However, if it was not expressed at the time of the original event, then the person is said to have 'unfinished business'. Psychotherapy seeks to finish that which has long remained unfinished. This finishing is more than catharsis, and it is the basis of the second principle. It not only allows for the purging of unexpressed emotion, but also for understanding and integration. When a person really connects with a traumatic event the memory becomes an emotion-free part of that person's history. Thus the second principle is the need to reconnect both physically and emotionally, thus reversing the split.

The third principle is that of the 'onion' with layers of defence surrounding a central, damaged core. Therapy does not slice through the layers, because that will damage the core. Human beings are really very vulnerable, and the therapist must create a safe relationship with the client. This relationship becomes one in which the client can remove his or her layers of defence, one by one, as and when he or she is ready to do so. These layers may be described graphically to the therapist by the client. One client described himself as living in a castle with walls 20 feet thick. He constantly patrolled the ramparts checking that all the machine guns were fully loaded and in working order. In fact the real man lived in a sealed room underground in the central keep, and would not come out until he felt totally safe.

In summary, it is my contention that psychological, physical and spiritual pain often cause serious problems in subsequent life so long as it remains unexpressed and unresolved. I further believe that some of the most far-reaching and intractable traumata occur in the womb during the first trimester. This notion requires further development, as the reader may reasonably question how a person can remember anything from the first 3 months in the womb. Although this is not yet fully understood, it seems certain that it is the case (Emerson, 1996). Somehow memories are encoded and replicated in every cell. Later in life, this encoded memory, which may be good or bad, influences behaviours in profound ways. This is illustrated very clearly in Hugh's story.

Spiritual pain and womb memory

The notion of spiritual pain is also fundamental to Hugh's story. It is the writer's belief that psychic pain and spiritual pain are one and the same. This is not to say that there is only one level of spiritual or psychic pain. Spiritual pain can arise from fetal experiences. For the fetus in the womb, the womb is God; it is the whole universe. If the womb rejects the fetus or gives the fetus a bad time, this tells the fetus a lot both about God and about him- or herself. Rejection is probably one of the hardest psychic/spiritual pains to bear. Following this line of argument, spiritual and psychic pain can be defined as that which has to do with how an individual relates to *being*. We do not fear death – what we do fear is annihilation or non-being. This is certainly what the writer means by 'spiritual'. I am not saying that religion is an illusion. For me, God is existence itself and therefore that in which everything else exists. Much confusion has been caused by asking whether we believe in God or not, that is, we ask 'Does *he* exist'? I say no, *he* does not exist; but *he is existence*. Hence spirituality is about our relationship to existence. That may sound impersonal, whereas in fact it is very personal and extremely apposite when speaking of how people relate to pain.

People accessing womb memory will frequently refer to how they perceive *her* to be feeling. The womb has a personality. It is the source of being, pain and pleasure. In the beginning it is God, although as we grow older in the world outside the womb our universe expands. However, I believe it is vital that our understanding of God/spirituality expands too, and we must find satisfactory ways of expressing our relationship with *being itself*. This is important therapeutically because it means that a particular religious stance becomes ultimately irrelevant. The fundamental question is how an individual relates to *being now* – which in therapy is usually in a painful way – and how that relationship can change to become a comfortable pain-free relationship. Sometimes it is not possible to free someone from physical pain, but only from psychic/spiritual pain. In this situation the physical pain may often be courageously borne.

It is clear to me that fetal, perinatal pains and pains experienced during the first year of life can have tragic consequences for individuals, families and society at large. It may well be that these pains are the root causes of much mental illness, psychosomatic illness, neurotic behaviour patterns and criminal behaviour.

Hugh's story

At this point the focus shifts to the life story of a specific real person whom we shall call Hugh. This is not his real name, but he has given his permission for his story to be told here.

Hugh's pains were both physical and emotional, although it was the emotional pain of depression that perhaps triggered the journey he made. Hugh's story does not necessarily unfold in chronological order, but develops by using his pain to frame the story. Hugh entered therapy in the spring of 1979. He was then a teacher in a fairly rough comprehensive school. Several bouts of depression had caused him to seek medical help. He was referred to a psychiatrist who informed him that he was manic-depressive and could be treated with lithium for the rest of his life. This diagnosis aroused Hugh to respond, saying inwardly *'not bloody likely'*. He came out of depression for a time, but sought help from an Anglican priest trained in counselling by the Clinical Theology Association (CTA), founded by Dr Frank Lake in 1962. The 'treatment' offered by the priest proved to be very fruitful and relied on regression via deep breathing. Through regression Hugh relived his childhood surgery for osteo-myelitis at the age of 6 years and 8 months. In particular he remembered the experience of 'going under' for his first anaesthetic. He reported that at first he did not know what was happening. As he lay on the floor breathing deeply he found himself making peculiar sounds as he exhaled. This 'just happened' and Hugh let it happen. Then he felt mild pain and discomfort in his jaw, he let this 'be', too. When he came out of what he now describes as a mild hypnotic state he found himself crying. He said that he was *'crying with happiness because I am alive. I didn't die when I went under'*. Clearly, Hugh's body and brain had recorded the anaesthesia event in precise detail. On a subsequent occasion he remembered in vivid detail 'coming to' in the theatre and seeing the nurse bandaging his left tibia with thick wads and splints. He remembered talking to her and looking around the theatre, which he can still describe in detail.

In the early autumn Hugh went with his counsellor/priest to a conference. One of the prime features of the conferences was the small group work in the mornings and evenings. Hugh's group of eight included a woman whose husband had recently died. After the third session Hugh retired to bed at about 11p.m. and awoke at around 1a.m. weeping. He cried with wracking sobs for one and a half hours or so. He told me that during the first half of this time he wept over his father's death which had occurred 24 years previously. During the second half of the time he wept for a friend who had died of meningitis when they were both 16 years old, some 34 years earlier. Hugh felt considerable relief as a result of this crying. He had not thought of his friend since his death, and told me he now realized just how much he had loved him. The following day one of the principal speakers conducted a 'fish bowl' – a small group working together with an audience looking in. This impressed Hugh mainly because of the release of real feeling among the participants. The speaker afterwards announced that he would demonstrate grief counselling in a sim-ilar fish bowl the following day and asked for volunteers. Hugh volunteered. Initially the leader asked each of the seven members why they had volun-teered. Hugh related very briefly what had happened in the early hours of the previous morning. The second time around when he came to Hugh the leader said, *'Now Hugh, you were saying about your father'*. Hugh began to respond, but before he could utter three words his still unexpressed grief poured out. He told me that he *'roared like a bull'* with his head down between his knees for several minutes. When he had finished the leader leaned forward with his open palms towards Hugh and asked him how he felt. Hugh said that he felt like a million dollars and as if he had just joined the human race. Shortly afterwards, the speaker, Frank Lake, passed Hugh and took him by the arm and said gently. *'It's in the first trimester, Hugh'*. At that stage Hugh did not have a clue what he was talking about.

Perhaps the foregoing account illustrates that we remember emotionally charged events and their unexpressed emotions in full detail. Hugh clearly experienced pain in the two situations. The pain in his jaw, which he experienced during regression, was a physical memory related to the anaesthetic/ surgery, while the grief expressed during the conference was certainly psychological and perhaps even spiritual pain.

Hugh joined the CTA and in 1980 went to one of Frank Lake's primal integration weeks in Nottingham. Here some 12 men and women gathered to work with their primal memories of pain under the guidance of Frank Lake, and with the help of his team of facilitators. I myself had attended one of these week-long workshops and I encouraged Hugh to go. Later, he reported to me what had happened to him. During the first 24 hours, the participants got to know one another and Frank Lake prepared them for the primal work. Then the participants met in small groups of four or five in two large adjacent rooms. Frank Lake sat in the doorway between the two rooms. From this position he could be heard by everyone. Those who were to work lay on a mattress in a fetal position. One member of each group operated a cassette recorder, a second member wrote down everything the 'subject' said and did, while a third was just supportively present and the facilitators sat close behind the subject. Frank Lake then began an induction in which he invited the subject to think of the circumstances of his or her conception, identifying first with Mother and the ovum which was to be part of him or her. Then Lake moved the subject on to identify with the Father and that one sperm which was to be part of him, and so on through the whole process of conception – first cell division and blastocyst floating on down the fallopian tube. The whole thing became real for Hugh as he experienced a blissful and beautiful floating and saw a lovely golden light and the furrowed lining of the tube. Implantation was vaguer and darker, followed by little or nothing until he came to birth itself. Quite suddenly and unexpectedly, as he remembers it, there is immense pressure and a moving forward in a very tight tunnel. Hugh is *'roaring like a lion'*. Then he is out and spitting (literally) into a bowl as he said 'get this stuff out of my mouth'. However, and this is significant, Hugh reported that *'I was spitting with such force that I felt I was knocking holes out of the bottom of the bowl. I felt so positive and victorious that I made it'*.

During the following session on the next day he felt that he was in his mother's arms and she was humming Brahms' lullaby – another blissful experience. Later in the process he stood up and punched a mattress that was strapped to the wall saying, 'I'm not a sissy. I'm not a sissy'. Apparently after the surgery at 6 years of age, he had to wear a full-length calliper for 9 months, and after that he was afraid to play rough games with the boys. Through his therapy he came to *know* that he was not a sissy.

Again Hugh had clear physical and emotional memories of key events in his life, and these could be worked with to help him face up to his pains and problems. By 1984 Hugh was coming for sessions every 2 or 3 months. Somehow he knew that there was more work to do. For one thing, he was still getting pain in his side. He had had this pain on and off since the age of 14 years. It was a stabbing and anxiety-provoking pain, and he had seen a heart specialist about it. Every 2 or 3 years he saw his GP about it. Always he was reassured that his heart was fine. In about 1990 he had a full cardiogram and was declared 'A1' although he continued to experience the pain.

At this time, in his therapy, he was talking about his parents and grand-parents. It became apparent that some of his pain was related to events that occurred at about 8 weeks gestation. It emerged that he was the fourth, or more accurately the fifth of six children, the first of whom had died at birth. He was the fourth living child – a crucial fact. His maternal grandmother's fourth child had died at birth. Hugh's eldest sister, who was 8 years old at the time of his birth, told him in 1994 how his grandmother had gone into his mum and dad's bedroom at 1a.m. early in the pregnancy, leapt on the bed and tried to strangle his father. Hugh then began to imagine what happened. He told me: 'I suppose that mother woke in terror with her adrenaline surging, leapt out of bed quickly to return to drag her mother off. Subsequently, peace was restored'. Having had these thoughts Hugh began to experience involuntary thoughts and imaginings. He thought, 'God is a sod!' – strong stuff for a Christian man! He also imagined himself with a bayonet ripping his mother open from vagina to throat. I suggested that perhaps he wanted to rip his way out from inside. That seemed more than probable to him. Many subjects of Frank Lake's (1981a,b) methods and his research show that, in regression, they feel as if a knife is going in at the navel (perhaps negative umbilical affect?). Hugh's primal response was to knife back. I believe this is worthy of careful research. That is to say, some criminal behaviour could well be related to early fetal distress (Lake, 1981a,b). Using very simple intuitive regression Hugh concluded that: 'It happened at about 8 weeks gestation. And the rush of adrenaline nearly did for me . . . . And I am just incredibly angry. I am in total rage about it'. I then invited him to take, in imagination, a bayonet to express his rage. He did this with 'mighty roars'.

From that moment he has never experienced the distressing and stabbing pain in his side. In addition, he now remembers both his mother and grand-mother with increasing affection, and moreover he says that now, at 67 years of age, he feels better, fitter and happier than at any time in his life. The process of healing involved knifing his mother back, virtually killing her. It was virtual reality. The result was that he understood both emotionally and cognitively that it was not his mother's fault. It was not even his grand-mother's fault. In fact, he now feels growing affection for both – although both have long been dead. Previously, doctors had repeatedly reassured him that his heart was fine and this information helped temporarily. Now, having con-nected with the root pain, he knows that his heart is fine, and importantly so much more is fine, too.

Hugh's story would not be complete without mentioning the time in 1986 when he woke in the early hours experiencing what he describes as the most intense, incredible and excruciating pain imaginable in his left tibia. This pain was not new, although the extent and intensity of it was. Between the ages of 7 and 17 years he had experienced bad night pain in his leg, but never anything like this. Moreover, after the age of 17 years, he experienced pain in his tibia when there were significant changes in barometric pressure and humidity. Since that one night of extremely intense pain in 1986 he has had no pain in his left tibia at all. Hugh's explanation for this was as follows: *'It was as if all the pain of my six operations came together and I felt it. My body had recorded it but never really felt it till that night in 1986. What a blessing to be free of it'*.

I have told Hugh's story at some length because it illustrates for me a number of crucial factors about pain. We remember everything, both subtle and raw.

Fetal memory: implications for Hugh and other people in pain

Much research has been done in Europe and North America on fetal responses to the kind of environment that is encountered in the womb. Obviously this relies on the existence of fetal memory. I accept that fetal memory is an established fact. The imprinting is stored in each and every cell – some would say from before conception, in the ovum and sperm. There is much evidence for this view in the case records of other psychotherapists. Then, once the synapses are present in the embryonic and fetal cortex, a more sophisticated remembering also develops. Lake (1981a,b) claims that fetal memory is beyond doubt. A vast body of subsequent research supports this view, and Hugh has no doubt about it whatsoever.

How do individuals survive a hostile womb environment? Some do not, and are aborted before implantation. Those that survive have the benefit of the organism's defence system to be able to cope. Bad events are split off – disconnected (Janov, 1970). 'Neurosis is a neurological event. The splitting leads to neurosis and the splitting is a neurological event'. Janov also said that neurosis is blocked feeling. The paradox is that originally the split saves one but in order to be healed one must reconnect. This is what Hugh did over the course of many years. In 1980, when he made his 'womb journey', he did not reconnect with the root event at 8 weeks into the first trimester. He was not yet ready, and his defences held firm. In 1995 he did reconnect. He was ready and he was healed.

Is this a spiritual dimension? That is to say, about the relationships between persons? There are many possible explanations. The therapist rarely knows which is the right interpretation. The client 'knows' the answer, but only when he or she is ready to access the truth. Meanwhile, it is locked up behind the defensive wall, which is a wall against pain. It was intolerable in its original context, but now with the support of the adult person and the therapist who remain alongside it might be tolerated. Breaching one's own defences can be extraordinarily difficult. Freud spoke of the 'flight from treatment'. Who would not flee from the jaws of hell? Many clients who finally find the resources to face their own fetal memories speak of their discoveries as hellish.

Lake (1981a,b) writes of Simone Weil's analysis of affliction, which Weil describes as a threefold pain composed of social scorn, a splitting mental pain and bodily anguish. Lake (1981a,b) states that 'I would say, with no fear of being wrong, that this tripartite terror is a direct result of transmarginal distress in the foetus, usually within the first trimester'. He further states that:

'Occasionally, an accidental near-miscarriage or attempted abortion in the third or fourth month can produce some of this affliction, as can a long and cruelly difficult labour'.

It is worth developing this theme. Life is, after all, a continuum from the moment of conception until death. The blueprint for our physical development and much of our mental development is in our genes, as is the potential for many diseases. We can further the nature vs. nurture debate by taking both the genetic inheritance and the womb environment of an individual very seriously. It is during the first 3 months that the foundations are laid. The human race has known this for several thousand years. The writings of the ancient Chinese and Indian civilizations include passages which stress the importance of making it possible for the pregnant woman to be kept tranquil and stress free. However, pregnancy in the West in the 1990s is often anything but stress free.

Verny (1991) made a number of positive and indeed dogmatic statements. For example: 'From the moment of conception babies in the womb are bombarded by chemical, physical and hormonal toxins'. The present author suggests that we can add psychological and spiritual toxins for many fetuses. Verny in fact says: 'As important as these external poisons are, my major interest lies in the exploration of the effects of internal emotional poisons on the unborn child'. He cites the myth of Oedipus to illustrate his point and says:

> If Freud had allowed himself to pay more attention to the events leading to Oedipus' birth then perhaps the Oedipus complex today would denote a person who suffered rejection and abandonment by both parents pre- and post-natally, and who as an adult exhibits severe sexual abnormalities and murderous rage'.
>
> (Verny, 1991)

Women ignore the babies in their wombs for a wide variety of reasons. Each form of ignoring has specific results. The fetus seems to have a remarkable ability to discriminate a subtle spectrum of its mother's emotions. Clients exploring these deep levels of memory come to a point where they know what she was feeling. Liley (1991) writes primarily of the physical activity of the fetus and its ability to hear and taste and to make itself comfortable. He states that 'Far from being an inert passenger in a pregnant mother, the fetus is very much in command of the pregnancy'. The fetus determines the duration of pregnancy and decides which way it will present in labour. Liley (1991) questioned the communication of maternal emotion to the fetus. To take this further, I would ask 'Can a fetus feel both his own and his mother's emotions and remember them in a way which can be accessed in maturity?' To begin with I am confident that mature adults do feel emotions which they do not understand as their own. Later in therapy they come to realize that the feeling is not theirs, but something which their mother felt during pregnancy. One such example is 'deep sorrow'. It is not uncommon for a client to report carrying a feeling of deep sorrow which sometimes causes them to weep copiously with no idea as to why, other than a profound sense of loss. Subsequently, it may come to light that their mother's mother died during her pregnancy. For the client, the realization that it is not their grief but their mother's gives total release. However, the encoded emotion of grief had been carried within the client from before birth right up to the time of release. Age is no bar. One client of mine, aged 42 years, literally danced with joy when the realization 'This is not my grief' came.

In the above example the 'knowing' is not very specific until the connection is made, when it then 'makes sense'. Again and again when a physical, psychological or spiritual pain makes sense it disappears. However, it must also be felt, given a voice and usually given an action as well. Hugh roared as, in fantasy, he ripped his way out of his mother. This is acting-in. The anger, sorrow or fear is focused in the right place. It is no longer projected or transferred. This perhaps has major implications for pain therapy.

Many doctors and nurses are becoming much more holistic in their approach. Surely this makes good sense in the light of our increasing knowledge of the complexity of human beings. Rossi (1993), for example, illustrates how certain biochemical compounds are transducers for communication between body and mind (and spirit). I watched him working with a woman with quite serious arthritic pain in her hands. She was in a mild hypnotic state, allowing the flow of images, thoughts, feelings and emotions to pass through her consciousness. She worked with Rossi for about 15 minutes. After about 10 minutes the pain in her hand had increased from about 3 to 9 on a scale of 1 to 10. By the time Rossi brought her out of her trance she was pain free and her hands were supple. At no time did Rossi suggest that the pain would go. There was no suggestion of any kind. He simply and gently encouraged her to go with the flow. Here it seemed to me that she felt her pain and it went, together with the inflammation in her hands.

Pain tends to increase as we resist or fight it. Hugh felt the pain of his operations in all its fullness one night. He is now pain free. Perhaps there is a sense in which what really hurts is the resisting – the trying to keep the floodgates closed against the enormous pressure behind them. Let the gates open and it does not hurt. Hugh says that when he was 'bellowing like a bull' in the fish bowl in 1979 he was not in any pain. His grief was just pouring out, and that did not hurt.

The day before that event Hugh participated in an imaginary journey in which he was to climb a mountain to the sunshine at the top. His mountain was made of jet black, jagged rock, totally devoid of vegetation. The path up it was narrow and dangerous with precipitous falls to one side. He never reached the top. After the fish bowl exercise he made the journey again. This time the mountain was ablaze with flowers all bathed in warm sunshine. The path was grassy and easy to walk, and he quickly reached the top. After feeling his grief the world was transformed. After the connection with the trauma at 8 weeks into gestation, the world was further transformed and Hugh is now totally pain free.

Much medical practice in relation to pain involves the use of drugs or surgery to alleviate or eradicate it. Obviously these procedures help, and often they are the only answer. However, intractable problems may leave the professions floundering. In some of these difficult cases neither drugs nor surgery work. In fact, the last state is worse than the first – the very treatment intended to heal or help can destroy. In a proportion of these cases the root problem is psychospiritual, with physical/functional consequences. This seemed to be the case with Hugh.

Hugh also told me that he became aware of huge anger towards the anaesthestist and nurse who put him 'under' at 6 years 8 months. He admits the illogicality of his anger. After all, these people seemed kind and they did save his life. It was not so much that they put him through terror – rather it was that they did not explain what he was about to experience. When he got in touch with this at the age of 55 years he says that his anger related directly to having been *betrayed* by not being told.

Thankfully – for Hugh and others like him – the profession is learning, and paramedics, surgeons and practitioners in every branch of medicine now routinely explain what they intend to do, and how and why. The benefits are obvious – patients are more relaxed and co-operative, and recovery times are shorter.

Conclusions

Any and every medical situation must seek to treat the patient with the utmost respect. This is surely a spiritual matter. That is to say, it is about relationships between people/beings. When ET said 'Home Elliott, home', it was about a common spiritual understanding – real communication. In my view an embryo, even a fertilized egg, needs to be regarded as a person. All of the potential is there in the beginning, profoundly affected by the psychosocial environment.

Perhaps medicine is becoming much more generally holistic. This means seeing a present illness or accidental injury in the context of the whole person and his or her whole life. It is not to say that doctors and nurses must know everything about a patient – that would obviously be impossible. It is more about an attitude of mind, and especially about a readiness to listen to a patient, and in a sense also to hear what they are not saying. This is the essence of respect.

Hugh's anger during the first trimester was about the way in which his world – the womb – was treating him. It had all but destroyed him. The whole experience was split off because it was literally intolerable. Later in life and in therapy work, he learned that anger, and even rage, were acceptable, and within certain rational limits he was able to express his fetal rage. Research within the last decade or so has shown that fetal human beings do understand tone of voice, and that they even enjoy Mozart! It surely follows that much 'pain' can be avoided. Health professionals have a vital and ongoing task. We are concerned not only with pain reduction, but also with pain prevention.

Physical pain is often unavoidable, whereas psychological and spiritual pain might be largely avoided. One of the most important implications of Hugh's story is that communication is of the very essence of life. Rossi (1993) develops the thesis that the development of biological organisms over the past four billion years has been about communication both within cells and between cells. What takes place between a psychotherapist and a client might be termed ideal communication. The therapist aims to be a facilitator of internal dialogue within the client. Typically, the therapist seeks to enable the client to hear what he or she is saying, thinking, feeling, sensing and imagining. In other words, it is about real inner communication. It is about knowing the truth, and about knowing what lies behind the walls of defence and the psychosomatic symptoms. In the practice of medicine, communication is vitally important. Patients who are fearful, anxious or distressed must have the opportunity to communicate these fears to a significant other. The terror must be respected – it must not be dismissed. For the patient it is very real, and appropriate support needs to be offered. When fear or any other pain is received, accepted and understood, it is considerably diminished.

Over a number of years, Hugh was heard by various helpers and so the layers of his 'onion' of pain were removed. Each layer removed was a significant healing, and made possible the removal of the next layer, until at last he could face the core. Each of his helpers played a part. No helper could have led him to the core alone, and each did his best for him. I know that Hugh is as grateful to the man who set him on the road as he is to the one who accompanied him for the last mile, and indeed all those who walked with him for parts of the journey in between. At the end of the road the onion had gone.

References

Emerson, W.R. 1996: The vulnerable prenate. *Pre- and Perinatal Psychology Journal* **10**, 125–4.

Janov, A. 1970: *The primal scream*. London: Abacus.

Janov, A. 1971: *The anatomy of mental illness*. London: Abacus.

Janov, A. 1975: *Primal man: the new consciousness*. London: Abacus.

Janov, A. 1980: *Prisoners of pain*. London: Abacus.

Janov, A. 1991: *The new primal scream*. London: Abacus.

Lake, F. 1981a: Fetal memory, fact or fiction? *BMA News Review* **7**, 12–19

Lake, F. 1981b: *Tight corners in pastoral counselling*. London: DLT.

Liley, A.W. 1991: The fetus as a personality. *Pre and Perinatal Psychology Journal* **5**, 191–202

Rossi, E.L. 1993: *The psychobiology of mind–body healing*. London: Norton.

Verny, T. 1991: Presidential address. *Pre- and Perinatal Pyschology Journal* **6**, 207–15.

Further reading

Autton, N. 1986: *Pain: an exploration*. London: DLT.

Maret, S.M. 1992: *Frank Lake's maternal–fetal distress syndrome. An analysis*. Oxford: Clinical Theology Association (obtainable only from CTA, St Mary's House, Church Westcote, Oxford OX7 6SF).

Odent, M. 1986: *Primal health*. London: Century.

Skevington, S.M. 1995: *Psychology of pain*. Chichester: Wiley.

Wasdell, D. 1994: *Mary. A study in primal integration therapy*. Meridian Monograph. London: Urchin.

Counselling in the management of chronic pain

Beatrice Sofaer

It is difficult for (other) people to understand what it is like to live with pain. My life is completely different now to what it was before the pain started. There is not now (in my life) that which I used to do. Beforehand I used to be a very fit active person. Now I have to confine myself to finding things that I can do indoors that don't require much energy. I am no longer able to work. It is almost like building a wall around oneself. Doctors are happy to see me, but it is almost as if they have written me off.

(Mrs M, a patient aged 38 years)

Introduction

The above quotation is from a woman who was medically retired from a government job because of chronic pain. It gives some indication of the sense of isolation that is felt by people who suffer chronic pain. Sometimes health professionals are at a loss in trying to help. This is because chronic pain is a very complex phenomenon and is difficult to treat.

The purpose of this chapter is not to provide definitive answers to a very complex issue, but rather to share with readers some ideas about the problems which often surface in patients who suffer from chronic pain. Multidisciplinary pain management units are now springing up in many parts of the world, and frequently patients will find that not only will they receive help and advice on the use of physical therapies such as analgesics and transcutaneous electric nerve stimulation (TENS), but they will be offered psychological help as well. Counselling is one approach that may be utilized in hospital, out-patient or primary care settings. It is a skill which many health professionals could use. Counselling can be practised at different levels. It can be used as 'part of work' or 'as work'. There are a variety of training courses available at certificate, diploma and postgraduate levels. It is important whenever counselling is practised that appropriate 'supervision' is provided and utilized. Supervision is the process whereby the counsellor has regular contact with another experienced counsellor and the process of counselling may be discussed. This mentor-type relationship is considered to be an essential part of the practice of counselling. Normally the term 'client' is used in counselling, but because this chapter is dealing with patients, for the present purposes the terms 'patients' and 'clients' will be used interchangeably.

Each person is different

It is important to understand that for each person the experience of pain is a different one, and that individuals each have their own 'autobiography' which influences how they will react to and give meaning to their pain. Culture, personality, environment, location and intensity of pain are all factors (among others) that will encroach on a person's lifestyle and life quality (Sofaer, 1998). Each person's behaviour may be influenced not only by the above factors, but by behaviours seen in others. Some people keep things to themselves, while others prefer to share their thoughts. However, when it comes to pain, particularly chronic pain, many people obtain 'relief' psychologically speaking when they realize that they are not 'going mad' but reacting to a situation which is making them feel out of control. Counselling provides them with the opportunity to regain control in their lives and to be able to cope better. Developing a therapeutic relationship with a counsellor provides the patient with an opportunity to discuss his or her feelings related to the pain, and is an important step in involving the patient as a partner dealing with psychological issues surrounding the pain.

Patients who suffer chronic pain are those who have had pain for 6 months or more. Frequently, people seem not to have been informed of a diagnosis. This is because sometimes no cause can be found for their continuous pain. Often these patients will have been seen by several doctors, have had many investigations and are at a loss to know why someone in the health profession cannot (a) tell them what the problem is and (b) take away the pain. A whole host of feelings then result, e.g. anger at the problem and with the medical profession, guilt because of being unable to contribute (socially and financially) to the family well-being, depression and/or despair due to being unable to see 'light at the end of the tunnel', and a huge sense of loss to do with all kinds of activities that they were previously able to engage in (Sofaer and Walker, 1996). Patients who suffer chronic pain on the whole feel isolated and dwell on the past. They feel that they are not getting anywhere and may blame the medical profession and 'the system'. A variety of therapies may have been tried in an effort to help them, sometimes partly succeeding and at other times not. Whatever the situation, patients frequently carry a burden of feelings linked with their pain and suffering, for which they need and appreciate having a person who will listen in a trusting professional relationship.

It is well recognized that in order to treat chronic pain effectively, a programme that includes medical and psychological strategies is most likely to meet a patient's overall needs. This has been referred to as the 'biopsychosocial model of pain management' (Waddell, 1992). Many pain management programmes do have a psychology service where psychologists will be asked by colleagues to work in collaboration with them to modify the cognitive, psychological or social behaviour of patients who are suffering pain, but as DeGood (1983) has pointed out, mutual understanding and co-operation between a psychologist and a medical patient may be difficult to establish because of a patient's pre-existing beliefs about the nature of psychology, and there may be a certain reluctance on the part of the patient to take part in therapy for a variety of reasons, including a lack of understanding of the reason for the referral (DeGood, 1983). Often fears can be dispelled by explaining to the patient that people who suffer chronic pain experience changes in their life which produce negative feelings about all kinds of things, and that this in turn may make them feel tense. Tension could exacerbate their pain and add to their suffering. Some of that tension could be relieved by talking over the issues with an experienced professional in a trusting and confidential environment.

What is counselling?

Counselling is one way of providing psychological help for patients. Often people perceive counselling as less threatening than 'psychology'. The practice of counselling is based on psychological theories but is seen as being more of a partnership rather than a treatment (although, of course, using counselling skills either overtly or covertly may be part of treatment). Counselling is a person-to-person form of communication which emphasizes the development of understanding best described as empathy. Counselling will focus on one or more of the patient's problems and is free from judgement or coercion. Counselling aims to encourage a person to decide on choices in their life, while respecting the individual's right to have and make a particular choice.

Counselling may take place at different levels, from the utilization of counselling skills as part of a health professional's role, to professional counselling sessions on a contractual basis (for a certain number of sessions). Stewart (1986) suggested that nurses, in particular, cannot avoid being drawn into using counselling skills, as their job demands it. In essence, listening is an essential part of counselling but to be effective it has to be active rather than passive. The skills which a health professional brings to counselling will depend on their experience in dealing with a particular problem and the depth of counselling that they are able to enter into with a patient. There are ethical issues which apply to all counselling situations. The British Association of Counselling (1993) has published a *Code of Ethics and Practice for Counsellors*, which considers such issues as client safety, terms of counselling, and the competence of the counsellor. The Code of Practice applies the values and ethical principles to specific situations in counselling and refers to issues of responsibility, counselling supervision, confidentiality, confidentiality in the legal process, advertising, research and conflicts between ethical priorities and other codes (those codes which relate to people who would not regard themselves as counsellors, but who do use counselling skills).

Counselling is based upon the utilization of several skills, including an awareness of individual differences, building rapport and empathy, and listening, questioning and reflecting. There are several models of counselling, but most of them emphasize the importance of listening, open-ended questioning, sincerity, warmth and reflection.

One approach which can be used is 'person-centred counselling'. This is perhaps the most appropriate style of counselling to use with people who suffer chronic pain. Developed by Dr Carl Rogers in the 1930s and 1940s, it was a departure from the analytical approach to therapy, and has as its core philosophy the idea that the client knows best what 'hurts'. Rogers saw progress as a way of working known as 'non-directive' counselling. The basis for this type of therapy and the way in which it 'works' are described in some detail by Mearns and Thorne (1988). Basically, the central assumption of person-centred counselling is that the client can be trusted to find his or her way forward if the counsellor provides the kind of encouragement in the client/counsellor relationship that will allow the client to feel safe enough to experience the beginnings of self-acceptance. For people who suffer chronic pain this is very important, because they have usually spent so much time hearing 'experts' telling them how to live their lives that their self-esteem is low. Constant pain has eroded their quality of life, interfered with their relationships and friendships, and their human spirit is depleted. Person-centred counselling should provide a background to the regeneration of 'self'. Empathic understanding should help to restore to an isolated individual a sense of belonging. There are three elements which the counsellor can offer in the therapeutic relationship, namely being genuine or congruent, offering unconditional positive regard and total acceptance, and feeling and communicating a deep empathic understanding (Mearns and Thorne, 1992).

Some examples of the use of counselling in the management of pain

Because there is a wide variety of problems encountered by people who suffer chronic pain, the counselling must be appropriate for the needs of the individual person. On the whole, though, it would seem that counselling is underutilized and perhaps could be offered more frequently to patients who suffer chronic pain. Sometimes the work will be aimed at improving communication, as in the case of Mr J, who needed to rehearse his potential encounters with staff when he had frequent admissions to hospital.

Mr J suffers from chronic pancreatitis. From time to time his condition worsens and requires him to be admitted to hospital. During the last couple of years his admissions have been a 'disaster', with staff not believing him and pain control being withheld or delayed. During counselling, Mr J disclosed that he felt the nurses were not hearing him and that when pain relief was delayed he began to feel out of control and bad tempered. This was accepted by the counsellor, and some work was undertaken in the counselling sessions to encourage Mr J to discuss this issue with staff. Following a rehearsal with his counsellor, he was able to feel 'more in charge' during the next hospital admission when, following an explanation to staff of his fears and worries about 'losing his cool', the communication difficulties were resolved and pain relief was not delayed.

At other times the work may be aimed at reducing isolation as, for example, in the situation of Mrs A, who spent all of her days at home watching television. It never occurred to her that she could do something useful to help others, even though she was unable to go out to work herself. In counselling she expressed the wish to find a way of distracting herself from the pain. This was accepted by the counsellor and she was encouraged to explore her options. After some time discussing these options, Mrs A decided that she would volunteer to read to a blind person.

Sometimes counselling is geared towards helping someone to come to terms with the sense of loss in their life and lifestyle, and the work is to help them to express grief which they may not have felt able to do previously. Once this work has been accomplished in a trusting relationship with a counsellor, frequently patients can 'ditch' the past and move on in their lives. This was the case with Mrs B, an elderly widow who came to the pain clinic reporting backache. No physical cause could be found for her symptoms, but she said that she would like to have some help with her feelings. At the first session with the counsellor she was invited to talk about herself. '*It hasn't been the same since my husband passed away*', she said. The following sessions were devoted to exploring her sense of loss, her feelings at selling her house, and finally her move into the home of her elderly brother, for whom she cared. She set herself some realistic goals and became determined to achieve them. Sometimes she would say how much her back hurt, but after about 6 months she reported how much better she felt and how she was coping better. '*Really I have little to grumble about, dear*' she would say to the counsellor. It seemed as if the loss exacerbated the pain and the pain had exacerbated the loss. So long as the door was left open for her to return to the pain management unit (if she wanted to), she felt able to move forward and she did.

There is little literature on counselling and pain relief outcomes. One author (Stewart, 1987) has given an account of how a patient with trigeminal neuralgia benefited from counselling and imagery, and Feinmann (1993) noted that counselling and medication were effective in 70 per cent of patients suffering facial pain. It has been noted by Rowlingson and Hamill (1991) that chronic pain patients are less likely to respond to long-term insight-oriented psychodynamic therapy than to counselling. It is suggested that patients who suffer chronic pain tend to express their psychological distress through their behaviour. Counselling which focuses on encouraging behaviour change, improving self-esteem and enhancing coping mechanisms can often help patients to come to terms with the fact that their pain may not disappear completely in response to medical interventions.

It might be useful for the reader to hear about an example of a situation in which counselling has proved to be successful (Sofaer and Lamberty, 1993). Anonymity has been respected, but written agreement was obtained from the patient for the publication of 'his story', which is one example of longstanding pain and stress suffered by a patient. In this instance, the amputation of a leg (below the knee) 47 years prior to seeking help from the pain management team was the problem. Brief excerpts from the 'life and pain' history are given in an attempt to demonstrate the value to a patient of communication within a counselling approach, and to demonstrate also that the management of chronic pain is a complex problem (a person-centred approach, as discussed earlier, was utilized).

Mr G's story

Mr G, a World War II veteran aged 69 years, was first seen in January 1991 with longstanding severe stabbing phantom limb pain. The pain occurred in bouts every 6–8 weeks and lasted for 6–24 h. No medication had been found to be effective. Carbamazepine was prescribed, and a diagnostic lumbar sympathetic block was planned. The patient was at his 'wits end'. It was suggested that he try counselling and guided imagery, and that he might learn deep relaxation. He took himself off the tablets without consultation. A *primum non nocere* axiom was employed and a postponement of nerve blocks agreed over the next few months while counselling and guided imagery took place and while the patient learnt deep relaxation. Ten hours of taped sessions followed. These sessions included a period of discussion using standard counselling techniques followed by guided imagery and deep relaxation (Sofaer, 1998).

The war experience

Being wounded: disbelief of self (session 1).   The clock was turned back to World War II. The patient recalled his thoughts at the age of 22 years before being bailed out over Arnhem. *'I couldn't really think that I would be badly wounded'*. He described the fight with the Germans. He lost his rifle and went to retrieve it. *'I said to the officer, "give me some cover". As I was coming back I was hit. It was a blow to my ego'*. It had never occurred to him that he would be wounded. He had 'supreme optimism', and being wounded came as a total surprise. He had expected to go to war, fight, win and return home safe and sound.

A prisoner of war.   *'I don't know the period of time I lay there, but eventually we were carried and put into lorries on straw and I was the only one amongst Germans. . . . The next day a doctor caused me excruciating pain by pushing a rag covered in ointment into the hole in my leg'*. He described the situation vividly and graphically. The memory was fresh in his mind as he talked in detail.

Amputation (session 2).   *'Later we were put into cells in a German civilian hospital. I became aware of a strange sensation. I'm sat in a pool of blood. A Russian orderly who was a prisoner of war got a tourniquet and applied it. The next day a French doctor came to me. "Bad news for you, I'll have to take your leg off"'*.

Incentive to live: a lack of faith (session 3).   *'Things began to get worse and one day I was put down in a little room on my own. A French padre came – "Let us pray, son."'* He recalls his thoughts at that moment. *'He bloody thinks I'm going to die'*. He clarified his thoughts on spirituality in the counselling sessions. His denial of faith is what he said kept him going. *'It wasn't the prayers'*. It was important for him that his lack of faith was totally accepted by the counsellor. It would seem that frequently people believe that it is a positive view of religion that offers strength and courage. In this instance it was not so. He recalled a dream that he had had when he was about 10 years old. In the dream he was being chased, and when the people in the dream caught anyone they would cut off their leg. *'They lowered me into the bath and of course the paper bandages came off, and I'd never seen this stump before and I looked down and there was the exact photographic picture of what I used to see as a young boy in those nightmares'*. He was intrigued by the fact that this dream was like a self-fulfilling prophecy, and he sought some explanation from the counsellor, who was unable to offer one. However, he himself was able to offer an explanation for the phantom pain: *'the physical part is taken away but the nerve centres that activate it, they go on to certain parts'*. His explanation of his phantom pain is interesting in that it is very much in keeping with current scientific thinking about phantom limb pain.

The bitter post-war years

Repatriation (session 4).   He was in a prisoner-of-war camp. He walked miles sharing crutches with others. Eventually he was exchanged in Switzerland for German disabled, liberated and sent home to a British army hospital. *'I saw this Major. I said "I'd like to go home, I don't know if my mother knows whether I am alive or dead". So I was sent home on the mail train. I arrived at 3 a.m.'*

The process of limb fitting.   In 1945, fitting of an artificial limb took place. *'I had to get used to it. One doesn't just put on an artificial leg and trot off down the road. It is a very painful and demanding process'*. He wore the limb to get married. Artificial limbs in 1945 were more cumbersome than in the 1990s, and it was with frustration that he recalled the experience.

Civilian life 1945–1979: distrust of people (session 5).   He experienced a long period of hardship. He was cycling miles to work as a signalman. He became unemployed. *'I had £1 a week disability pension to compensate me for all the pain and discomfort . . . which I thought was extremely unjust'*. This period was a very bitter time. He fathered two children, but the effect of his leg on his lifestyle severely hampered family activities. There was some marital conflict. Various jobs followed until disability forced his early retirement in 1979. It became obvious that the bitterness of these years had a profound effect on his life and on his perception of pain and suffering. He told the story with an air of despair at the memory. During deep relaxation he was requested to imagine both legs 'warm and heavy and tired and numb'. Guided imagery was used so that he could imagine himself in a place where he wanted to be. He responded well and said that he was able to imagine this. During the fifth session with the counsellor he felt pain in his phantom instep. The therapist suggested that he talk to it. *'How will I address it other than in rage? I've so desperately begged it to leave me in the past'*. He thinks quietly for several minutes. *'I've suffered so much in the past, why have I got to go on suffering?'* He talks (silently) to the leg, and there is silence in the room. *'The pain has gone'*. What did you do? (asks the counsellor). *'I think I was just asking it nicely to leave me'*. These moments when Mr G relinquished his pain were moving and touching moments both for himself and for the counsellor. There was a feeling of humility and surprise on the part of the counsellor, and for Mr G there were feelings of relief, but also fear that the effect might not last.

Retirement (session 6).   This session centred around eight very difficult years. His wife became ill *'with a fleshy growth'*. There were frequent hospital-izations. They both knew it was cancer, but when it was nearly *'the end'*, they were not informed. *'Nobody told me she was terminal. I just casually kissed her good-bye and said "I'll be up in the morning, dear". She was dead by 3 a.m.'* He was informed of her death by a policeman knocking on his door at 8 a.m one morning. This was a period when he felt a huge sense of loss which he relived in the sessions with the counsellor (*'I have told nobody else about this'*). The whole family was incredibly bitter at the lack of sensitivity of the medical and nursing professions. This bitterness was reflected in Mr G's distrust of the doctors who were dealing with his phantom limb pain. It was therefore crucially important now for him to be heard by someone who accepted what he was saying and listened empathically to him. *'I became rather more cynical than I should have been and I don't think that has helped me'*. He contrasted the constant huge loss of life and limb in World War II with minimal losses in the Gulf War.

Relinquishing the pain

This patient's story of 47 years was vividly told, and it reflected experiences to do with lack of faith – in himself, in God, in people and in the medical and nursing professions. In a trusting relationship with the therapist he finally relinquished his pain. Four subsequent sessions were geared towards helping him to relinquish his fear that the pain might return, and dealing with the aftermath of living a life free of pain! Eighteen months after the first visit to the pain management unit he said *'I came in considerable pain. Now the pain is gone. I look younger and I feel younger'*. Two years later he was leading a creative and productive life and had a hobby of wood turning. He presented the counsellor with a clock he had made. In reflecting back 5 years later (in 1996) with Mr G about his perceptions of how life has changed, the counselling process was discussed. He said, *'it changed the negative thinking to positive thinking. Drugs are for some people but not for me – they didn't help'*. In relation to the present time he said *'I am quite happy now, I can't think of anything I could worry about. One lives a more relaxed life now. I don't have the threat of pain hanging over me. That is quite something. I used to warn people that I might be caught in pain. Now this is not necessary. Pain was a phase of my life which is in the past'*.

Conclusions

For people who suffer chronic pain, the idea that it may eventually become part of their past is initially seen as being very far away from reality. However, with help and encouragement from a supportive and non-judgemental team of health professionals, people can often make improvements to their quality of living. In all counselling situations, as in the situation cited above, the relationship between counsellor and patient is important. For Mr G, it was the very first time he had felt able to trust a member of the health profession. Building that trust meant careful listening by the counsellor, complete acceptance of what he said, and the conveying by her of appreciation that he had invested his trust. A heartfelt respect was felt by the counsellor during the sessions.

Coping with pain in partnership with a counsellor who is working in collaboration with other health professionals can really make a difference. Counselling could play a more major part in the multidisciplinary treatment of pain. It is hoped that this under-used and under-researched skill will find its place at the forefront of pain management in the future.

Acknowledgements

The author wishes to acknowledge the contribution of colleagues in the Pain Management Unit, Brighton Health Care NHS Trust, towards the multidisciplinary management of pain with patients, and also to express her thanks to her counselling supervisor.

References

British Association of Counselling 1993: *Code of ethics and practice for counsellors.* Rugby: British Association for Counselling.

DeGood, D.E. 1983: Reducing medical patients' reluctance to participate in psychological therapies: the initial session. *Professional Psychology: Research and Practice* **14**, 570–9.

Feinmann, C. 1993: The long-term outcome of facial pain treatment. *Journal of Psychosomatic Research* **37**, 382–7.

Mearns, D. and Thorne, B. 1988: *Person-centred counselling in action.* London: Sage Publications.

Rowlingson, J.C. and Hamill, R.J. 1991: Organization of a multidisciplinary pain center. *Mount Sinai Journal of Medicine* **58**, 267–72.

Sofaer, B. 1998: *Pain: principles, practice and patients,* 3rd edn. Cheltenham: Stanley Thornes.

Sofaer, B. and Lamberty, J. 1993: *47 years of phantom pain. 'I don't need it anymore!'* *Counselling in pain therapy.* Poster presented to seventh World Congress on Pain, Paris, 22–27 August 1993.

Sofaer, B. and Walker, J. 1996: *Pain careers: experiences of chronic back pain patients.* Poster presented to Eighth World Congress on Pain, Vancouver, British Columbia, Canada, 17–22 August 1996.

Stewart, W. 1986: *Counselling in nursing: a problem-solving approach.* Lippincott Nursing Series. London: Harper and Row Ltd.

Stewart, W.S. 1987: Counselling and pain relief. *British Journal of Guidance and Counselling* **15**, 140–9.

Waddell, G. 1992: Biopsychosocial analysis of low back pain. *Ballières Clinical Rheumatology* **6**, 523–57.

Pain: a feminist perspective?

Angela Cotton

> It is as difficult to think about pain as about love; both are charged with associations going back to early life, and with cultural attitudes wrought into language itself. Yet pain, like love, is embedded in the ideology of motherhood, and it has so much depth of allusion for all women, mothers or not, that we need to examine its meaning more closely.
>
> (Rich, 1977, p.157)

Introduction

Within this chapter I shall present a number of interrelated and interdisciplinary themes which feminist scholars and activists have explored, relating to the experience of pain. I shall draw upon ideas which, I believe, make an indirect impact upon the contemporary discourse on pain, and I shall include an eclectic consideration of how feminists have recognized and made explicit the significance of the body for social theory.

In order to illustrate some of these ideas, I have chosen to focus upon specific areas of women's experience. The meanings of the painful preparation of girls' and women's bodies for heterosexual relationships, and the regulation and medicalization of women's experiences and their concomitant iatrogenic consequences will be presented for thought. I shall also consider the implications of the regulation of women's bodies through painful surgical procedures, and how being in pain may ensure that women never forget about their bodies. The discussion will also allude to how pathologizing the everyday painful sensations associated with women's bodies – menstruation, giving birth, menopause – may be said to encourage an alienated sense of being 'out of control' of our bodies, and indeed may foster dependence upon medical intervention.

Why a feminist perspective on pain?

Why a feminist perspective on anything? One could perhaps be forgiven for thinking that the feminist arguments and agendas of the last 25 years have been resolved, that they are now somehow irrelevant, or that they seem strangely 'out of step' with contemporary discourses in the late 1990s. There is a proliferation of ideas vying for attention, an unprecedented knowledge explosion impacting on academia and the media, an abundance of theories of post-modernist, post-structuralist and post-feminist persuasions (Farganis, 1994). Yet many of the issues which have concerned and been addressed by feminists remain topics of unresolved debate. It would seem that feminism is now a 'post-' phenomenon but, despite the rhetoric, there are still structures in existence which women and other marginalized groups find oppressive. The ways in which Western society is structured have a history, and have meanings situated in a specific moment. Feminists have critiqued the shaping of this history, pointing to how male interests have defined both the events them- selves, and the telling and re-telling of those events. Feminists would say that the interests of men form the basis of androcentric, malestream, patriarchal thought. Medicine is one such institutional structure – historically misogynist, paternalistic in approach, and with a dualist, Cartesian philosophical tradition. In view of this, when pain is considered as a topic for feminist scrutiny, it is likely that more questions will be raised than answered.

I acknowledge, furthermore, that there are many facets to this discussion which, due to limitations of space, are not considered here. For example, the notion of pain as an experience that is possibly life-enhancing for women, and perhaps self-actualizing (e.g. painful self-improvement through surgery lead- ing to increased self-confidence, raised self-esteem, or feelings of being 'in control' of one's body), is not considered. Nor are the complexities inherent in notions of self-inflicted pain held up for reflection. Questions related to moti- vations for painful self-improvement are further areas which the reader may wish to consider further.

There is a notion that 'feminism' is more than a 'perspective', if a per- spective is a way of seeing – it is also an epistemology, a way of knowing, and, in addition, an ontology, a way of being in the world (Stanley and Wise, 1990). Oleson (1994, p. 158) has pointed out that 'there are many feminisms, hence many views, some conflicting (Tong, 1989; Stanley and Wise, 1990; Reinharz, 1992; Devault, 1993)'. However, these many voices share the outlook that it is important to focus upon and make problematic women's diverse situations and the institutions and frames that influence those situations. The examina- tion of problematics with reference to the theoretical, policy or action frame- works in the interest of realizing social justice for women is a further aspect of this shared outlook (Eichler, 1986; Oleson, 1994).

Elam (1994, p.4) is wary of offering definitions of feminism, because doing this tends to crystallize meaning, threatening to function like final answers whose status becomes unshakeable – rarely, if ever, being interrogated. She talks of feminism as having a 'disciplinary uncertainty' or 'ambiguity' – a 'cross-discipline' with the potential to expose the thoughts and actions which are contained within ivory towers. Applying the ideas of Derrida (1976), she sees feminism as deconstructive – a narrative, but not a single coherent story- line. I introduce this to acknowledge my own linking and narration of events and issues, as they seem to me to illustrate my own construction of feminism and its contribution to the discourse on pain. Like Elam, I am wary of seem- ingly fixed ideas, preferring to encourage readers to think for themselves. The proliferation of feminist thought and theory, and its increasing tendency to permeate and influence ideas, is becoming a widespread and commonplace phenomenon. Feminists have addressed almost the gamut of human experience, opening to scrutiny and challenge both mainstream and esoteric thought and ideas within the fields of science, philosophy and the arts.

Harding (1991), among others, has critiqued the virtues of scientific inquiry and found it wanting in many ways. She suggests how feminist challenges can reveal the questions that are asked and those that are not asked, and makes the point that scientific explanation of any area, when this is merely from the perspective of bourgeois, white men's experiences, can only lead to partial, and sometimes even perverse understandings of social life. The distinctive feature of feminist research and feminist perspectives is that problematics are generated from women's experiences, with women revealing for the first time what these experiences are.

However, Harding (1991) does stress that there is no 'woman's experience', in the same way that there is no universal 'man' – only culturally different men and women within every race, class and culture. Thus there are feminists who propose that there should be talk of 'feminisms', since there is no one set of feminist principles or understandings beyond the very general ones, and this leads to the need to explicate one's own cultural identity, assumptions and beliefs. My own approach is inextricably rooted in my academic, professional and personal experiences, as a woman who is a mother, a mental health nurse, an educator and a feminist.

Pain – pleasure and the beautiful body

The preparation of girls' and women's bodies for heterosexual relationships, through painful and often laborious practices and procedures, may be understood by considering ideas surrounding embodiment. Feminists and others have paid significant attention to how dualist, Cartesian philosophies have come to associate human characteristics and qualities with female and male bodies – pain/pleasure, mind/body, logic/intuition, are all examples of this dualism. Women's bodies, historically, have been associated – through experiences such as childbearing and menstruation – with pain (Ehrenreich and English, 1988). It may thus be useful to consider some related ideas which enable us to think about the experiences of women's painful bodily self-improvement in the quest for a beautiful body.

There is an increasingly prolific literature which addresses the sociology of the body (Turner, 1984, 1992; Jacobus et al., 1990; Featherstone et al., 1991), yet as Nettleton (1995) points out, feminists were the first to recognize and make explicit the significance of the body for social theory. She points to these feminist analyses of women's bodies as being illustrative of how the medical and scientific descriptions of biology were socially constructed, and how this work could be used for ideological purposes such as maintaining gender inequalities.

The way in which women's bodies have been regulated and controlled by a male-dominated medical profession is a well-established and well-documented phenomenon (Nettleton, 1995). Feminists have also drawn attention to the political status of the body, with women's bodies frequently being the sites of exploitation.

The notion of the beautiful body, with its androcentric standards of the ideal feminine form, has received considerable critique from feminists as being oppressive, exploitative and objectifying (Galler, 1994). There have been insightful analyses which have addressed the ways in which women have attempted to live up to these standards, resorting to depersonalizing their selves, and subjecting their bodies to painful, often humiliating, surgical procedures (Morgan, 1994).

Morgan reflects upon the need for feminists to understand why 'actual, live women are reduced and reduce themselves to "potential women" and choose to participate in anatomizing and fetishizing their bodies' – especially in view of the growing market and demand which 'can and do result in infection, bleeding, embolisms, pulmonary edema, facial nerve injury, unfavourable scar formation, skin loss, blindness, crippling and death' (Morgan,1994, p.240). Dworkin (1994), taking a more structural approach, is equally critical: 'In our culture, not one part of a woman's body is left untouched, unaltered. No feature or extremity is spared the art, or pain, of improvement' (Dworkin, 1994, p. 217).

From 1990, the most frequently performed kind of cosmetic surgery has been liposuction, and the second most frequent has been breast augmentation (Morgan, 1994). The tolerance of the pain associated with these 'improvements' has been cited by Dworkin (1994) as being a deliberate and integral aspect of the heterosexual grooming process from pre-adolescence. Eyebrow plucking, armpit shaving and hair dyeing are perhaps more common, but still painful and laborious, and are endured in the name of beauty. She observes how 'no price is too great, no process too repulsive, no operation too painful for the woman who would be beautiful' (Dworkin, 1994, p. 219).

Dworkin feels that the preparation for the tolerance of and habituation to pain is romanticized into pain happily suffered, preparing women for lives of childbearing, self-abnegation and husband-pleasing. Because all value is placed upon the woman's body, then she as an adult becomes totally oriented around embodiment, 'willingly' paying the price for a perfect body – undergoing painful cosmetic surgery. Morgan (1994) contrasts with this view by considering the significance of undergoing surgical procedures, anaesthetics, postoperative drugs, and predicted and lengthy pain. She suggests that a woman may 'choose' this option as her only means of self-determination, if her access to other forms of power and empowerment are, or seem to be, limited. Her Foucauldian (see Foucault, 1979) analysis considers women's meanings regarding cosmetic surgery – and addresses the paradoxes of choice inherent in surgical interventions. She talks of how women's bodies are pathologized to such an extent that we cannot but feel alienated from anything less than perfection – leading to a painful sense of inadequacy. Thus a Roman nose indicates the need for a 'nose job', folds and curves benefit from 'nips and tucks', sagging chins need 'a lift' – the surgeon's knife makes him (*sic*) a sculptor in flesh, with all of the pain that this surgery entails written out of the deal (Morgan, 1994, p. 250).

Featherstone *et al.* (1991) have pointed to the cult of the body in consumer culture as being an increasingly important dimension of post-modern societies, and view the commercial and cosmetic interest in the body as a concern with the regulation of bodies. I would suggest that the regulation and control of women's bodies is an intensely complex phenomenon, with individual women constructing their own meanings when they make choices regarding their bodies. However, I would also contend that there is considerable resonance in Jaggar's (1994) observation that, despite the variability of women's situations, and the uncertainty over the achievements of a quarter century of feminist activism,

> Women are still evaluated primarily by a standard of sexual attractiveness that prizes youth, slenderness, blondness, and the absence of visible disabilities. We are stigmatised if we are not perceived as heterosexual and, to a lesser extent, if we lack a partner.
>
> (Jaggar,1994, p. 5).

Dualism and alienation: the pathology of womanliness

The notion of the medicalizing and pathologizing of women's bodies is a familiar theme within feminist work. In view of this, I wish to revisit Morgan's (1994) idea of feeling alienated from one's body to such a degree that the pain of improvement is perceived by women to be a viable option. The way in which cosmetic surgery is increasingly being 'normalized' as an acceptable alternative for women, and the raising of the level of intolerance with specific 'parts' of our bodies, could be said to be colluding with the dualist philosophy that separates mind and body – having a body rather than being a body (Berger and Luckman, 1967; Plessner, 1970).

Bendelow and Williams (1995) have pointed out how the essential ambiguity of human embodiment is expressed as both personal and impersonal, objective and subjective, social and natural. Their suggestion is that there is value in focusing upon bodies as both objective and subjective, with 'pain' as an 'embodied' experience which transcends both. It is interesting also to consider Leder's (1984/85, 1990) work in relation to the pain of bodily improvement. Leder's philosophical investigation into the 'absent body' draws attention to how our bodies are normally phenomenologically absent from view: 'Whilst in one sense the body is the most abiding and inescapable presence in our lives, it is also characterised by absence. That is, one's own body is rarely the thematic object of experience . . . the body, as a ground of experience . . . tends to recede from direct experience' (Leder, 1990, p.1).

However, this mode of bodily experience tends to be profoundly disrupted in the context of factors such as pain, disease and death, whereby the body becomes central to experience, contrasting with the phenomenologically absent body: '. . .there is a *sensory intensification* which pain brings into play, its *episodal temporality* and the *affective call* which it establishes'. This leads to a 'peculiar hold it has over our attention' and is ultimately *'a matter of being-in-the-world'* (Bendelow and Williams, 1995, p. 143; their emphasis). This 'sensory intensification' makes the person intensely aware of their body, making the body acutely present to be emotionally engaged with. Bendelow and Williams (1995) show how this pain re-organizes our lived space and time, and our relationships with others and with ourselves.

When these ideas are applied to the pain and discomfort of cosmetic surgery and other bodily improvements a woman may undertake, the 'peculiar hold' over her attention, with the accompanying focus upon her 'being-in-the-world' as an embodied female, would give her considerable meaningful awareness of herself. The significance which this painful experience would perhaps have in shaping her 'lived space and time', and her 'relations with others (and herself)' (Bendelow and Williams, 1995, p.144) is considerable.

The experience of pain, inflicted in the name of patriarchal beauty, would thus never let a woman be 'absent' from her body (Leder, 1990), able to transcend embodiment (de Beauvoir, 1989). This flies somewhat in the face of the feminist notion of women being more than sexual and reproductive objects in a patriarchal world.

The 'temporality' alluded to by Leder (1984/85) is also interesting, in that women tend to be only too aware of the passing of time, the ageing face and the drooping flesh. If pain endured can somehow enable the cheating of time, then it is worth enduring. Time given over to pampering the body and indulging in pleasurable bodily experiences, cosmetics and the taking care of ourselves on the surface seems like a good option, but the flipside shows the coercion and the pain/pleasure dichotomy for women when they take pleasure in painful improvements – the social approval of looking good. A further dualistic notion which perhaps has some relevance here relates to the idea of the cultured body, artifice in the face of 'natural' woman – who is hairy, animal and threatening. There is an additional interesting temporal factor related to being preoccupied with painful (and pleasurable) bodily regulation and beautifying concerns, in that this ensures that women never forget their biological identity. The time needed to pamper the body leaves little time for more empowering activities.

If women's experience of their bodies is indeed partly characterized by painful processes and procedures which regulate and contain them (for example, periods and childbearing, cosmetic improvement), then it is not surprising that women may be preoccupied with having and being their bodies, rather than with transcending and being disembodied, an 'absent body' who operates freely without constraint. Being a 'good enough' woman, without surgical intervention or artifice, takes considerable courage within this climate, particularly if one holds with the view that femininity is socially constructed. The sanctions imposed by being 'fat' or 'plain' or 'on the shelf' within Western culture bring their own pains – and women go to such lengths either to rationalize their bodies, or to 'do something about' their weight (Schmidt,

1994, p. 220), rather than 'let themselves go', because a man '. . . likes a woman who takes care of herself' (Dworkin,1994, p. 220).

Surgical interventions have a history within medicine, and raise some important issues for women. Feminists have been wary of the 'experts' within patriarchy, because of the roles which medicine and other institutions have played in defining women's experiences, from a masculinist perspective, in ways that have been oppressive to women. The rise of scientific knowledge within medicine, as I alluded to earlier, has had a significant influence upon women's lives. Ehrenreich and English (1988) give a detailed account of this influence, and document how, historically, women were disenfranchised from healing and there evolved an increasing dependence upon medicine. The mistrust which followed this is inherent in women's knowledge of their bodies. This, together with the cultural acceptability of visiting doctors with distresses, and the medicalization of daily life (Illich, 1976), are significant factors in women's dissatisfaction with their bodies, and the seeking of a medical strategy to 'do something about it' (Schmidt, 1994, p.220). The medicalization of normal female life events such as menstruation, birth and menopause has been vigorously critiqued by feminists (e.g. Oakley, 1993). The rendering of wrinkles, fat and hairiness as cause for medical concern, with its invasive technological intervention and associated painful and sometimes iatrogenic consequences, I would suggest, is cause for similar critique. Questions arise as to the notion of why this happens, whether it is demand led and if so, why do women do it?

An additional feminist concern lies with the personalizing, individualizing quality that is inherent in cosmetic surgery and its associated pain and trauma. The meanings women have for choosing surgical intervention, if taken on an individual level, have the effect of making the experience invisible – a private, personal choice, subject to secrecy and embarrassment. Only by considering the collective experience, and its attendant political implications can the issues be held up to scrutiny. The romanticization of pain which Dworkin describes, and individuals' desires for the 'rewards' of beauty, ensure that women take part and collude.

Conclusions

The meaning and cultural shaping of the discourse of pain for women is multifaceted, and the historical perception of women as 'Other' (de Beauvoir, 1989) is integral to this. As I mentioned earlier, there are dualisms within Western culture which have a considerable bearing upon the structuring of society (Bendelow and Williams, 1995; Shuster, 1996) and these dualisms – mind/body, rational/emotional, pain/pleasure, woman/man – have internalized associations for people, and have historically favoured men within a patriarchal society (Turner, 1992).

Medicine, as a patriarchal institution concerned with the uses of scientific knowledge to promote healing, has played a large part in the regulation of bodily disease, pain and illness, founded upon dualistic, Aristotelian assumptions (Wakefield, 1995).

Feminists have been wary of the work of 'experts' who set themselves up as the authority upon a particular aspect of experience. They state that too often experts, whether they are medical professionals, academics or anyone else, have frequently served their own interests before those of their clients, audiences, etc. The notion of healing is perhaps dichotomous with regard to the surgical interventions for cosmetic reasons, and encourages the view that women's (and increasingly men's) bodily 'imperfections' are legitimate areas for medical concern. The pain endured in the name of the 'ideal' notion of perfect femininity – i.e. patriarchal femininity – clean, deodorized and tamed, thus has many facets. The idea that pain makes bodies 'present' that are usually 'absent' (Leder, 1990) would also perhaps serve to legitimate the presence of (only perfect) women.

Woodhead (1996) has observed how throughout human history there have been moral and social anxieties and threats associated with women's bodies, with female sexuality being a particular target for religious and magical practices that aim to restrain women and control their sexuality. It is interesting to speculate on the sanitization, through painful cosmetic surgical and other interventions, of women's bodies in a similar way. Sontag (1988) talks of how diseases and illnesses may become metaphors for societal concerns – could women's pain experience, medicalized and pathologized, in the pursuit of beauty be a metaphor for the threat of transcending femininity?

References

Bendelow, G.A. and Williams, S.J. 1995: Transcending the dualisms: towards a sociology of pain. *Sociology of Health and Illness* 17, 139–65.

Berger P. and Luckman T. 1967: *The social construction of reality.* London: Allen Lane.

de Beauvoir, S. 1989: *The second sex* (translated by H.M. Parshley). New York: Vintage Books.

Derrida, J. 1976: *Of grammatology* (translated by G.C. Spivak). Baltimore, MD: Johns Hopkins University Press.

Devault, M.L. 1993: Different voices: feminists' methods of social research. *Qualitative Sociology* 16, 77–83.

Dworkin, A. 1994: Gynocide: Chinese footbinding. In: Jaggar A. (ed.), *Living with contradictions. Controversies in feminist social ethics.* Oxford. Westview Press, 213–20.

Ehrenreich, B. and English, D. 1988: *For her own good. 150 years of the experts' advice to women.* London: Pluto Press.

Eichler, M. 1986: The relationship between sexist, non-sexist, woman-centered and feminist research. *Studies in Communication* 3, 37–74.

Elam, D. 1994: *Feminism and deconstruction.* London: Routledge.

Farganis, S. 1994: *Situating feminism. From thought to action.* London: Sage.

Featherstone, M., Hepworth, M. and Turner, B.S. 1991: *The body: social process and cultural theory.* London: Sage.

Foucault, M. 1979: *Discipline and punish: the birth of the prison* (translated by A. Sheridan). New York: Pantheon.

Galler, R. 1994: The myth of the perfect body. In: Jaggar A. (ed.), *Living with contradictions. Controversies in feminist social ethics.* Oxford: Westview Press, 234–9.

Harding, S. 1991: *Whose science? Whose knowledge? Thinking from women's lives.* Ithaca, NY: Cornell University Press.

Illich, I. 1976: *Limits to medicine: medical nemesis – the expropriation of health.* London: Marion Boyars.

Jacobus, M., Fox Keller, E. and Shuttleworth, S. 1990: *Body/politics: women and the discourses of science.* London: Routledge.

Jaggar, A. (ed.) 1994: *Living with contradictions. Controversies in feminist social ethics.* Oxford: Westview Press.

Leder, D. 1984/85: Toward a phenomenology of pain. *Review of Existential Psychiatry* 19, 255–66.

Leder, A. 1990: *The absent body.* Chicago: Chicago University Press.

Morgan, K.P. 1994: Women and the knife: cosmetic surgery and the colonization of women's bodies. In: Jaggar, A. (ed.), *Living with contradictions. Controversies in feminist social ethics.* Oxford: Westview Press, 239–56.

Nettleton, S. 1995: *The sociology of health and illness.* Oxford: Basil Blackwell.

Oakley, A. 1993: *Essays on women, medicine and health.* Edinburgh: Edinburgh University Press.

Oleson, V. 1994: Feminism and models of qualitative research. In: Denzin, N.K. and Lincoln, Y.S. (eds), *Handbook of qualitative research.* London: Sage, 158–74.

Plessner, H. 1970: *Laughing and crying: a study of the limits of human behaviour.* Evanston, IL: Northwestern University Press.

Reinharz, S. 1992: *Feminist methods in social research.* New York: Oxford University Press.

Rich, A. 1977: *Of woman born.* London: Virago.

Schmidt, C. 1994: Do something about your weight. In: Jaggar, A. (ed.), *Living with contradictions. Controversies in feminist social ethics.* Oxford: Westview Press, 220–23.

Shuster, E. 1996: For her own good: protecting (and neglecting) women in research. *Cambridge Quarterly of Healthcare Ethics* 5, 346–61.

Sontag, S. 1988: *Illness as metaphor.* Harmondsworth: Penguin.

Stanley L. and Wise, S. 1990: Method, methodology and epistemology in feminist research processes. In: Stanley, L. (ed.), *Feminist praxis: research, theory and epistemology in feminist sociology.* London: Routledge & Kegan Paul.

Tong, R. 1989: *Feminist thought: a comprehensive introduction.* Boulder, CO: Westview.

Turner, B.S. 1984: *The body and society.* Oxford: Basil Blackwell.

Turner, B.S. 1992: *Regulating bodies: essays in medical sociology.* London: Routledge.

Wakefield, A.B. 1995: Pain: an account of nurse's talk. *Journal of Advanced Nursing* 21, 905–10.

Woodhead, L. 1996: Religious representations of women. In: Cosslett, T., Easton, A. and Summerfield P. (eds), *Women, power and resistance. An introduction to women's studies.* Buckingham: Open University Press, 125–35.

Suffering, emotion and pain: towards a sociological understanding

Eileen Fairhurst

Introduction

The greeting, 'How are you?' provides the starting point for this chapter. Conventionally, stock responses may be either 'Fine, thanks' or 'Well, thanks'. We routinely respond to this question in terms of a concern for our welfare and, in particular, in relation to how we are feeling. Irrespective of whether we 'honestly' reveal our feelings, we take it for granted that the question refers to our physical health or our emotional state – how we currently view our 'selves'. In this sense, allusions to matters of pain, suffering and emotion are part and parcel of our everyday experiences and life.

In such everyday talk it is not incumbent upon parties to it to specify whether the enquiry is directed to 'the mind' or 'the body'. The phrase 'How are you?' invites us to home in on whichever one of these we choose. Ideas about 'being/wellness', then, are commonsensically taken to mean that the enquiry embraces either or both of these matters. It is in our reply that we make clear to which we are referring: 'I'm feeling low today' or 'My back's playing me up'. It is the content of the response itself which enables the hearer to recognize that a distinction between mind and body has been made. This simple if seemingly banal statement provides the analytical pivot and pervasive theme of this chapter. Indeed, to pose as separate matters the two questions 'What do you think pain is?' and then 'What do you think suffering is?' may lead to some puzzlement as to whether the enquiry is about the mind or the body. Pain may be identified, for instance, as consequent upon breaking a leg and, as such, linked to the physical and thereby to the body. Having cancer, however, may entail suffering as a result of being in pain. Pain and suffering, therefore, may be seen either as separate entities or as inextricably linked.

Reference to such matters allows the introduction of two analytical issues which underpin this chapter. First, the use of the prepositions 'to' and 'in' in the above examples carry theoretical import. Describing a broken leg as having painful consequences 'to' or 'for' the body suggests that the body has an ontological existence. This separateness/thing-likeness of the body confines to it the experience of physical pain. On the other hand, 'being in pain' from cancer implies an affective state engendering emotional feelings and suffering which are expressed in social interaction. The concern here is not to make imperialistic claims for the supremacy of either the 'physical' or the 'emotional' in understanding pain and suffering, but rather to show how such differences reside in language usage.

Secondly, concepts of pain and suffering have no intrinsic meaning. It is only with the furnishing of a context that pain and suffering make sense. To introduce them 'out of the blue' and to make them the focus of discussion is to invite puzzlement. That the meaning or sense of language is not an inherent matter is the central premise of ethnomethodologists. On the contrary, one of their bedrock assumptions is that the meaning or sense of language is obtained from the context in which it is used or situated. Garfinkel and Sacks (1970) refer to this as the indexicality of language. A consequence of this is that a priori claims are not made that actions or events to which language refers always and inevitably have the same sense or meaning – to do so would invite advocacy of a correspondence theory of reality.

The brief reference above to how we may talk about pain and suffering illustrates the relevance of viewing language as an indexical matter. The questions were posed to a group of health workers. They specified pain and suffering in terms of a 'broken leg' and 'cancer', respectively. The point is that to make sense of the concepts 'pain' and 'suffering' they supplied the context in which to situate them. The context used was that of health care, in which they were employed and, which was therefore familiar to them. The significance of their choice of context as a sense-making procedure was not lost on them. They noted that it was because they were nurses that they saw pain and suffering in this way, but acknowledged that others would not necessarily share these views.

When it comes to the realm of the professional, however, no such permeability of mind/body is recognized – a clear boundary between mind and body is seen to exist. Nowhere is this more apparent than in the distinction made by Western systems of medicine between physical and mental illness – the former relating to the body and the latter to the mind. This distinction pertains to an assumed specific entity. The genesis of such thinking will be elaborated upon subsequently.

This chapter aims to offer a particular perspective on matters of pain and suffering. Women's experience of the menopause provides the substantive realm for the elaboration of analytical and theoretical issues pertinent to pain and suffering. Arguably, the menopause is an ideal matter in which the problematics of the mind/body distinction are revealed and can be examined. It is indisputably a physiological event in which hormonal and other bodily changes occur. A biological and social consequence is the end of a woman's reproductive cycle.[1] In Western cultures the ending of reproduction together

---

[1]However, the advent of new reproductive technologies affords the possibility of childbearing beyond the menopause.

with its potential occurrence with other social events, such as children leaving home, results in the menopause sometimes being pictured as signalling the end of a woman's 'useful life', to which she may respond by psychological upset. A focus on the menopause therefore potentially lays bare for examination the conundrum of the mind/body distinction.

Initially, sociological literature which addresses the legacy of the Cartesian dualism between mind and body will be considered. Such literature seeks, by calling for the incorporation of specific conceptual frameworks, to supplement this dualism. Nevertheless, a consequence of that dualism – that is, how the mental, the private, is made knowable – remains unresolved. An ethnomethodological approach, resting upon the situated use of language, will be applied to discuss the menopause. More importantly, this discussion will be employed as a topic for analysis in its own right. Such data will be used to demonstrate that concepts of pain and suffering are constituted in language usage.

Contrastive and oppositional categories and the Cartesian legacy

It is Descartes to whom the origins of the mind/body split in Western medical systems are attributed. For Descartes, the human organism consisted of two classes of substances, namely 'palpable *body* and intangible *mind*' (Scheper-Hughes and Lock, 1987, p.9). Descartes' attempts to reconcile material body and divine soul meant that he was able to preserve the soul as the domain of theology and to legitimate the body as the domain of science' (Scheper-Hughes and Lock, 1987, p.9). As Scheper-Hughes and Lock emphasize, an underpinning commitment of Western science and clinical medicine has been to distinctions between spirit and matter, mind and body, and real and unreal. Moreover, not only are these matters contrastive, but they are also oppositional categories.

For Scheper-Hughes and Lock, the Cartesian legacy to Western medicine and social science has been 'the rather mechanistic conception of the body and its functions and a failure to conceptualise a "mindful" causation of somatic states' (Scheper-Hughes and Lock, 1987, p.9). They argue that, even within psychoanalysis and psychsomatic medicine, there is still a tendency to maintain contrastive categories so that aetiology is depicted as 'either wholly organic or wholly physiological in origin: "it" is *in* the body, or "it" is *in* the mind'.

According to Scheper-Hughes and Lock, the mind–body dualism is linked to other dichotomous categories in Western epistemology, such as nature and culture and individual and society, and is evident in the work of social thinkers. Thus, for Durkheim 'The body was the storehouse of emotions that were the raw materials, the "stuff", out of which mechanical solidarity was forged in the interests of the collectivity' (Scheper-Hughes and Lock, 1987, p.10). Freud's theory of dynamic psychology pictured the individual as being at war within himself. Marx argued that it was through human labour that nature was domesticated, and in this way humans differentiated themselves from animals. Human labour transformed the natural world, which had an objective external existence.

Scheper-Hughes and Lock note that, despite the assumed predominance of these ideas within Western philosophy, there are other ontologies. For instance, where culture is said to be 'rooted *in* nature' then 'mind collapses into body'. For some reductionist biologists (Ornstein, 1973) the oppositional categories identified are natural categories of thinking, since they are cognitive and symbolic manifestations of human biology. The brain's left hemisphere dominance accounts for the cognitive and symbolic domains of mind over body, culture over nature, and so on.

However, such oppositional categories of Western philosophy are neither universal nor 'natural'. Scheper-Hughes and Lock refer to alternative epistemologies in non-Western civilizations in which connections amongst entities are conceptualized in monistic rather than dualistic terms. Relationships of parts to the whole are emphasized. In ancient China the whole of cosmology rested on the idea of dynamic equilibrium between moving poles of yin and yang, masculine and feminine, light and dark, and hot and cold. Such ideas informed concepts of health, so that it rested on balance in the natural world, and the health of individual organs depended on their relationship to all other organs. Scheper-Hughes and Lock note that 'In ancient Chinese cosmology the emphasis is on balance and resonance: in Western cosmology, on tension and contradiction' (Scheper-Hughes and Lock, 1987, p.12).

Moreover, the Western philosophical concept of an 'I', a mindful self independent of the body and separate from nature, is a further consequence of Cartesian dualism which is quite different to Buddhist philosophy. Within Buddhism, subjectivity relates to the natural world so that the latter is a product of mind. Meditation is the means through which individual minds merge with the universal mind.

The attribution of palpability to the body and intangibility to the mind led to Descartes' proposal of a specific pain system that carried messages from pain receptors in the skin to pain centres in the brain. It is perhaps noteworthy that, via this theory, the mind is transformed into the brain – the two appear to be synonymous. The specificity theory of pain held sway until Melzack and Wall's (1988) criticism, in which they developed the original theory in terms of a gate control theory of pain. This proposed that psychological and cognitive variables have an impact on physiological processes involved in human pain perception and response. Melzack and Wall introduced the idea that pain has cultural and psychological components, and they suggested multidisciplinary approaches to the understanding of the phenomenon of pain. However, Bendelow and Williams (1995) argue that, despite Melzack and Wall's attempts to widen the study of pain, and their implicit confrontation of the mind/body dualism, the biological predominates at the expense of the cultural. The former authors contend that 'scientific medicine reduces the experience of pain to an elaborate broadcasting system of signals rather than seeing it as moulded and shaped both by the individual and their particular socio-cultural context. (Bendelow and Williams, 1995, p.140). They go on to conclude that:

the elevation of sensation over emotion in traditional medical and psychological approaches results in the lack of attention to subjectivity, which in turn leads to a limited approach towards suffering and a neglect of broader cultural and sociological components of pain. In other words, a far more sophisticated model of pain is needed; one which locates individuals within their social and cultural contexts and which allows for the inclusion of feelings and emotions.

(Bendelow and Williams, 1995, p.146)

Bendelow and Williams are concerned to offer a conceptual and methodological examination of pain which will move away from a reductionist emphasis on pain and sensation to one that embraces the social. They suggest that a way forward to confront the impasse of the mind/body distinction is to emphasize ideas about the self and the subjective experience of illness. They draw upon the work of Bury (1982) and Williams (1984) and their use of narratives in furthering our understanding of the experience of chronic illness. Bendelow and Williams argue that such an approach would allow for an examination of suffering. For them, pain is concerned with sensation and suffering with emotion. They seek to emphasize the meaning of pain.

Bendelow and Williams, in attempting to offer a sociological perspective on pain and suffering, propose an emphasis on the social as opposed to the biological. In doing this, they overlay a further dualism onto the already existing one of mind/body. Despite efforts to eschew the particular dualism of mind/body, paradoxically such boundaries are evidenced. Moreover, additional boundaries are evident by the introduction of different kinds of contrastive categories, such as objective/subjective, self/other and inner/outer. In this sense their argument can be located in the Western philosophical tradition discussed by Scheper-Hughes and Lock (1987).

Irrespective of this, however, further points can be made. Bendelow and Williams call for the meaning of pain to be the proper concern of sociological examination. The entrées into revealing such matters are narratives and subjective accounts of illness. Now Scheper-Hughes and Lock (1987) issue a note of caution about such pursuits. Whilst intent on offering a critique of Cartesian dualism in their medical anthropological programme to provide an innovative epistemology and metaphysics of what they term the mindful body and of the emotional, social and political sources of illness and healing, they note a potential pitfall, that of a 'Cartesian anxiety', the fear that in the absence of a sure objective foundation for knowledge we would fall into the void, into the chaos of absolute relativism and subjectivity' (Scheper-Hughes and Lock, 1987, p.30). Since Bendelow and Williams do not appear to acknowledge this possibility, their exercise in addressing the implications of Cartesian dualism paradoxically leaves them with a methodological problem.

This methodological issue links with Silverman's (1993) critique of some sociologists' use of accounts based on the individual's experience. Such an approach is often advocated in opposition to positivism and its use of the survey approach. Whereas the latter is depicted as relying on the a priori categories of the researcher, the former embraces those of the researched, so that the individual's own perspectives are paramount in the analysis. As Silverman argues, however, a consequence of this view is that the individual's own experience was assigned a privileged status. Furthermore, experience provided validity – capturing experience, of itself, was a guarantee of authenticity and thereby of validity. In a similar way, Bendelow and Williams follow such a path by assuming that, of themselves, subjective accounts and narratives will solve the problematic issues of pain and suffering.

Finally, Bendelow and Williams propose that narratives and subjective accounts are used as the resource in their analysis, rather than the appropriate focus of enquiry. Narratives and subjective accounts, then, are not regarded as topics for analysis in their own right. In this way such materials are located within a correspondence theory of reality, for they are taken to stand on behalf of reality and are distinguishable from and have an existence apart from the text. A coherence theory of reality, by contrast, emphasizes how individuals or members actively produce, through talk, social and moral activities. By making the account a topic for analysis in its own right, such matters may be laid bare. It is this approach which provides the point of departure for an examination of language usage in enabling the study of such cognitive issues as pain, emotion and suffering.

Language usage and the mind/body dualism

For some sociologists, language is a topic the use of which may be examined in particular social settings. For ethnomethodologists, however, language is a topic worthy of study for its own sake. As Sharrock and Watson (1989) note, 'language is not only the medium of social life' but also constitutes 'primary data for most sociological inquiry'. They identify three major assumptions of ethnomethodologists: first, that language is not only a social phenomenon but also a social practice; secondly, that other social phenomena are analysable as a way of talking; and thirdly, that sociology itself is a natural language endeavour using a range of natural languages. A consequence of these matters is that ethnomethodologists consider that much sociological inquiry treats linguistic phenomena as a means to an end. Sharrock and Watson argue:

> sociological analysis treats linguistic materials as *transparent*, one can see social phenomena in them and through them, but one need not ask how linguistic interchanges are organised to exhibit the social phenomena that they show. Just *what* features of a verbal exchange give it that characteristic that sociological analysts attribute to it, just *what* things? Rather than regarding the linguistic exchanges as a 'neutral' and transparent medium for the conduct of social life, then, ethnomethodology invites the examination of linguistic data to discover in what its transparency consists: how do we learn from talk those things that we do, undoubtedly, learn from it?
>
> (Sharrock and Watson, 1989, p.437, emphasis in original)

Thus, in relation to the concerns of this chapter, what can we learn about pain and suffering from talk about the menopause? This is not to deny that the mind/body distinction is not a boundary like any other. However, in contrast to Bendelow and Williams (1995) and Scheper-Hughes and Lock (1987), the concern here is to look at the distinction that resides in language. Distinctions between mind and body are contextually produced. More importantly, language is not a transparent way to get into mental predicates, but rather such matters – in general those pertaining to the mind – are public matters which are linguistically constituted.

It is such a standpoint that Coulter has utilized and built upon in his explorations of cognitive matters. For Coulter, cognitive matters, unlike their conventional attribution to the inner workings of the mind and their depiction as private and their consequent inaccessability to empirical investigation, are socially organized accomplishments. He advises us to 'treat the "mental" properties of persons as generated from situated, constitutive practices' (Coulter, 1983, p.128). A particular interest of Coulter's is in memory. Recently he has linked a 'storage' view of memory to the Cartesian dualism of mind and body – memories are stored in the mental space of the mind and retrieved by a search process. According to Coulter, materialist philosophers would argue against the Cartesian perspective and for our brain being the location of storage, retrieval and remembering, so that memories are depicted as *themselves neurally encoded phenomena*' (Coulter, 1991, p.188). Given that, for Coulter, all cognitive phenomena are properties of persons, then the former cannot of themselves have an ontological existence.

Ostensibly this matter of language has not been ignored by others in their examination of the mind/body distinction. For instance, Scheper-Hughes and Lock refer to this matter when they contend:

> We lack a precise vocabulary with which to deal with mind–body–society interactions and so we are left suspended in hyphens, testifying to the disconnectedness of our thoughts. We are forced to resort to such fragmented concepts as the bio-social, the psycho-somatic, the somato-social as altogether feeble ways of expressing the myriad ways in which the mind speaks through the body, and the ways in which society is inscribed on the expectant canvas of human flesh.
>
> (Scheper-Hughes and Lock, 1987, p.10)

On close examination, however, we can see that firstly, reference to vocabulary/language is syntaxical and, secondly, that again mind and body are assigned an ontological existence. In particular, reification is evident where reference is made to the 'disconnectedness' of our thoughts and mind 'speaking' through the body. In terms of Sharrock and Watson's standpoint, Scheper-Hughes and Lock regard language as the means to an end – as the conduit for the revelation of mind.

Pain, suffering and experiencing the menopause

Wowk's ethnomethodological explorations of emotions in relation to the experience of a mastectomy are salient to the substantive concerns here. Parallels may be drawn between a mastectomy and the menopause. Both are matters affecting the body which may engender physical pain and have implications for cultural ideas about femininity and physical attractiveness. However, there is an important difference between the two. Noting Smith's (1978) point that the apparent seriousness of a situation provides the grounds for the extent or degree of emotional upset, Wowk (1989) demonstrated how typically a mastectomy is taken to be so serious that women may be allowed, if not expected, to be seriously emotionally upset by the surgery. The menopause, however, perhaps because it is experienced by all women, does not typically come within the category of a serious matter warranting serious upset. The very inevitability of the menopause assigns it to the category 'not serious'. Paradoxically, however, the absence of such seriousness, as will be demonstrated below, may be the source of suffering, and emotional upset for women.

Before showing how distinctions between pain and suffering reside in language usage, some comment is required on the purposes of the original study. It sought to compare the experiences of 'well women' and those attending a menopause clinic.[2] It might be expected a priori that, since the latter group had sought help for bodily experiences/changes, there would be clear differences between the two groups' experiences and, consequently, those of pain and suffering. On the contrary, whilst the same physical feelings were experienced by both groups of women, they were not inevitably seen as painful or as the source of suffering. When women talked about their own experiences they turned to ideas about a normal or typical menopause. This category served as a baseline against which women assessed their physical and mental feelings. Moreover, the putative manifestation of the menopause assumes a pivotal position in everyday theories of middle-aged women's actions. Prior to the perceived onset of the menopause, taken-for-granted matters have reliably informed a woman's actions, but at its onset these are fashioned in a problematic mould. Such matters are situated in everyday theories of middle-aged women's behaviour. I shall show how these inform women's talk about their own menopause.

A normal menopause

Women's conversations with other women, their husbands, kin and doctors, together with media sources, such as television programmes, newspapers and women's magazines, enabled women to build up a picture of what might typically be expected. They provided the means through which women could map out their own model of a normal menopause. This embraced both physical and emotional feelings. How women respond to physical feelings rests upon their use of the notion of a normal menopause. Cessation or irregularity

[2]The study was undertaken in an industrial town in north-west England and used tape-recorded, thematic interviews with women and, where possible, with their husbands. The experiences of a small group of 'well women' were compared with those of a small group attending a menopause clinic. In all, 34 women and 24 husbands were interviewed. The women were in their fiftieth year of age, and both middle and working class backgrounds were represented.

of menstruation and hot flushes were identified as symptoms which normally occurred in menopausal women. Depression and/or general emotional feelings occupied a much more ambiguous place than physical feelings in women's depiction of a normal menopause.

So taken for granted is the idea that hot flushes are a dramatic and obvious manifestation of the menopause that their absence or perceived insignificance to women led them to question whether they were 'really' experiencing the menopause. On the one hand, lack of such typical feelings was a cause of confusion to some women but, for others, their inability to cope with them was seen as an affront to their self-identity as someone who could cope with life (see Fairhurst, 1980; Fairhurst and Lightup, 1981).

Whilst the category of a normal menopause operated as a kind of boundary maintenance mechanism to enable women to make sense of their experiences, its constituent parts showed different degrees of salience. They varied according to women's current and prior experiences. Contact with workmates, memories of a mother's own menopause and neighbours' experiences provided contexts against which to compare and assess experiences. On the basis of such matters, women isolated one feeling as inextricably linked with the menopause and one as likely to be the source of great distress to them. When the expectation was not reflected in reality, women assessed their own experience in a favourable light, so that feelings that were expected to be painful and 'to be suffered' were not so described.

So much importance was attached to a specific feeling that it overshadowed all others. This is not to say that women did not experience any other feelings, but those feelings were assigned a minor, almost insignificant, part that scarcely merited comment, in their accounts. Here workmates' experiences of hot flushes are identified as the predominant feeling for comparative purposes. Having identified those experiences as *'where they get into bed and they're burning all over'*, a woman described her own experiences:

> *I've never experienced anything like that. . . . We talk at work about these things. Some of them do have these hot sweats. Most of them do. I don't understand why I don't you see. I mean I've never had any reason to go to the doctor. I should imagine I have gone through it (the menopause) with flying colours.*

In relation to her workmates' experiences, this woman's experiences were untypical and prompted her puzzlement and wonderment about the absence of hot flushes. By implication, others' experiences were of such severity that they merited a medical consultation. The fact that she had not pursued a similar course of action offered further grounds for the insignificance of her own experience. The combination of these two matters furnished the assessment of no pain or suffering. Going through an experience with 'flying colours' suggests that the experience itself is likely to be 'testing' or 'arduous' and carries connotations both of success and of being unscathed by untoward matters.

In the data extracts that follow, headaches are linked to childhood memories of a mother's behaviour during the menopause: *'Well I thought it (the menopause) would be worse than it was. I thought I'd be having to go to bed every week or something like that, you know with monstrous headaches and stomach pains and God knows what.'*

Now we all may experience headaches, but we do not routinely 'take to our beds'. Headaches are not normally regarded as incapacitating. It is only those of particular severity that warrant such action. Indeed, the assumed very 'ordinariness' of headaches may hinder their identification as a serious matter about which 'something needs to be done'. In the case of meningitis, for instance, such lack of attention may have dire consequences. Furthermore, not only are headaches during the menopause seen to be a serious matter, but also they are regular and frequent occurrences requiring the same action every week. In this sense, therefore, a specific physical feeling pervades everyday life and becomes linked to a particular life-stage category – that of a menopausal woman. Headaches are not normal outside this particular stage of life, but paradoxically they are normal in middle age. It is in this way that the woman situates the physical feeling of a headache as a painful matter to be endured during the menopause.

The data extract goes on to focus on the woman's childhood memories of her mother being unwell and the implications of these memories for her expectations for her own menopause:

> *I was too young to understand these things. I was terribly innocent as a kid and I didn't know what my mum was going through until my sister told me, because she seemed to be crying a lot and had those terrible headaches. She would have to go and lie down and when my sister explained what happened, explained what happened to women, well ever since then, if I thought about it, I thought I would probably go through the same sort of pain and upset.*

The significance of the mother's crying and headaches for the woman described here are to be understood in terms of children's typifications of mothers. Whilst mothers are not immune from being upset or having headaches, they are expected to 'soldier on' regardless of their physical or emotional feelings. It was precisely because the woman's mother did not conform to such typifications that the action of 'lying down' was connected not only to physical and emotional feelings but also, thereby, to the category of menopausal woman. The unusualness of the mother's actions enabled puzzlement to be expressed by the daughter about her mother's response to physical and emotional matters. Indeed, the woman's identification of herself as 'innocent' points to her lack of chronological years and serves to emphasize the 'indelibility' of the experience. For the woman it was inevitable that her menopause would mirror that of her mother's.

In this next data extract we can see how a woman's youthful experience of her neighbour's depression had acted as a pointer for possible problems in her own menopause:

> *You read about people who are affected. They are depressed. I remember someone at home when I was young, vaguely. Maybe this impressed me, I don't know, but she committed suicide and it was put down that she sort of got very depressed.*

But it was only listening in to other people's conversations. Probably that did make me feel it might be worse than it was but that's all I know.

Depression may not be in the same category of ordinariness as headaches, but some kinds of depression may be regarded as more 'normal' than others. Hence the distinction that is sometimes made between reactive depression and clinical depression – depression associated with a bereavement falls into the former category. In this extract the fact that the depression was not normal is highlighted by noting its possible consequences. The identification of suicide as a response to depression not only emphasizes the seriousness of the depression, but also links it to a specific life-stage category – that of menopausal woman.

These data extracts demonstrate how women used others' experiences as the baseline for the model of a normal menopause, and then used the baseline to assess their own experience. The absence of certain physical and emotional feelings, namely hot flushes, headaches and depression, to which they had previously assigned specific importance, led them to depict their own experience as 'trouble free'. Contrary to their expectations of a troublesome menopause, this was not reflected in their own experiences.

Whilst the concept of a normal menopause offered women a necessary yardstick, of itself it was not always sufficient to account for their own particular experiences. In these circumstances, women referred to a notion of individual normality as well as that of a normal menopause. Both women who were attending the menopause clinic and those who did not do so had recourse to a view of individual normality in assessing their own experiences. These women had clear ideas of what they were normally like – they had a definite idea of themselves as individuals. In talking about what was happening to them they referred both to ideas about what was normal for all women going through the menopause and what was normal for them as individuals, irrespective of the physiological event. It was only when women saw their thoughts and actions as being untypical of what they were usually like and beginning to approximate to those of other women who were said to have had, for example, 'nervous breakdowns' that they decided to 'do something':

The reason I'd gone to the doctor was I'd begun to feel suicidal and for me that is quite unusual because I am an optimist. I am not a pessimist by any means and when you start thinking about chucking yourself off railway bridges and under buses, well I thought it is time to do something.

The source of this woman's suffering lay in the declared incongruity between her normal optimism and her current pessimism. As a consequence of such an assessment process, she sought medical help.

The problematic status of endowing (irrespective of language usage) physical or mental feelings with some kind of objective entity warranting the label pain or suffering is evident when considering how the well women who were interviewed employed ideas about individual normality when assessing their own menopause. Idiosyncratic features of their normal selves were those very matters which, in other contexts, could be pinpointed as adverse feelings often associated with the menopause.

In the following data extract, a woman identifies premenstrual tension from which she had long been a sufferer as harbouring portents for her own menopause:

It (pre-menstrual tension) used to drive me up the wall. You could feel yourself losing control and there's nothing you can do about it. I used to throw the children's toys out of the window. I used to run down the road rather than stay in the house and do something I'd regret. I mean I'd always recognised that I'd had these difficulties with this tension and this sort of thing so I viewed the menopause with horror. I thought, well if I'd had this tension normally, you know, I was going to have all my hot flushes and what have you. . . . It was a sort of non-event really as far as I was concerned. I've always felt that those two D and Cs did me good, in some shape or form. I think if I hadn't had them I might have had a very agonising time, you know, with the periods. I've always slightly suspected they removed something and they never said; but maybe not. I don't know.

The ways in which emotional feelings may be situated in terms of suffering are evident here. Typically mothers are not expected to throw their children's toys out of the window but, above all, the ability to control one's temper or anger is a prerequisite for being a 'good mother'. This typification had consequences for the woman's behaviour because, in order to avert actions that she might regret subsequently, she used to remove herself from such potential situations. These emotional feelings led her to predict that her menopause would be 'horrible' and 'agonising' and something to be suffered. On the contrary, the absence of feelings of tension resulted in the assessment of her menopause as a 'non-event', and thereby devoid of suffering.

Below we can see how, whilst hot flushes are acknowledged as part of a normal menopause, in the context of this woman's individual normality, they were not regarded as being of great relevance:

Well I think when I had that feeling in the supermarket I was probably feeling a bit warm but I have always been an easy blusher. I mean I colour up very easily with heat or drink or eating too much or if I find myself doing three different things at a time in the kitchen and also leaning over a hot oven or something. I suppose if I felt flushed a little I'd just say I was jittery about something and I'd think no more about it.

This woman links routine, everyday activities, such as eating, drinking or busying herself in the kitchen, with blushing and feeling hot. As such, these feelings were not unusual for her. Nevertheless, in the context of an interview about her experience of the menopause, they warranted comment. She links physical feelings with emotional ones by accounting for the former in terms of being 'jittery'.

Furthermore, the kind of emotional talk reported in this extract allows an interesting contrast to be made with that found in the previous extract. We have instances here of gradations of suffering – of how different emotional feelings may be contextualized as more serious suffering. Hence describing emotions as 'agonising' conveys much more suffering than those referred to as being 'jittery'.

Everyday theories of middle-aged women's behaviour

In contrast to the approach of Scheper-Hughes and Lock (1987) and Bendelow and Williams (1995), physical and emotional feelings have been used as a topic for analysis rather than a resource in that analysis. In doing this, it has been possible to demonstrate how, through their usage in language, physical and emotional feelings may be situated as issues of pain and suffering. These processes of situating pain and suffering are further amplified by typifications of middle-aged women's behaviour. These matters were most apparent in those women whose expectations of having a straightforward and trouble-free menopause were not matched by reality.

The woman whose experiences are detailed in the data extract below believed that she had started her menopause when she was aged forty. She thought that this had accounted for the deep depressions which had pervaded her experience.

> When I first went there (to the clinic) I felt this is the end of the line. I thought I've been to ante-natal clinic, post-natal clinic and all sorts of clinics. Now this is the end – menopause. I said to a woman, 'Is this the end of the line – menopause clinic?' 'No', she said. 'There's a geriatric clinic'. I said, 'I feel awful coming here. Do you?' So she said, 'Well I did but my friend told me the gynaecologist's quite pleased by the type of women that are coming to the clinic. It was a new thing when he started it and he's noticed that they're all intelligent women that want to do something about it'. That boosted me a bit because I felt very down when I went, as if I was giving into something.

This woman identifies a trajectory for women which links physiological events to particular life stages – pregnancy and childbirth precede the menopause. It is within this trajectory of life-stage categories that the woman situates her talk about the pain and suffering she experienced during her menopause. The contrast that is made between women attending the clinic as 'intelligent and wanting to do something about it (the menopause)' and women who 'give in' points to an underlying pattern of the categories of 'rational' as opposed to 'emotional' women. By implication, intelligent women see attending the menopause clinic as a means to an end, and have arrived there as a consequence of making a choice. However, 'emotional' women lack such control and 'give in' by reacting to matters. On her taking hormone replacement therapy she stated:

> I would never have thought for one moment I ever would have needed it because I'm really a hard person. I had the children without any problems. . . . When breastfeeding my first child I used to wake up wet through because the milk had burst out and my breasts were so painful and hard but I could always put up with things. I've never been one for really going and complaining to the doctor so when I watched that hormone transplant (on a television programme) I would never have thought I would have to go on such things. I was quite surprised really when I realised that all my problems have been hormone deficiency.

Female life-stage categories are returned to in order to locate and emphasize the pain and suffering experienced by this woman. Her ability to cope with the pain from the retention of breast milk is called upon in her self-categorization of being able to endure pain. She saw herself as being 'a hard person' and not 'a complainer'. The implied moral weakness of the category 'giver in' is tempered by the account of her depression and emotional feelings in terms of a physiological matter – 'hormone deficiency'.

In this final data extract, the woman is comparing her experience with her expectations of the menopause. The former did not reflect the latter.

I suppose something that could never happen to me because, as I say, I've not been all that sympathetic with those people who seem to enjoy bad health and I thought I wasn't one of them. . . . If anything, women went mad on the change. They didn't all go mad on the change but if anybody went mad, it was on the change. And I used to wonder what they did when they went mad. In fact I did have a bit of a breakdown. I didn't think it was a breakdown. I just left them all (her family) to it. It surprised me really because I didn't know what you did when you had a breakdown. I thought you threw things or you ran up the street naked or something mad.

Again, ideas of moral weakness and how it may be connected with a particular response to suffering are evident here. Women identified as 'enjoying' bad health are by implication deemed not to be deserving of 'sympathy.' Menopausal women's responses to suffering, then, may be morally evaluated in terms of being either a 'strong' or a 'weak' person. The former categorization rests on enduring and the latter on enjoying emotional upset.

These data extracts reveal how assessments of mental and physical feelings that are typically associated with the menopause are situated in everyday categories of middle-aged women's behaviour. At this time of life, women are unlikely to overcome mental and physical feelings, but rather allow them to pervade all aspects of their life. Not only do they tend to complain and 'go on' about their situation, but they also enjoy it. Such matters may also tip the balance of a woman's emotions so that she becomes mentally unstable. Moreover, the fact that women are not expected to be seriously upset by physical and mental feelings at this stage of their life presents a dilemma to those who are, and it is in talking about this problem that suffering is contextualized.

Conclusions

This paper has focused on the Cartesian dualism between the mind and the body, and its linkage with the concepts of pain and suffering. Recent anthropological and sociological literature in this domain has been examined. Although both Scheper-Hughes and Lock (1987) and Bendelow and Williams (1995) claimed to offer solutions to this dualism, it was argued that both were characterized by adherence to a correspondence theory of reality. In contrast, a coherence theory of reality was suggested as an alternative way forward, for this eschews concerns with distinctions between mind and body and pain and suffering as ontological entities in favour of differences that reside in language usage. A further consequence of such a path is that pain and suffering were seen as topics for analysis in their own right. Using an ethnomethodological approach to the examination of talk, data from a study of women's experience of the menopause were employed to demonstrate how the categories of pain and suffering were situated in language usage. It was possible to show how the same physical and mental feelings could be differentially assigned to the categories of pain and suffering.

Acknowledgements

I would like to acknowledge the comments made by students on the part-time degree course in Health Studies at the Manchester Metropolitan University, and their contribution to the ideas contained in this chapter.

References

Bendelow, G. and Williams, S. 1995: Transcending the dualisms: towards a sociology of pain. *Sociology of Health and Illness* 17, 139–65.

Bury, M. 1982: Chronic illness as biographical disruption. *Sociology of Health and Illness* 1, 167–82.

Coulter, G. 1983: *Mind in action*. Oxford: Polity Press.

Coulter, G. 1991: Cognition: cognition in an ethnomethodological mode. In Button, G. (ed.), *Ethnomethodology and the human sciences*. Cambridge: Cambridge University Press.

Fairhurst, E. 1980: *A preliminary study of the meaning of the end of the reproductive cycle in women*. Final Report to the Social Science Research Council (now the Economic and Social Research Council) grant no.HR 6156. Manchester: University of Manchester, Department of Geriatric Medicine.

Fairhurst, E. and Lightup, R. 1981: *The notion of normality and the interpretation of physiological events: the case of the menopause*. Paper presented to the Third International Conference on the Menopause, Ostend, 9–12 June 1981.

Garfinkel, H. and Sacks, H. 1970: On formal structures of practical actions. In McKinney, J.C. and Tiryakian, E.A. (eds), *Theoretical sociology: perspectives and developments*. New York: Appleton- Century- Crofts, 337–66.

Melzack, R. and Wall, P. 1988: *The challenge of pain*. Harmondsworth: Penguin.

Ornstein, R. 1973: Right and left thinking. *Psychology Today* May, 87–92.

Scheper-Hughes, N. and Lock, M. 1987: The mindful body: a prolegomenon to future work in medical anthropology. *Medical Anthropology Quarterly* 1, 6–41.

Sharrock, W. and Watson, D. 1989: Talk and police work: notes on the traffic in information. In Coleman, H. (ed.), *Working with Language*. The Hague: Mouton, 431–44.

Silverman, D. 1993: *Analysing qualitative data*. London: Sage.

Smith, D. 1978: 'K is mentally ill'. The anatomy of a factual account. *Sociology* 12, 23–53.

Williams, G. 1984: The genesis of chronic illness: narrative reconstruction. *Sociology of Health and Illness* 6, 175–200.

Wowk, M. 1989: Emotion talk. In Torode, B. (ed.), *Text and talk as social practice*. Dordrecht: Fons, 51–71.

Pain management: training and education issues

J. Edmond Charlton

Introduction

Control of pain is a basic humanitarian right, and the symptom of pain is that most commonly encountered by all specialists when their help and advice is sought. It is the symptom that takes patients to see their doctors more frequently than any other, and there is a widely held belief that pain can be controlled with ease. Why then, should there be a need for a specialty that calls itself 'pain management'? The simple truth of the matter is that pain management is not easy, nor is it well understood by many health care professionals. Pain that needs treatment can be acute, such as that following surgery or an injury, or chronic, arising from a wide variety of causes, or it can be the pain that may accompany malignancy and terminal illness. Clearly, pain arising from such a wide range of potential causes is unlikely to be simple to treat.

Every physician or surgeon believes that they know how to treat pain – they have, after all, been treating it since the time of Hippocrates. Many generations of treating pain their way has led to certain prejudices which may manifest themselves when faced with a growing, and at times, vocal group of individuals who believe that they can carry out pain management more effectively. Proof that change is required in the way in which pain is managed by all health care disciplines can be found in the large numbers of patients on the wards and in the clinics for whom pain control simply is not good enough. This would seem to indicate that training in the skills and arts of pain management could be improved for everyone graduating from medical and nursing schools.

Teaching pain management

Organizations and special interest groups concerned with pain relief and pain management are a recent phenomenon. The Pain Society was founded (as the Intractable Pain Society) in 1967. It was not until 1974 that an international body, known as the International Association for the Study of Pain (IASP), was founded. Both bodies are multidisciplinary in nature and both share common aims, and the Pain Society has become a chapter of the IASP, although retaining independence over all its actions in Great Britain and Ireland. Members of the Pain Society have always been active on the Council and committees of the IASP, and have taken a leading role in formulating policy.

One of the major roles of both bodies is in education. In 1988, the IASP published an undergraduate curriculum for teaching pain. This was perceived by the authors to be a bare outline of the knowledge necessary for the effective management of pain. The curriculum consisted merely of subject headings and covered less than a side of paper. The subjects covered ranged from basic neuroanatomy and neurophysiology, through many forms of practical management to behavioural factors and ethics. This important initiative led on to a series of curricula for various disciplines which have been immensely popular with the membership. The curricula have proved be a tremendously important tool for introducing the teaching of pain throughout the world.

Since this initial effort other curricula have been introduced, including: undergraduate dentistry (1991), nursing (1991), pharmacy (1993), physical and occupational therapy (1995) and psychology (1998). All are different and all are provided with key references in the relevant literature. The medical post-graduate curriculum has just been revised and re-issued as a second edition (1995). Although many clinicians from Great Britain and Ireland have contributed to these texts, little has been achieved in introducing them to teaching practice at either undergraduate or postgraduate level within these isles.

Undergraduates

Clearly the place to start is at the undergraduate level, yet no core curriculum exists for training in pain management. The General Medical Council has no prescribed view on this, individual medical schools being free to include as much or as little training as they see fit. In general lip service is only being paid unless individuals lobby hard to convince Deans and curriculum committees that the need is great. Personal experience suggests that the effort is worthwhile and that effective teaching can be introduced. The ideal format is for aspects of acute pain management to be introduced at the very beginning of clinical teaching. Frequently this can be combined with symptom control and basic concepts of palliative medicine. Small blocks of teaching can then be given each year which extend knowledge and introduce basic science and practical management of acute and chronic pain, with separate teaching of behavioural aspects.

The importance of teaching pain management in medical school is reinforced by the need to include a substantial section on pain control in each pre-registration house officer orientation course. Two of the most worrying prospects for the new medical graduate are the thought of needing to carry out resuscitation and having to treat patients in pain. Effective training and reassurance by anaesthetists at this stage have been found to be very helpful. It can be argued that these skills should already have been acquired. Alas! There is no agreement by Deans of medical schools that the acquisition of such skills should be mandatory. Whilst it might be argued that this is special pleading, there is already plenty of this within medical teaching where entrenched interests maintain that it is necessary to devote a disproportionate amount of teaching time to rare neurological diseases or complex surgery performed upon tiny numbers of the population. The teaching of pain management in at least one medical school in Great Britain has increased only because of the persistent demands of final-year students and pre-registration house officers for more such teaching to be given.

Things are little better in the USA. Despite great efforts, particularly by those concerned with the management of cancer pain, the overall management of pain by medical students appears to be suboptimal. An abstract presented at a meeting of the International Anesthesia Research Society in Washington in 1996 showed that final-year students close to qualification were able to assess pain reasonably well, but only a minority were able to manage pain adequately. There are no comparable data for Great Britain and Ireland, but the suspicion must be that the same situation pertains. National bodies cannot influence medical schools, and it appears that the IASP is powerless to help in such matters – only local effort effects change, and that, in simple terms, means Pain Society members lobbying in their local medical schools. In brutal terms it may mean doing surveys and demonstrating ignorance among graduating doctors, but it certainly means local action.

Postgraduates

The key to postgraduate educational projects in pain management is the second edition of the International Association for the Study of Pain publication entitled *Curriculum for Professional Education in Pain*. This was first published in 1991, and a revised version was issued in 1995. This consists of a simple list of topics covering all aspects of pain management from basic sciences to advanced techniques, each accompanied by a list of references to introduce the reader to key literature on the topic. It is this type of endeavour that should form the basis for national training programmes, but no medical postgraduate body has such a programme at present, nor do any of the statutory bodies responsible for training other health professions.

The Royal Colleges of Anaesthetists and Psychiatrists are the only medical postgraduate bodies in Great Britain that include the treatment of pain as part of their postgraduate curriculum. There is a mention of pain in the syllabus of some specialist surgical Fellowship examinations. In practice, only anaesthetists are likely to receive formal training in pain management and to be examined in order to assess their competence and knowledge. This is likely to concentrate upon the management of acute pain. Questions on chronic pain can form part of the examination for Fellowship of the Royal College of Psychiatrists.

How can training in pain management be introduced and improved? If one is medically qualified and wishes to be recognized as a specialty, one must have an approved training programme. In the UK this has to be administered by one of the medical Royal Colleges. Because pain is multidisciplinary, it might be thought that there would be competition among the Colleges to claim it as part of their sphere of interest. Not so. By default it has been given to the Royal College of Anaesthetists to sort out. In 1993, the Conference of Medical Royal Colleges and their Faculties approved the approach from the Royal College of Anaesthetists to develop pain management as a specialty within anaesthesia, and a curriculum for training has now been agreed upon by the Council of the Royal College.

As part of this process, the College saw and initially rejected the IASP core curriculum as being far too complicated. Indeed, the fairly crude IASP undergraduate curriculum is, in truth, much more comprehensive than the pain management section of the curriculum published 8 years later by the Royal College of Anaesthetists for the Fellowship of that College. This is disappointing, as pain management is one of the major specialist interests of anaesthetists, and over 90 per cent of physicians practising within the subspecialty of chronic pain management have anaesthesia as their initial specialty.

The syllabus for the Primary and Final examinations for Fellowship of the Royal College of Anaesthetists has 48 pages, and a single page is devoted to pain management (Table 11.1). Candidates are expected to have a detailed knowledge of the control of acute pain in the context of postoperative and post-traumatic conditions, and 'an understanding of the principles' of chronic pain management in a pain clinic setting. It seems curious that a broad theoretical knowledge is required for such a subject. It looks even more odd when placed alongside training requirements for other parts of anaesthetic practice that are resplendent in vast detail, or that insist on statutory amounts of training time being allocated to subspecialties, such as cardiac and neuro-anaesthesia, which are practised by only a handful of practitioners throughout

Table 11.1 Syllabus in pain management: Royal College of Anaesthetists

A detailed knowledge of the control of acute pain in the context of postoperative and post-traumatic conditions will be expected, as will an understanding of the principles of chronic pain management in the pain clinic setting

- Anatomy, physiology, physiology and basic pharmacology relevant to pain management
- Assessment and measurement of pain – with special reference to children and the elderly
- Investigation and diagnosis in the pain clinic
- The place of drug therapy, including management of substance abuse
- Stimulation-produced analgesia including transcutaneous techniques and acupuncture
- The role of and indications for neural blockade: peripheral nerve, plexus, epidural and subarachnoid blocks; techniques of sympathetic blockade: neurolytic agents and procedures; implanted catheters and pumps for drug delivery
- Symptom control in terminal illness
- The organization of pain management services
- Principles of ethics of pain research

Source: Royal College of Anaesthetists. Reproduced with permission.

the country. More recently, the Royal College of Anaesthetists has taken a dramatic and positive step by approving the 1995 IASP core curriculum for training anaesthetists intending to specialize in pain management. The syllabus in pain management for the fellowship of the Royal College of Anaesthetists remains the same.

Ideas for change

The Pain Society is in a unique position to provide an impetus to training for all disciplines with an interest in the effective treatment of pain. Many of the statutory bodies concerned with education in the UK and Ireland recognize that they have insufficient expertise to bring training programmes up to date, and will welcome the introduction of something like the core curriculum as an aid to this process. As the British and Irish Chapter of the International Association for the Study of Pain, and as a multidisciplinary body, the Pain Society possesses an interest and enthusiasm for this subject which can be harnessed in the education of colleagues. The obvious place to start this process is with the education of pain management specialists with a background in anaesthesia. This would follow lines already proposed for intensive therapy, where a set period of formal training would be followed by a formal assessment, and successful candidates would be awarded a registerable qualification denoting specialist knowledge of that subject.

North American experience

Elsewhere in the world other bodies are offering extensive educational programmes, and the eventual aim should be to reproduce similar programmes for the UK and Ireland. In addition, educational programmes using a core curriculum are being introduced for many different subspecialties and disciplines.

The societies and bodies listed in Table 11.2 offer extensive postgraduate educational courses which are designed to fulfil virtually every requirement for Continuing Professional Development (CPD) credits for doctors, as well as similar requirements for nurses, psychologists and pharmacists. Dentists are catered for, but to a lesser degree. Clearly this arrangement would be desirable for all professional bodies, and there is a need for postgraduate education in

Table 11.2 Bodies offering pain education courses based on a core curriculum[a]

International Association for the Study of Pain
European Society for Regional Anaesthesia
American Pain Society
American Society for Regional Anesthesia
Canadian Pain Society
Australian Pain Society

[a] Specific pain-related CPD credits are available for physicians, nurses, psychologists and pharmacists at meetings held by these bodies.

pain management in the UK and Ireland to be placed on a firm and logical basis. At present there is no structure to this, and in particular there are no plans for assessment of those delivering the teaching or those being educated.

Registration and certification in medicine in every component state of the USA requires mandatory re-certification at regular intervals. It is subject to rigorous audit, is dependent on presenting satisfactory evidence of continuing medical education, and it contains compulsory elements. These are not great at present but the potential for expansion is there, and the trend is for more and more regulation as a method of ensuring quality of practice. The health care delivery system in North America is changing, and the concept of managed care has been developing rapidly. The likelihood is that a similar philosophy will be introduced into Europe, too.

Faced with the rising cost of health care, insurers in the USA have turned to a system not unlike that provided by the National Health Service. This involves a restricted choice on the part of patients as to where and by whom they can be treated, modifying the clinical behaviour of doctors and others with guidelines and protocols, and emphasizing primary care. Having instituted these controls, those responsible for the delivery of health care can apply the three essentials of disease management:

- a knowledge base that quantifies the economic structure of the disease problem and describes care guidelines;
- a delivery system that co-ordinates all carers – primary, secondary and social; and
- a quality improvement system to audit performance against evolving standards.

Part of the process involves re-certification, and this is dependent upon both CPD and qualifying examinations at appropriate intervals, usually 5 years. In addition, they have in place continuing assessment and professional testing of all those who are examiners. There are two examiners on Specialty Boards in the USA – one to assess the candidate and the other to assess the examiner. If the examiner starts to fail, he or she is out. There are plans to introduce similar requirements for other professional groups within health care.

In the USA, for medical practitioners to be certified as having an approved training in pain management there are two possible routes that can be followed. Ominously, these routes are not compatible and at present are not recognized mutually. For anaesthetists they should have passed the appropriate specialist Board examination after a period of approved training. After that they can obtain added or special qualifications by completing a further period in a recognized anaesthesia training programme which also offers training fellowships in pain management. These training fellowships have to apply to be recognized, and the fact that they have to be anaesthesia-based has led to some very well-known pain clinics that were based on neurosciences or behaviourally based being ineligible to have pain fellowships that lead to additional qualifications. Anaesthetists taking an additional qualification in pain management had to have completed an approved training post, or to have fulfilled a requirement that they had spent the equivalent of 2 years of full-time practice in pain management, or 50 per cent for 4 years and pro rata. This was in addition to being certified by the American Board of Anesthesiology, having a current state medical licence and having satisfied all of their CPD requirements, including the mandatory components. These are criteria that only US anaesthetists could fulfil, so there is no chance that non-US doctors could take these examinations as a method of demonstrating their experience and knowledge of pain management.

There is a need for doctors with a background in other disciplines to show evidence of their experience and knowledge of pain management. This role has been taken on by the American College of Pain Medicine, which is a multidisciplinary body that examines in pain medicine and thus satisfies the requirements for medical practitioners of disciplines other than anaesthesia to have a qualification. Their method of establishing an examination was interesting and deserves wider recognition. First, they appointed liaison and commissioning committees of senior clinicians who, in essence, invented an examination. They did this by surveying a very high proportion of their membership and establishing what was current practice. Then they constructed an examination which wisely took the entire IASP curriculum as its base, but which emphasized current practice. Interestingly, they gave the pilot examination to their committees and Council, although they did not award them pass marks. Indeed, no one knows how they got on!

Training specialists

Clearly, this has lessons for those who wish to start professional examinations in pain management. In introducing any assessment in pain management we must include examination of the knowledge and interests of all concerned. Thus both the knowledge base and the examination process must be multidisciplinary and, in addition, they should represent current opinion and practice. This will meet the concerns of special interest groups and will increase the skills and knowledge of all concerned.

The introduction and establishment of a new specialty requires time, enthusiasm and prodigious effort. A starting point in that process is the introduction of a specialist qualification. Because of the large numbers involved it has to be an examination for physicians, as it is probable that added qualifications in pain management will lead to improved standards and status. It shows that we mean business, and it may even lead in the fullness of time to a separate faculty for medical pain specialists. At present, because the majority of pain management specialists are anaesthetists, the appropriate home is the Royal College of Anaesthetists. When members of other disciplines want to go down this route the Royal College of Anaesthetists would be in a position to help their equivalent colleagues at the Royal College of Nursing or other statutory body.

The ideal for teaching at any level would be to have a joint curriculum. If one's base is the same, this means that duplication of effort is limited. The interpretation and marking of examinations may be different, but there is no reason why we should not use the same database. This could apply to any qualifications throughout the UK or Europe, or further afield if needed. The questions remain the same, but the level of answer that satisfies the examiners may vary according to location, and for this reason reciprocity would seem unlikely.

Training others

Synchronous with moves to establish a postgraduate medical pain management qualification should be a concerted effort to improve education in undergraduate medical and nursing training. A 'package' approach involving acute, chronic and palliative medicine should be evolved. This should be centred on a generic curriculum based on those that are currently available. Learning materials should be offered as part of this process to make it easy for curriculum committees to assimilate what for them will be a new departure. A similar package should be developed for pre-registration house officers, covering those aspects of beginning medicine that present the most problems – namely acute and chronic pain relief, death, dying and breaking bad news, resuscitation and obtaining consent for various procedures and operations. It is a fact of life that recruitment into and retention of staff within any discipline are dependent upon early and positive contact. Making structured efforts to help and educate colleagues at the beginning of their training will pay dividends later on.

Further efforts can be made to promote awareness throughout each hospital by introducing regular 'pain days'. These would be open to all and run by a wide variety of people from the pain services. They should cover all aspects of pain management and should have a varying format. These, too, should be based on standard learning materials. The innovative concept of distance learning can be applied to the teaching of pain management to any professional group, and again this is where the use of an IASP core curriculum comes into its own. These curricula are to be updated on a regular basis, but it is important that they be reviewed and modified in order to put a European 'spin' on the recommendations and associated literature citations.

After training ourselves we need to train others. The Royal College of Anaesthetists has been identified as being important to the future development of pain management. The next necessary step is to identify and support advisers to other statutory bodies. We also need to encourage these bodies to appoint specialist advisers, both nationally and locally. We also need to help the statutory bodies to identify individuals who can train and who can assess training, and we need to find a way of making some sense of the diplomas and degrees that are currently on offer. Few of them appear to have any relevance except as commercial enterprises. In particular, we need to avoid problems like those extant within palliative medicine, where over 50 separate diplomas and an increasing number of degree courses are being offered without any overall supervision or assessment of their value. A desire to do good is simply not a good enough guarantee of quality.

Training the decision makers

Changes to training in any discipline mean a political change. This means medical politics, nursing politics, and the equivalent in other professions, and it means political politics. We have a golden opportunity if we care to take it. Every group has a story to tell, and members of that group want the public and those in power to hear that story, to take notice and to do something about it if needed. For other pressure groups, such as Greenpeace, or political groups the message may form part of a media event, a demonstration, a television or radio show, a newspaper story or a dinner. There are dozens of ways of being heard. Those of us in the mainstream healing professions have, historically, shunned the spotlight. We saw ourselves as humble public servants and did not advertise or call undue attention to ourselves. We felt that if we did a good job, were conservative and non-aggressive in our approach to others and took care of our patients as well as possible, then we would be respected and have our opinions respected by patients, politicians and the public at large.

We now know that not only are our opinions not respected by those individuals who take decisions, but we are not allowed to look after our patients in the way we want because of restrictive actions and policies of other health care workers, employers, insurance companies, bureaucrats and politicians. The issue of looking after patients is being taken away from the professions and handed to bureaucrats. Sunrise specialties such as pain management, without an established place within the hierarchy and without lobbying power, are soft targets for cost-cutting and resource restriction. At the very time when we need increased resources there is a world-wide movement to put a lid on the costs of health care.

We have to build up political muscle, and we can start by trying to put in place policies that stress the need to relieve pain – either acute or chronic. There is no good fairy or magic bullet as far as political clout is concerned. Health care is never going to be able to muster the firepower that law and order matters can produce in any legislative body. Lawyers love becoming politicians. Because of this, the law has usually found it easy to look after its own interests, whereas health care has few advocates within most legislatures, and is an easy target. Because we cannot rely upon a powerful network of support within politics, we must start to work harder to involve ourselves more fully in the wider political process, both centrally and locally.

Audit and research

We have to start with management. Increasingly, power and the ability to make decisions about clinical matters are being handed over to administrators, business principles are becoming paramount, and patient care and service development are being left to individuals who have no clinical experience in the health care sector. We have to be able to provide a sound case to ensure that our needs are met. We need to be able to show that pain management works, and regrettably we cannot do this on the strength of humanitarian concern and shroud waving. We must have data on cost-effectiveness and outcome to show that it works. We need to get away from the philosophy of treatment that judges quality by the thickness of the carpet and the number of flashing lights on the equipment. This means audit and it also means research.

Up until now research on pain-related topics has been of poor quality, sporadic and disorganized, with a few notable exceptions, particularly the work of the group in Oxford conducting systematic reviews of pain management. The opportunity to improve this situation has presented itself with the publication of the Culyer Report (1995), which proposes the centralization of research and development funding and resources. There is still funding for regional research, and at a regional level the Directors of Research and Development will be the focal point. They will have a significant role in commissioning and managing research and development, and will co-ordinate local research interests of both purchasers and providers. Research does not have to be 'blockbuster' in nature, and the Culyer Report recommends that pre-protocol work, curiosity-driven research and similar activities should continue to attract support from the NHS where outside funding is not obtainable. Funding is to be dependent upon performance. Full criteria are not available, but it seems likely that research and development money will go, at least initially, to those with a proven track record who are receiving funding already.

Pain management needs to become organized if research is to be commissioned and funded under the new system. Unless we can institute successful research projects in pain management, there will be no further funding and we will be left with anecdotal research that offers no prospect of improving the status of our specialty. One solution is to list all current research. Areas where research needs to be undertaken should be targeted and brought to the attention of research and development commissioning units. The best prospects for success with research and development funding applications may well be those that are multidisciplinary in nature and involve effective pain management (acute or chronic) as a method of reducing health costs.

Greater emphasis should be placed upon the elucidation of the causes of pain and pain behaviour, using epidemiological methods. Data on unmet need and on 'achievable benefit not achieved' should be collected in order to advance the quality and quantity of pain services. The presentation of reliable hard data on what can be achieved with existing resources is always impressive to legislators, and the burden of proof is always going to lie with us. In this context, it is vital to co-ordinate all of the professions involved in the delivery of pain management, and to ensure that they are all singing the same song.

Getting money and resources out of people is difficult. Probably the best selling tool that we possess is our passion and zeal for our speciality. What we need to know is how to harness that passion and how to instil it into the other professionals and persuade them to donate their expertise, as nothing is more certain than the fact that money is needed to achieve things. Charities and fundraising for good causes are a huge business which must be undertaken professionally, and this will form part of our training philosophy in the same way that we need guidelines for strategy, business plans and market research.

What must be emphasized is that a strong belief in what one is doing is far more important than all the marketing techniques in the world. Getting the basis of our specialty legitimized, if you like, is a sensible way forward.

Conclusions

Training must start with education of those currently engaged in pain management. It must be followed by training for those who administer our specialty, for professional colleagues, for legislators and finally for the public. We must start with a series of goals that are achievable, as success encourages people to set new targets, whereas lack of success leads to disillusionment.

We need to see who we can get on our side, and then use them to enlist others. Then we need to ensure that a consistent message is being sent out. Politicians like to be known to have special interests, and it is a good idea to remind politicians of their personal responsibility to the people who elected them, and that includes medical politicians and local politicians, too. The advocates we use must be slick, available and have a sense of humour. Other lobbyists will be keen to label us as a fanatic or fringe group. It is a beauty contest and we must never forget that. This makes it important to have young, bright and articulate spokesmen who will present in a positive manner. Presenting reams of doleful data is a certain way to lose one's target audience, and will result in accusations of fanaticism. The subject has to be made glamorous, with an emphasis on boosting efforts directed at research and training. Above all, it has to be a team effort with representatives from all disciplines interested in pain management evolving a common theme to present.

What is needed is the David philosophy. David beat Goliath because he had moral rectitude and a carefully laid out plan of campaign. He won by patience and a careful aim.

Further reading

Culyer, A.J. 1995: *Supporting research and development in the National Health Service.* London: HMSO.

Fields, H.L. 1995: *Core curriculum for professional education in pain*, 2nd edn. Seattle: IASP Press.

International Association for the Study of Pain 1994: *Curricula on pain for medical, dental, pharmacy, nursing, psychology and physical therapy/occupational therapy schools.* Seattle: IASP Press (available from the International Association for the Study of Pain, 909 NE 43rd Street, Suite 306, Seattle WA 98105–6020, USA).

Royal College of Anaesthetists 1996: *Primary and final examinations for the FRCA. Syllabus.* London: Royal College of Anaesthetists.

Royal College of Physicians of London 1995: Report of a meeting of the 1942 Club, January 1995. The recommendations. *Journal of the Royal College of Physicians of London* 29, 216–24.

Organizing acute pain management

Ramon Carlo Pediani

Introduction

This chapter describes the development and current role of hospital-based acute pain services. Elsewhere in this book topics such as the assessment and treatment of pain are covered in detail, but for the purposes of this chapter it is important to consider how they formed the bedrock upon which the organized approach to pain management was founded. This chapter will explore the following areas:

- the inadequacies of pain management which were increasingly identified from the 1970s and 1980s up until the present day;
- why newer techniques, such as 'patient controlled analgesia' (PCA) and 'epidural infusion analgesia' (EIA), were developed and recommended for general surgical wards, but not accepted into widespread usage;
- the development of organized acute pain services;
- the acute pain service model recommended for the UK by the Royal College of Surgeons and College of Anaesthetists Working Party Report (1990) on Pain after Surgery.

In this way the reader will be presented with a historical account of the evolution of acute pain services (APS).

Originating in the USA, acute pain services have developed as organized multidisciplinary teams working as a division of anaesthetic departments, with the intention of improving the quality of pain relief for the post-surgery patient. This co-ordinated service model has been taken up in many countries around the world, and since the late 1980s has been developing in UK. There are at the time of writing (December 1997) over 250 acute pain services in the UK, ranging from those run by a single doctor or nurse to multidisciplinary teams consisting of medical, nursing, pharmacist, psychologist and physio-therapist input. Their focus is primarily on acute postoperative pain but, increasingly, they are reaching out to all departments within a hospital where acute pain may be being experienced, regardless of its aetiology.

The anaesthetic consultant is a logical choice for the medical lead for an acute pain service, because anaesthetists have a working knowledge and experience of the physiology, pharmacology and anatomical pathways involved in the modulation of acute pain (Hord and Kelly, 1992). However, such anaesthetic-led services often rely heavily on nurse specialists for their day-to-day running at ward level.

Through a co-ordinated service, new technologies such as patient-controlled analgesia (PCA) and ward-based, continuous epidural infusions can be safely and effectively utilized. This demands a large education and training commitment as well as a defined clinical workload for the specialist nurse. The future of the acute pain service seems to be one of expansion into areas such as medicine, radiology and trauma nursing, using the organizational weight behind the pain service to institute changes where individuals may previously have been unsuccessful. Hospital-wide prescribing guidelines, standardized protocols for Entonox usage and intramuscular analgesia algorithms (Gould *et al.*, 1992) are just some of the large-scale developments to come into being under the auspices of a multidisciplinary, authoritative team. The acute pain service is not only an easily accessible, rapid-response service for acute pain problems, but it also has a more fundamental role as a planning and co-ordinating service for large-scale policy developments.

Many hospitals are now recognizing that, by virtue of the specialized clinical techniques at their disposal, acute and chronic pain services are in a position to be able to offer all patients optimum care at any stage in their treatment, or in the progression of their condition. Acute pain teams as described in this paper generally focus their attention solely on the hospital setting, but can often offer advice to community services on particular pain management problems.

Pre-acute pain services

It is an indictment of modern medicine that an apparently simple problem such as the reliable relief of postoperative pain remains largely unsolved

(Anonymous, BMJ Editorial, 1978).

The above statement serves to remind us that the problem of postoperative pain is not new. The control of pain has received considerable attention from writers and researchers within the professions of medicine and nursing over the past 30 years. Many of the conclusions and suggestions resulting from this work bear a striking similarity to current strategies for the relief of pain, as many of the same problems are still seen to be present – poor prescribing and administration habits, lack of pain assessment, lack of awareness of the problem, and the general inflexibility of the hospital organization. The recent changes in hospital management of acute pain, i.e. the setting up of acute pain teams, coupled with developments in the understanding of the pharmacology of analgesics and the development of new technologies for administering them, have begun to raise the standard of analgesia provision. This may in part be because postoperative pain control is no longer seen as a luxury, or about simply being 'nice' to people. Important as the humanitarian dimension of acute pain care is, the therapeutic value of good pain relief is now recognized as being an integral part of ensuring a good recovery from surgery and early restoration of normal functioning.

Pain assessment

One of the factors that has perhaps hindered the successful tackling of the acute pain problem is that pain itself is not a clearly defined entity. As Sofaer (1983) has said, pain is a complex phenomenon, known to many but defying definition. McCaffery (1983) simply stated that pain is what the patient said it was. This of course is true, but unhelpful. However, it does serve to remind us that, although we may learn about the physiology and pharmacology related to the topic, only the person experiencing the pain can truly know its reality. Acute pain is often associated with a distinct disease or injury and the duration of the pain is assumed to be limited to the time required for healing of the damage (Mitchell and Smith, 1989).

If pain is difficult to define, it is especially difficult to measure. Many tools have been developed to try and obtain some objective measure of the patient's pain (Schofield, 1995), but these can only ever be approximations and cannot be directly compared between individuals. The reason for this is that pain is an 'unverifiable personal experience' (Harrison, 1991). Many factors will affect the patient's perception of their pain and their ability to cope with it. Such factors may include the patient's cultural background, his or her previous experience, and the nature of the pain. The assessors, too, have their own biases and, in addition to their own cultural background, also belong to a professional subculture which has its own values and norms. We can see that the complex mix of factors which govern a patient's responses to a given situation, and the complex factors that affect the professional's perception of the patient's pain, do not make for good communication. It is not surprising, therefore, that many studies have shown that nurses generally underestimate patients' pain (e.g. Dudley and Holm, 1984; Seers, 1987).

The degree to which any one factor plays a part in any particular nurse/patient interaction may be impossible to predict. For example, Levine and De Simone (1991) showed that male subjects under-reported their pain to female researchers as compared to male researchers, yet male patients often receive more analgesia than female patients (Simmons and Malabar, 1995). It would be practically impossible to design a pain assessment tool that could take into account all of the possible variants and interactions, but perhaps, for short-term clinical purposes, that is not what is required. Simply taking the trouble to ask the patient may be all that is needed. A simple score, which to some extent makes compromises between validity and reliability in favour of ease of use and general applicability, may be appropriate if the goal is to ensure that the patient is not restricted in his or her ability to expectorate and co-operate with physiotherapy postoperatively. A simple pain score system, however crude, if used regularly should show whether the pain is getting better or worse and give some impression of how it is affecting mobility. Accuracy of pain assessment is only as useful as the contribution it makes to the 'appropriate utilisation of measures to relieve pain' (Zalon, 1993). The use of a pain assessment chart has been shown not only to improve the provision of analgesia for the postoperative patient, but also has benefits for the staff as well (Scott, 1994).

It can be difficult to ensure common goals for pain relief between nursing and medical staff, among whom different values may be held, and between acute and chronic pain conditions (Hockley, 1988). This compounds the problems associated with trying to titrate analgesia to effect as there is often no clearly defined endpoint (Mitchell and Smith, 1989). Yet despite the inherent difficulties of the topic, within the nursing, medical and paramedical professions, the relief of pain should be one of the most important and challenging issues. In particular, with the 24-h close patient contact of nursing teams, nurses should recognize their role as 'pain managers' (Wells, 1985).

Opioid administration

Gould *et al.* (1994) showed that newly qualified house officers have a poor knowledge of analgesia regimes. Hatcher and Peacock (1995) supported this finding, claiming that gaps in knowledge 'jeopardise basic standards of safe prescribing'. Harmer (1994) in an editorial in the journal *Anaesthesia*, suggests that there is a role for the acute pain service in the education of future house officers. The arguments for pain service involvement are supported by studies such as a survey by Bruster *et al.* (1994) of 5150 hospital patients, in which it was found that 61 per cent suffered pain, 87 per cent of whom had severe or moderate pain.

There has long been present among both medical and nursing staff a fear of causing addiction in patients supplied with opioid drugs for the relief of their pain. This fear is 'common and misplaced' according to Lipman (1984). It overshadows the therapeutic benefits of analgesia and the potential for pain-induced complications following surgery, such as deep vein thrombosis, chest infection and pulmonary emboli (Cuschieri *et al.*, 1985). This concept is evident today as Walco encapsulates in his statement that 'an overestimation of the risk of analgesic-induced addiction leads to an underestimation of the harm of untreated pain' (Walco *et al.*, 1994). Lack of knowledge was regarded as one of the main obstacles to good patient care. Hosking (1985) found that nurses were not giving analgesia until patients were already in considerable pain, rather than keeping them comfortable and pre-empting painful activities. Hosking assumed that this was because the staff were unaware of the rationale of pain prevention. Watt-Watson's study of Canadian nurses was typical of many which found that nurses lacked knowledge of pain assessment and opioid administration (Watt-Watson, 1987).

In a seminal paper, Cohen (1980) found that over 75 per cent of post-surgical patients had experienced moderate or 'marked pain distress'. Despite the fact that analgesia had been prescribed, patients received less than optimal amounts. One of the key difficulties had been a lack of formal pain assessment. This resulted in miscommunication between patients and nursing staff; but in addition female patients received less analgesia than male patients. Cohen found that 'choices of analgesic medications seemed irrational, and knowledge of the drugs was inadequate.' She recommended better education for nurses in pharmacology and better pre-operative information for patients, so that they might feel free to request analgesia and not try to 'be brave.'

Assessing and recording the pain experience of an individual in some fashion is not simply good record-keeping – just as a diabetic patient may have their blood glucose level assessed as a method of titrating their insulin supply, a patient's current level of pain can be a guide to titrating the provision of analgesia. Fry (1979) described hourly pain and respiratory rate assessment as a criterion by which to gauge intravenous opioid administration. Papaveretum was administered via a continuous infusion, but nursing staff were able to give additional top-ups on the basis of their assessment. This technique was shown to be superior to intermittent intramuscular analgesia as it relieved pain more quickly and reliably, and it maintained a more even level of analgesia over the postoperative period.

Rutter *et al.* (1980) showed that morphine could be safely administered by continuous intravenous infusion. This method of opioid delivery achieved superior pain relief for patients undergoing major surgery when compared to intermittent intramuscular injection. The total dose of drug required was also seen to be reduced. Rutter suggested that continuous intravenous infusion of an opioid should be the method of choice for postoperative pain control. Yet intramuscular injections remained the method in widespread use, despite the inherent limitations of fixed dosage regimes and poor administration practices. Cartwright *et al.* (1991), in an audit of 735 patients who had been prescribed intramuscular injections following surgery, found that such prescriptions are 'poorly complied with, since 80 per cent of patients received only 0, 1 or 2 doses'.

Epidural analgesia had been shown to reduce postoperative pain significantly. The infusion of analgesics into the epidural space in particular was shown to do much more than merely relieve the suffering associated with surgical wounds. Cuschieri *et al.* (1985) demonstrated that, in addition to superior pain relief, when compared to the use of intravenous or intramuscular morphine, epidural analgesia significantly improved pulmonary function and reduced the respiratory complications of thoracic surgery, such as chest infection. This may prompt the question of why, if epidurals can achieve both humanitarian and therapeutic goals, they should not be more widely used? For Cuschieri, the technique appeared to be limited to selected cases where recovery-room facilities and personnel experienced in regional analgesia were available. In the majority of hospitals at that time such facilities were simply not widely available.

Hobbs and Roberts (1992) showed that an epidural infusion of combined low-dose local anaesthetic and diamorphine was a 'highly effective method of providing postoperative analgesia after intrathoracic, intra-abdominal, and major lower limb surgery in appropriate patients'. Although no mention is made of organizing the ward-based epidural regime under the control of an acute pain service, key points are raised, namely the need for nurse education and a standardized monitoring protocol. In this way, Hobbs and Roberts suggests, the technique need not be restricted to intensive care or high-dependency units. The pain assessment method described in Hobbs and Roberts' paper is almost identical to that described by Wheatley *et al.* (1991), which has become the score most commonly used by acute pain services – a scale of 0 to 3 which takes into account pain at rest and on movement (see Figure 12.1 for an example of a postoperative audit chart).

Patient-controlled analgesia

In response to the clinical problems associated with the variation between individuals in their tolerance of pain, and the variability in the pharmacokinetics of analgesics, a system was developed which allowed the patient to be the judge of the amount of analgesia necessary to control the pain intensity to their satisfaction. This system is known as patient-controlled analgesia (PCA).

The basic design of the system allows the patient to self-administer a small intravenous bolus of an opioid analgesic. One dose is too small to cause any major opioid-related problem, such as respiratory depression or excessive sedation. The system has a 'lock-out' period built into it – this makes the patient wait long enough for each dose to be evaluated properly before another bolus can successfully be requested. Unlike intramuscular regimes, the gap between doses is measured in minutes rather than hours. A typical regime would be a bolus dose of 1 mg of morphine available intravenously, with a 5 minute waiting period between successful demands.

Most of the papers written in the medical and nursing literature about PCA have been published over the past 6 years. However, the concept of patient-controlled analgesia was described many years earlier. Sechzer (1971) started experimenting with an analgesic demand system in 1965, and saw the system as a laboratory method of measuring pain and the relative efficacy of analgesics, a means of conducting psychological studies on pain, and also as an excellent method of postoperative pain relief since 'the relief is usually achieved with relatively low total drug dosage and patients are generally satisfied with the results.' It has been noted that for patients using PCA there can be a large variation in opioid requirement. The dose range 24 h following surgery has been observed to be 2–200 mg of morphine (Hunter, 1991).

If patients become sleepy as a result of the PCA-administered opioid, their ability to make further presses of the demand button is reduced. It is therefore difficult to self-administer to the point of overdose. As a method of opioid delivery PCA is judged to be a safe system (White, 1987). PCA has been shown to produce less postoperative hypoxaemia than either intermittent intramuscular injection or extradural opioids (Wheatley *et al.*, 1990). However, there are safety considerations, such as the potential for air leaks to cause siphonage. Deaths have been reported due to whole syringefuls of opioid being allowed to free-flow. The use of anti-siphon and non-return valves in the giving set, and placing the machine no higher than the patient, is recommended (Elcock, 1994).

Notcutt and Morgan (1990) introduced PCA to a district general hospital and presented their analysis of the first 1000 patients treated. 'Teething prob-

---

(Affix Label or Enter)

Hosp No

Name

DOB/Age

Sex

ANALGESIC TECHNIQUE:-	SPECIALITY	INCISION SITE
....	0. Unknown	0. No Incision
Principal Opioid Used:	1. General Surgery	1. Upper Abdomen
....	2. Gynaecology	2. Lower Abdomen
2nd Opioid:	3. Genito-Urinary	3. Peripheral
LA Used:	4. Orthopaedics	4. Thorax
Antiemetic:	5. Trauma	5. Thoraco-Abdominal
Operation:	6. Obstetrics	6. Upper & Lower Abdo
Emergency: Y / N	7. Thoracic	7. Head & Neck
Urinary Catheter in Theatre: Y / N	8. Vascular	8. Spine
Doctors signature:	9. ENT/Dental	9. Perineum
....	10. No Operation	10. Abdo Perineum
	11. Cardiac	11. Sternum
	12. Groin	

PROTOCOL PRESCRIPTIONS:
PCA
Analgesic: Morphine
Concentration: 1mg / ml
Bolus Dose: 1 mg
Lockout Time: 5 mins
Droperidol 2.5 mg Y / N

WARD: ....   LOCAL BLOCK: Y / N   NSAID: Y / N

RETURN FROM THEATRE TO: WARD ☐ ICU ☐ CSU ☐ HDU ☐

EPIDURAL
250 ml of 0.125% Bupivacaine + Diamorphine 10 mg
Diamorphine added ....mg
Above T8 @ 2 - 5 cc/hr
Below T8 @ 4 - 8 cc/hr
Bolus 2 cc - 20 min lockout

LEVEL OF INSERTION		SUGGESTED ANTIEMETIC REGIME
Above T8	☐	PCA:- Droperidol 2.5 mg in syringe + Cyclizine
T8 - T12	☐	25 - 50 mg 8 hrly PRN breakthrough
T12 - L2	☐	EIA:- Regular Cyclizine 25-50 mg TDS + Stemetil
L2 - S1	☐	OR IM 12.5 mg 8 hrly PRN breakthrough
Caudal	☐	* Please write all drugs on prescription chart *

	PAIN		SEDATION		POSTOP NAUSEA + VOMITING (PONV)
Score = 0	No pain at rest / No pain on movement	0	None (fully alert)	0	No nausea or vomiting
Score = 1	No pain at rest / Mild pain on movement	1	Mild (easy to arouse)	1	Mild nausea, but no vomiting
Score = 2	Intermittent pain at rest / Moderate pain on movement	2	Moderate (Drowsy or asleep but can be woken	2	Moderate nausea and/or occasional vomiting
Score = 3	Continuous pain at rest / Severe pain on movement	3	Severe (Somnolent or difficult to arouse)	3	Severe nausea and/or frequent vomiting

WARD STAFF PLEASE ROUTINELY CHECK HEEL CIRCULATION IN EPIDURAL PATIENTS AND REPORT EXCESSIVE LEG BLOCK IMMEDIATELY

DATE	TIME	RESP RATE	PAIN SCORE	SED' SCORE	PONV SCORE	BP	PCA TRIES	PCA TOTAL	EPI RATE	EPIDURAL TOTAL	IM or ORAL	SIGNATURE

Figure 12.1   Victoria Hospital Post-Operative Audit Chart

lems' were experienced with slow respiratory rates, monitoring and equipment difficulties and ward management. This led to the identification of 'specific hazards and management problems' which improved the system's safety. The technique was judged to be successful and became the standard method of pain control for postoperative pain. It was clear that staff education, protocol development, pain and sedation scoring underpinned the safety and success of the technique. Sedation level monitoring has been shown to be a better indicator of potential opioid overdose than simple respiratory rate counting (Ready et al.,1988).

PCA has been shown to be an effective method of controlling pain, and has the added benefit of breaking the reliance on painful intramuscular injections. The patient, by titrating his or her own analgesia within safe limits, could use more or less opioid depending on the activities being undertaken at the time, e.g. physiotherapy or bed bathing. However, problems have been experienced with patients being poorly prepared for the technique and not fully understanding how to get the best maximum benefit from it (Aitken and Kenny, 1990). PCA systems have also been found to be a safe and effective means of providing analgesia in paediatric patients (Rodgers et al., 1988).

More consistent analgesia may provide better pain relief, but opioid-induced side-effects such as postoperative nausea and vomiting may be made worse. This may be in part because the patient is able to maintain higher opioid concentrations than an intramuscular injection would have allowed. Another factor may be that nurses would previously have given a prophylactic anti-emetic at the same time as an opioid injection, but for patients on PCA they will wait until the patient complains of significant nausea, or actually vomits, before they administer an anti-emetic. The concept of PCA itself is generally seen as a method to spare the patient the discomfort of injections (Thomas, 1993). To improve on the provision of anti-emetic medication it has been shown that adding an anti-emetic directly to the PCA morphine gives better symptom control (Sharma and Davies, 1993).

It might have been expected that new ideas and new technologies would not fare any better than the ideas and methodologies put forward in past years, but the acute pain service (APS) model which began to evolve gave some organizational structure on which to build new practices, and changes began to be reported in the medical (primarily anaesthetic) and nursing literature.

The acute pain service

Ready et al. (1988) described the development of a postoperative pain management service at the University of Washington School of Medicine. The goals for the APS were to improve postoperative analgesia, to train anaesthetists in methods of acute pain management, to apply and advance new analgesic methods and to conduct clinical research. It was recognized that PCA and epidural analgesia had been held back in clinical practice due to fears of respiratory depression and a lack of structured training programmes. Ready's APS set about extending the advantages of these techniques to larger numbers of postoperative patients. A joint education programme was developed with the anaesthetic and nursing departments with the aim of safely administering opioid epidural analgesia on general surgical wards.

Medical staffing was provided by the anaesthetic department, conducting daily clinical rounds with the clinical nurse specialist. On these rounds every aspect of the analgesic technique was considered, from the condition of the indwelling epidural catheter to the incidence of side-effects and quality of pain relief. All of the data collected were entered into a computer database. Continuous audit is a feature of many pain services. It can be instructive to look at the distribution of activity of the service, and the relative success of pain management in different surgical specialities. Such audit data can lead to changes in practices and a refinement of techniques. Audit can also be conducted as part of a wider quality assurance programme, making possible improvements in such areas as the treatment of postoperative nausea and vomiting, and extending the scope of nursing actions (Pasero and Hubbard, 1991).

Standard protocols were developed by Ready for PCA and epidural regimes, including nursing and medical care. An important area of APS responsibility is to check that protocols are closely followed in order to ensure consistency and some degree of predictability. An anaesthetist using a vastly different PCA regime could confuse attending medical and nursing staff in the event of a clinical problem. Many regimes can be equally effective, but a standardized regime has the advantage of familiarity.

A 'nurse-based, anaesthesiologist-supervised' model of pain management in Sweden has been described by Rawal and Berggren (1994). The success of this model is attributed to the provision of in-service training for ward nursing staff, the optimal use of opioids and the development of local anaesthetic and patient-controlled analgesia techniques. The policy of routine pain assessment and recording of treatment efficacy is claimed to be the 'cornerstone' of this model. An 'acute pain' nurse specialist makes daily rounds of the surgical areas and reports problem patients to the anaesthetist. This is an important manpower consideration, as an appropriately trained and experienced nurse can offset most of the ward problems, and screen for those that need more medical intervention – thus reducing the workload of the anaesthetic department, which has to provide ward pain control cover in addition to emergency theatre and resuscitation cover.

The 1990 working party report (WPR)

The treatment of pain after surgery is central to the care of postoperative patients. Failure to relieve pain is morally and ethically unacceptable.
(The Royal College of Surgeons of England and College of Anaesthetists, 1990)

This working party consisted of representatives from the fields of surgery, anaesthetics, nursing and pharmacy. It considered the failings – highlighted in many studies over the years – of postoperative pain management, and concluded that the management of pain after surgery in the UK was unsatisfactory. The report advocated the introduction of acute pain teams, such as that described by Ready et al. (1988) in the USA, in all major hospitals performing surgery in the UK. The main aims and recommendations of the report can be summarized as follows:

- improve hospital staff education and challenge traditional attitudes;
- routine and systematic pain assessment, involving the patient where possible;
- a named consultant to be responsible for pain relief policies;
- the establishment of acute pain services in all major hospitals;
- continuous audit and appraisal of the service;
- appropriate standards of monitoring and resources for pain management;
- the safe introduction of new methods.

The working party report was not a technical or detailed publication. It spoke simply of common-sense measures, and cited key works which would be instrumental in assisting the design of effective pain services. However, the report was to have far-reaching consequences, and has become one of the most quoted sources in recent acute pain literature.

The development of the acute pain service in the UK

It was recognized that the use of more sophisticated, technical methods of acute pain control were well developed in the USA, but had not become widespread in the UK. This, it was suggested by Mitchell and Smith (1989), was because the development of techniques such as PCA and epidural infusions may be time-consuming and their correct application requires 'specialist skills and knowledge'. Other personnel in addition to the anaesthetist in charge need to be familiar with the techniques in order to maintain them safely throughout the postoperative period. Their introduction requires careful planning, and must include a comprehensive training programme for all relevant staff (Notcutt and Morgan, 1990).

Rawal and Berggren (1994) comment that the solution to the problem of inadequate postoperative pain relief lies not so much in the development of new techniques as in the development of a formal organization for the better use of existing techniques. This has not always been found to be so straightforward, as Cartwright et al. wrote:

> One approach to improve the situation is to use existing well tried drugs and techniques and, after operation, to follow up and monitor patient comfort closely. This may appear a simple, logical step, but it is fraught with difficulties, prejudices, practical constraints, communication problems and involves hard work.
>
> (Cartwright et al., 1991)

The introduction of new technology for pain management may provide a focus around which a hospital can organize its resources for training and policy changes, and so gain leverage to streamline all practices related to pain control. However, it is important that an acute pain service is not seen as being solely about the acquisition of new technology. 'It is about a change in the attitudes and emphasis by all staff towards the patient in pain' (Swallow, 1994). It is a feature of many APSs that they introduce pain assessment as a routine systematic observation where this had not previously been the case (Hiscock, 1993). Acute pain teams can promote the concept of using pain relief, by whatever method, as a means of enhancing patient mobilization and return to normal functioning. Kehlet (1994) argues that, until there is sufficient research data on 'expensive and elaborate' pain treatment methods, 'we may expect the combination of increased education, use of pain assessment and conventional opioid treatment to be the most widely used techniques.'

Cartwright *et al.* (1991) reported that the 'most difficult barrier' to the introduction of a smooth-running pain service in fact concerned the mundane practicalities of what ward nursing staff were allowed and not allowed to do. Nursing managers had to be persuaded that prescribed variable opioid infusion rates were in principle no different to *pro re nata* (PRN) intramuscular regimes, where the dose and timing can be within prescribed limits, or variable insulin infusion regimes, titrated to blood sugar assessments. The expertise of hospital pharmacists can be useful and influential (Lipman, 1984; Ashby and Taylor, 1994), and they are essential members of the multidisciplinary team.

An anaesthetic-led multidisciplinary team based on the model described earlier by Ready *et al.* (1988) was set up in York. An account of the first year's experience of that acute pain team was published in 1991, a year after the WPR recommendations. The purpose of the team was clear – to improve the management of acute pain throughout the hospital by taking responsibility for: 'the training of medical and nursing staff, organisation of services to provide adequate levels of care, audit and evaluation of new and existing methods of treatment and undertaking clinical research into postoperative management' (Wheatley *et al.*, 1991).

The York team were aware that restriction of new techniques such as PCA and continuous epidural infusions to intensive-care or high-dependency units would result in little improvement for the majority of patients. To ensure the safety and efficacy of these techniques, the service was organized such that standardized treatment regimes were used for both PCA and EIA, the acute pain sister had responsibility for written procedures and in-service training, and there was 24-h availability of an anaesthetist, with designated consultant cover. The introduction of routine pain assessment was described, and the 0–3 scale validated with respect to visual analogue recordings. The daily audit of the service, the use of new technologies, and the greater use of non-steroidal anti-inflammatory drugs (NSAIDs), opioids and regional techniques were all seen to have led to a more consistent standard of postoperative care.

This model of acute pain management has also been adopted in specialist children's hospitals. Each hospital develops its service to suit local requirements, but the overall strategy is the same – a named consultant takes responsibility for the development of the service. Lloyd-Thomas and Howard (1994) list three broad aims of a paediatric acute pain service:

- the safe and successful provision of analgesia;
- training; and
- research and development.

The clinical nurse specialist

It may be unrealistic to expect busy medical or nursing staff to be able to devote the clinical time required to fine-tune analgesia regimes to individual patient responses in a wide range of clinical settings. In view of the variability in patients' analgesia requirements, and the degree of specialist knowledge required by the practitioner, Dodson made the suggestion that: 'There is probably a place for the nurse with a specific responsibility for pain relief who can more carefully use established methods, top-up epidurals and investigate new methods, trying to tailor treatment to the patient' (Dodson, 1982).

The acute pain specialist nurse's role has been strongly associated with the medical interventions, and in particular with the introduction of new technologies such as PCA. Swallow (1994) stated that, in response to difficulties in co-ordinating the use of PCA, such as selecting suitable patients, a member of staff who showed a particular interest 'took on the unofficial role as Acute Pain Nurse.' However, the pain nurse's remit goes much further than simply being a 'pump attendant.'

Mather and Ready claimed that the UK was falling behind America's lead in pain management for two reasons: 'they have acute pain teams and there is greater nurse involvement and education in new analgesic techniques. In the UK we have the technology but not always the ability to apply it' (Mather and Ready, 1994). This statement recognizes that the anaesthetic/medical strides that are possible with new technologies cannot realize their true potential unless the environment in which they must operate – the general postoperative ward – is staffed and supported by knowledgeable, appropriately skilled nurses. Mather and Ready identify the key position that nurse specialists hold in developing the general nurse's ability to care for patients in acute pain.

If ward nurses are to be supported, educated and work within agreed policies and protocols, the clinical nurse specialist (CNS) must be largely involved in this area. In so doing, techniques such as PCA and epidural infusions can be safely and widely used on general surgical wards, as they must if postoperative pain is to be managed more successfully (Carr, 1992). It has also been asserted that the education role of the pain nurse is vital if ward nurses are not to be deskilled – being blindly led into new practices. To some extent this is also true for junior medical staff. It is important that they are not excluded from the decision-making processes of the pain team. This may result in ongoing ignorance of pain management methods, persistent problems and 'damaged relationships between patients and their front line carers' (Austin,

1992). Many pain nurses are actively involved in education programmes, both in the higher education institutions and in smaller ward-based groups.

Unlike chronic pain services, which may require a senior physician's referral to the pain consultant, acute pain services, organized at the ward level through the pain nurses, provide a rapid-response service. This is of course entirely suited to the patients' requirement for prompt treatment of their acute pain. What makes this system work is that the most junior nurses on a ward can feel encouraged to make contact with the pain nurse, who is after all a nurse colleague. This easily accessible system of referral should result in prompt assessment and action by the pain team. If the pain nurse feels that conditions warrant interventions at a higher level, the full weight of the pain services can be brought to bear.

A description of the roles of the acute pain service clinical nurse specialist at the University of Washington Hospital was given by Carr (1992) following a visit there. These included the following:

- establishing and evaluating standards of care in the acute pain management area;
- planning and implementing educational programmes for nurses and medical staff;
- co-ordinating patient care – education and monitoring;
- collection of pertinent data;
- acting as a consultant and resource to all members of the team.

One of the first UK acute pain nurses, working within an acute pain service, to write an account of her area of work was Debbie Hunter (1991). The role she describes is essentially the same as the US pain nurse's role described earlier. The driving force for the creation of her post appears to be strongly linked to the introduction of PCA, as there had been dissatisfaction with the traditional intramuscular analgesia techniques' inability to cope with individual requirements.

The experience of nurse Michelle Hiscock, Pain Control Co-ordinator at the Royal Brompton National Heart and Lung Hospital is similar (Hiscock, 1993). Hiscock describes being made responsible for the introduction of PCA. This was done with the involvement of representatives from nursing, medicine, physiotherapy and pharmacy. Standards for pain control were set and a baseline audit carried out. Education programmes were organized and PCA was successfully introduced. The creation of a specialist nursing position in response to the introduction of new technology following the recommendations of the WPR may be a common experience of many of the recently created UK pain nurses' posts. Lloyd-Thomas and Howard (1994), in a description of the development of a paediatric acute pain service that has introduced PCA and 'nurse-controlled' analgesia, stated that nurse specialists are essential members of a pain service:

Nurse specialists are pivotal to the success of an acute pain service, because they motivate ward nurses, develop nursing protocols for specific analgesia techniques, institute ward nurse education, and supervise the development of patient observation. These are the most important factors enabling safe management of analgesia in general paediatric wards.

(Lloyd-Thomas and Howard, 1994)

Other forces such as quality assurance initiatives, and changes to the scope of professional practice for nurses (United Kingdom Central Council, 1992), while not directly calling for new methods of pain control or specialist nurses to organize them, lend weight and guidance to the role development.

Without the introduction of PCA, clinical nurse specialist development in this field may have evolved, albeit at a slower rate, in response to existing criteria such as the longstanding need for better education in pain management and the need for improvements in quality of care as a response to quality initiatives. CNS development may also have drawn more heavily on the experience of, or been more deeply rooted within chronic pain care, rather than being more narrowly focused on postoperative pain. Anaesthetic department-led postoperative pain management strategies, as the driving force for new technology, may have given the nursing profession the boost it required to realize the creation of a new style of specialist nursing post. It is interesting to note the rank order of major forces which the International Council of Nurses lists as giving impetus to the nursing specialization movement:

1. new knowledge;
2. technological advances; and
3. public needs and demands (International Council of Nurses, 1992).

Perhaps medical intentions and requirements for clinical support should be added to this list.

The way forward

If new technology – the actual hardware and the logistical support required for the medical staff introducing the technique – has been instrumental in bringing about a new speciality within nursing, we must ask where the post will lead in the future. If, as has been shown, there existed nursing and medical research questioning the quality of all aspects of pain management over many years, then the pain nurse's agenda will encompass more than simply PCA provision. It must logically follow that for the pain nurse post to remain viable once PCA is at the top of its growth curve – that is, has become as commonplace as injectable opioids – the concept of the CNS for acute pain must have laid down roots in the culture and practice of nursing.

It has been recognized that there is a role for acute pain services in the training of junior doctors in the art of logical and effective analgesia prescribing. Many pain services have developed hospital-wide prescribing guidelines. Pain nurses are increasingly called upon to advise medical staff on the fine-tuning of analgesia prescriptions. As pain nurses work largely on their own, the reliance on medical staff to sign for changes to the analgesia regime may 'build delays' into the changes recommended (Hahu and Adams, 1995). This may lead to the development of prescribing protocols for pain nurses, working within their consultants' guidelines, to make changes to patients' treatments in response to their efficacy. *The Medicinal Products: Prescription by Nurses, Midwives and Health Visitors Act* (Department of Health, 1992) allows community nurses and health visitors, who have completed a special course, prescribing rights from a limited formulary. This is a very different situation, and in fact hospital protocol development is already covered by existing laws and codes of conduct (United Kingdom Central Council, 1992), but such a move will represent a shift in the ward staff's concept of the role of the specialist nurse, and may risk further deskilling of junior medical staff.

Acute pain teams, once they have made fundamental changes in the practices related to acute pain, must forge stronger links with chronic pain services. Acute pain that is being experienced in non-surgical areas is in need of special consideration. The technical knowledge base and staff management skills honed in the postoperative field can be brought to bear wherever there are acute pain problems. Once the new approaches have become routine, the pain service organization must take on a much wider remit.

Summary

The inadequacies of pain management were increasingly identified during the 1970s and 1980s. Newer techniques such as PCA and EIA were developed and recommended for use on appropriately staffed general surgical wards, but these techniques were not accepted into widespread usage at that time. This was due to a combination of factors, including the cost and reliability of new equipment, and the lack of an identifiable champion to take responsibility for co-ordinating new practices, and fears for safety. The US experience of organized acute pain services and new techniques was described in the medical literature. This model of organization was used in other countries – fledgling services developed in the UK with pioneering champions such as Wheatley in York, Harmer in Cardiff, and Notcutt in Great Yarmouth.

This model was recommended for the UK by the Working Party Report – in particular, that a named consultant should be responsible for a multidisciplinary team which included, ideally, a pain nurse, a pharmacist and a psychologist. Through the organizational weight of such a team, standardized drug protocols and protocols for monitoring patients could be instituted. The routine assessment of pain could take place on a wider scale. Anaesthetic staff can provide out-of-hours ward cover to ensure the availability of on-hand advice on pain relief and patient safety. Ward nursing staff can work at their full potential through policy and training initiatives.

The impact of commercially available, portable and reliable analgesia pumps cannot be overstated (Counsell and Gosling, 1993), but pain teams are about much more than new technology – which is just another means to an end. The employment of specialist acute pain nurses is a logical step to realizing the potential of an acute pain service. Having made profound changes in the management of postoperative pain, and having – through audit and research – been able to demonstrate the effectiveness and safety of the techniques, the way forward for pain services now is to use their organizational abilities and branch out further into the hospital environment to improve the provision of pain relief for all patients who are experiencing acute pain. In addition, closer links need to be forged with chronic pain services in order to provide all patients with high-quality care.

References

Aitken, H.A. and Kenny, G.N.C. 1990: Use of patient-controlled analgesia in postoperative cardiac surgical patients – a survey of ward staff attitudes. *Intensive Care Nursing* 6, 74–8.

Anonymous 1978: Postoperative pain. *British Medical Journal* 6136, 517–18.

Ashby, N.J. and Taylor D.M. 1994: Patient-controlled analgesia and the hospital pharmacist. *Hospital Pharmacist* 1, 38–41.

Austin, J. 1992: Something for your pain, dear? *British Journal of Theatre Nursing* 2, 4–6.

Bruster, S., Jarman B., Bosanquet N., Weston, D., Erens R. and Delbanco, T.L. 1994: National survey of hospital patients. *British Medical Journal* 309, 1542–6.

Carr, E. 1992: Pain-free states. *Nursing Times* 88, 44–6.

Cartwright, P.D., Helfinger, R.G., Howell, J.J. and Siepmann, K.K. 1991: Introducing an acute pain service. *Anaesthesia* 46, 188–91.

Cohen, F.L. 1980: Post-surgical pain relief: patients' status and nurses' medication choices. *Pain* 9, 265–74.

Counsell, D.J. and Gosling, A.S. 1993: Evaluation of the Provider 5500 infusion pump for ward-based epidural infusions: resource and manpower implications. *Today's Anaesthetist* 8, 68–70.

Cuschieri, R.J., Morran, C.G., Howie J.C. and McArdle, C.S. 1985: Postoperative pain and pulmonary complications: comparison of three analgesic regimes. *British Journal of Surgery* 72, 495–8.

Department of Health 1992: *Medicinal products: prescription by nurses, midwives and health visitors Act.* London: HMSO.

Dodson, M.E. 1982: A review of the methods for the relief of postoperative pain. *Annals of the Royal College of Surgeons of England* 64, 324–7.

Dudley, S.R. and Holm, R. 1984: Assessment of the pain experience in relation to selected nurse characteristics. *Pain* 18, 179–86.

Elcock, D.H. 1994: Overdosage during patient-controlled analgesia. *British Medical Journal* 309, 1583.

Fry, E.N.S. 1979: Postoperative analgesia using continuous infusion of papaveretum. *Annals of the Royal College of Surgeons of England* 61, 371–2.

Gould, T.H., Crosby, D.L., Harmer, M. *et al.* 1992: Policy for controlling pain after surgery: effect of sequential changes in management. *British Medical Journal* 305, 1187–93.

Gould, T.H., Upton, P.M. and Collins, P. 1994: A survey of the intended management of acute postoperative pain by newly qualified doctors in the South West region of England in August 1992. *Anaesthesia* 49, 807–10.

Hahu, C.E. and Adams, A.P. (eds) 1995: *Patient-controlled analgesia.* London: BMJ Publishing Group.

Harmer, M. 1994: Editorial: back to basics? *Anaesthesia* **49**, 749–50.

Harrison, A. 1991: Assessing patients' pain: identifying reasons for error. *Journal of Advanced Nursing* **16**, 1018–25.

Hatcher, L.S. and Peacock, J. 1995: Knowledge of commonly used postoperative analgesic regimens in two groups of house officers. *Anaesthesia* **50**, 96–7.

Hiscock, M. 1993: Setting up a patient-controlled analgesia service. *British Journal of Intensive Care* **3**, 144–52.

Hobbs, G.J. and Roberts, F.L. 1992: Epidural infusion of bupivacaine and diamorphine for postoperative analgesia. Use on general surgical wards. *Anaesthesia* **47**, 58–62.

Hockley, J. 1988: Setting standards for pain control. *Professional Nurse* **3**, 310–13.

Hord, A.H. and Kelly, P.M. 1992: University-based acute pain treatment service. In Sinatra, R.S., Hord, A.H., Ginsberg, B. and Preble, L.M. (eds), *Acute pain mechanisms and management*. St Louis, MO: Mosby Year Book, 532–8.

Hosking, J. 1985: Knowledge and practice. *Nursing Mirror* **160**(Suppl.), ii–vi.

Hunter, D. 1991. Relief through teamwork. *Nursing Times* **87**, 35–8.

International Council of Nurses 1992: *Guidelines on specialism in nursing*. Geneva: International Council of Nurses.

Kehlet, H. 1994: Postoperative pain relief – what's the issue? Editorial. *British Journal of Anaesthesia* **72**, 375–7.

Levine, F.M. and De Simone, L.L. 1991: The effects of experimenter gender on pain report in male and female subjects. *Pain* **44**, 69–72.

Lipman, A.G. 1984: Pain management. In Herfindal, E.T. and Hirschman, J.L. (eds), *Clinical pharmacy and therapeutics*, 3rd edn. Baltimore, MD: Williams & Wilkins, 823–44.

Lloyd-Thomas, A.R. and Howard, R.F. 1994: A pain service for children. *Paediatric Anaesthesisa* **4**, 3–15.

McCaffery, M. 1983: *Nursing the patient in pain*. London: Harper & Row.

Mather, C.M.P. and Ready, L.B. 1994: Management of acute pain. *British Journal of Hospital Medicine* **51**, 85–8.

Mitchell, R.W.D. and Smith, G. 1989: The control of acute postoperative pain. *British Journal of Anaesthesia* **63**, 147–58.

Notcutt, W.G. and Morgan, R.J.M. 1990: Introducing patient-controlled analgesia for postoperative pain control into a district general hospital. *Anaesthesia* **45**, 401–6.

Pasero, C.L. and Hubbard, L. 1991: Development of an acute pain service monitoring and evaluation system. *Quarterly Review Bulletin* **17**, 396–401.

Rawal, N. and Berggren, L. 1994: Organisation of acute pain services: a low cost model. *Pain* **57**, 117–23.

Ready, L.B., Oden R., Chadwick, H.S. *et al.* 1988: Development of an anaesthesiology-based postoperative pain management service. *Anaesthesiology* **68**, 100–6.

Rodgers, B.M., Webb, C.J., Stergios, D. and Newman, B.M. 1988: Patient-controlled analgesia in pediatric surgery. *Journal of Pediatric Surgery* **23**, 259–62.

Royal College of Surgeons of England and College of Anaesthetists 1990: *Commission on the Provision of Surgical Services: Report of the Working Party on Pain After Surgery*. London: HMSO.

Rutter, P.C., Murphy, F. and Dudley, H.A.F. 1980: Morphine: controlled trial of different methods of administration for postoperative pain relief. *British Medical Journal* **280**, 12–13.

Schofield, P. 1995: Using assessment tools to help patients in pain. *Professional Nurse* **10**, 703–6.

Scott, I.E. 1994: Effectiveness of documented assessment of postoperative pain. *British Journal of Nursing* 3, 494–501.

Sechzer, P.H. 1971: Studies in pain with the analgesic demand system. *Anaesthesia and Analgesia* 50, 1–10.

Seers, K. 1987: Perceptions of pain. *Nursing Times* 83, 37–9.

Sharma, S.K. and Davies, M.W. 1993: Patient-controlled analgesia with a mixture of morphine and droperidol. *British Journal of Anaesthesia* 71, 435–6.

Simmons, W. and Malabar, R. 1995. Assessing pain in elderly patients who cannot respond verbally. *Journal of Advanced Nursing* 22, 663–9.

Sofaer, B. 1983: Pain relief – the core of nursing practice. *Nursing Times* 79, 38–42.

Swallow, D. 1994: The development of an acute pain service in a specialized Plastic Surgical and Burns Unit. *Today's Anaesthetist* 9, 145–7.

Thomas, N. 1993. Patient and staff perceptions of patient-controlled analgesia. *Nursing Standard* 7, 37–9.

United Kingdom Central Council 1992: *Standards for the administration of medicines.* London: United Kingdom Central Council for Nursing, Midwifery and Health Visiting.

Walco, G.A., Cassidy, R.C. and Schechter, N.L. 1994: Pain, hurt and harm. The ethics of pain control in infants and children. *Pain* 331, 541–4.

Watt-Watson, J. 1987: Nurses' knowledge of pain issues: a survey. *Journal of Pain and Symptom Management* 2, 207–11.

Wells, N. 1985: Responses to acute pain and the nursing implications. *Journal of Advanced Nursing* 9, 51–8.

Wheatley, R.G., Sommerville, I.D., Sapsford, D.J. and Jones, J.G. 1990: Postoperative hypoxaemia: comparison of extradural, I.M. and patient-controlled opioid analgesia. *British Journal of Anaesthesia* 64, 267–75.

Wheatley, R.G., Madej T.H., Jackson, I.J.B. and Hunter, D. 1991: The first year's experience of an acute pain service. *British Journal of Anaesthesia* 67, 353–9.

White, P.F. 1987: Mishaps with patient-controlled analgesia. *Anaesthesiology* 66, 81–3.

Zalon, M.L. 1993: Nurses' assessment of postoperative patients' pain. *Pain* 54, 329–34.

Developing best practice through comparison and sharing

Judith Ellis

Introduction

Identification of what constitutes best practice with such a complex phenomenon as individuals' pain experiences is far from easy. However, pain assessment and management is an area of practice in which all members of the multidisciplinary team, and indeed the patient, would have little difficulty in reaching agreement on the outcome sought. Clinical effectiveness is the 'extent to which specific clinical interventions when deployed in the field for a particular patient ... do what they are intended to do' (National Health Service Executive, 1996). Effective practice in pain control could be seen as interventions which ensure that pain is at a level acceptable to the patient. This outcome appeals to the compassionate nature of individuals involved in care delivery, as few are unmoved by the sight of suffering, but translating this concern into actual and consistent changes in practice requires more than mere good intent. Indeed, a systematic approach is required to develop practice where, having identified and reached agreement on the outcome required, the processes involved in achieving such an outcome are clearly identified and executed with correct allocation of resources.

In many areas of practice there are examples of isolated developments that have arisen in immediate response to problems giving rise to 'pockets' of good practice. The perpetrators, or indeed innovators, of such practices are unaware that if the national picture is considered, it becomes apparent that their effort is being repeated elsewhere. Although ownership of developments is important and recognized as a motivator for change (Wilson, 1992), it is interesting to consider how much further practice could develop with a more co-ordinated effort. Indeed, the primary purpose of the NHS is, as stated in the *Promoting Clinical Effectiveness* (National Health Service Executive, 1996) document, 'to secure through the resources available the greatest possible improvement in the physical and mental health of people'. If developments had been shared, this might have released resources and innovative vigour for other areas.

Co-ordination of effort must also include interdisciplinary working in order to prevent repetition of effort or contradictory developments that may inadvertently occur. For example, nurses should, as with any area of development, work in '. . . an open and collaborative manner with health care professionals and others involved' recognizing and respecting everyone's contribution (United Kingdom Central Council, 1992). This requires members of the interdisciplinary team to problem-solve beyond the confines of their particular knowledge base (Diller, 1990). Such sharing of knowledge and expertise in turn requires professionals to value not only others' input, but also good interprofessional communications. However, there is little evidence to suggest that teams generally '. . . adopt collaborative , integrated styles of working . . .' (Poulton and West, 1993), and indeed research performed to consider interprofessional working between nurses and doctors would suggest that such a relationship is rarely seen (MacKay, 1993; Walby and Greenwell, 1994).

Economic considerations may also threaten the interdisciplinary team involved in caring for a patient with pain. For example, the fewer professionals that are involved in care, the cheaper it may become. Many providers are being asked to justify the employment of professionals allied to medicine, as well as complementary therapists, e.g. acupuncturists. Research into the effect of such intervention upon outcomes is required. Clients and their carers are now also seen as part of the caring team. Working in partnership with clients and their carers is accepted as being desirable (National Health Service Executive, 1995), not only for supporting the delivery of individualized care but also in allowing the identification of patient-focused best practice (London, 1993) which actually meets customer requirements (Carr-Hill, 1992). It is evident that the current move towards focusing the required outcome for best practice or quality care upon the patient, and not professional group practice, has supported the move towards co-ordinated developments that will prevent unnecessary repetition and correctly channel health service energies.

The development of a market system has also supported the drive towards effective pain assessment and management. Most purchaser specification documents include in their quality requirements reference to effective care in this area, not only to the benefit of the patient's actual experience, but also in recognition that poor pain assessment and management may affect the length of the patient episode and thus have cost implications. Whilst purchasers are being encouraged to demand effective care (National Health Service Executive, 1996), concern may arise that, within such a competitive system, innovative developments may not be willingly shared, as good practice may provide a winning edge when competing for contracts. However, for professionals seeking to 'act at all times in such a manner as to safeguard and promote the interests of individual patients and clients' (United Kingdom Central Council, 1992), and for compassionate individuals, such withholding of developments in practice is unjustifiable. A charge may be made for the sharing of specific material, but colleagues must still be supportive in developing practice. Indeed, open sharing and thus resultant comparison may be just the catalyst that is required to develop practice, not only for practising professionals who do not wish to lag behind, but also supporting the identification of necessary resources to develop an adequate service.

The development of best practice in pain assessment and management will benefit all, winning contracts and preserving jobs, but most importantly benefiting the patients. The patient focus must not be lost.

Identifying best practice

Practitioners must fully utilize all available sources of information and support in order to identify best practice. It can be suggested that any development must ensure provision of evidence-based care, and indeed if sound research is available then it should be used. However, various problems exist for practitioners who wish to develop research-based practice. Since the move into higher education some of them no longer have local access to a library, and many have neither the time nor indeed the skills to carry out a systematic review of the literature (Bassett, 1992).

Another issue that needs to be addressed is research that is not shared. It may never have been published, or it may have been published in journals that are infrequently accessed by practitioners. Indeed, as Nolan and Behi (1995) have stated, it may be written in academic or research jargon as a 'shorthand way of conveying complex ideas', but a language that 'may seem unnecessarily obscure'. If research is to be useful in the development of best practice, the 'language of theory' must not be 'divergent from the language of practice' (Tolley, 1995). These problems are increasingly being recognized, and services now exist that aim to meet this need. The Cochrane database, for example, coordinates global systematic reviews, and the Centre for Reviews and Dissemination compiles reports in a user-friendly format.

Some national organizations – for example, the Royal Colleges – have gone a step further and released their own guidelines on effective pain assessment and management. However, these tend to err towards the 'overall achievable', seldom striving for best practice, but looking at what is the minimum acceptable practice by all providers. Many providers use such national guidelines to support them in compiling local standards and guidelines. However, these also err on the side of the achievable minimal standards, rarely pushing back the boundaries of care but mainly being utilized as a monitoring tool, with comparison and therefore support for development only possible within the provider unit. The most useful national guidelines in the development of best practice are those compiled by consumer groups speaking on behalf of the clients and their carers. For example, in paediatrics the organization Action for Sick Children produced a leaflet entitled *Children and Pain* (Action for Sick Children, 1992). It is also useful locally to consider the views of the Community Health Councils as to what constitutes a good service, as these bodies should be responsive to local needs assessment, e.g. cultural issues in care provision.

All opportunities for gaining the patient's viewpoint on what constitutes best practice should be utilized, e.g. by collecting information from patient satisfaction surveys and creating opportunities for joint discussions. Eventually, however, having sought the views of national organizations, research, patients and carers, it is also vital to utilize to the full the vast experience of the professionals. National guidelines may be limiting, research data may not be available, valid or applicable, and patient requests may not be viable within the organizational context of care delivery.

Professionals must be encouraged to draw upon their own experiences, ensuring that professional and not personal considerations are utilized. Increasingly, practitioners are being asked to reflect upon their own professional practice (Atkins and Murphy, 1993), and through the formative function of clinical supervision it is envisaged that this will develop not only their own practice but that of the professions (Butterworth and Faugier, 1992). Indeed, it could be argued that the wider the professional viewpoint the more valuable the consensus view reached, and in fact the greater the sharing that can occur, with wide external comparison achievable. Organizations such as the King's Fund, through its Nursing Development Network, the Centre for Reviews and Dissemination, the Clinical Outcomes Group and the colleges, all assist in this effective network, supplying on request details of others involved in developing practice in an area such as pain control. In addition, the National Centre for Clinical Audit can provide useful information and also comparative data that enable effective sharing of developments.

Using all of this data widens the experiences available to help professionals to reach agreement on what constitutes best practice. The process of reaching such a consensus may be fraught, but it provides a valuable statement that can in itself open up avenues for future research, for example by identifying areas that need researching in order to promote beneficial changes in practice (Department of Health, 1993).

Once best practice has been identified, this can be used as a benchmark against which to compare practice (Lam, 1994; Ellis, 1995), so that those who are achieving can not only share their successes, but also support others in the development of practice.

A benchmark of best practice is therefore reached when the following have been considered:

- research base;
- national guidelines/standards;
- consumer requirements;
- professional consensus.

The identification of a benchmark of best practice is followed by systematic benchmarking. Benchmarking allows structured comparison and sharing (Lam, 1994; Ellis, 1995), and is widely used in industry (Lipsky, 1992), the health care services in the USA, and increasingly by the UK health service. However, benchmarking effort within these organizations even if set in a particular clinical arena appears to focus upon organizational issues (McKeown, 1996), e.g. staffing ratios, and many have clear resource implications (Aspling and Lagoe, 1996), e.g. reduction of waiting times, which will attract contracts, and shorter patient episodes, which will reduce episode costs. Clinical practice benchmarks remain rare, and again could appear to focus upon not only patient-centred focused quality care but also areas with clear resource implications, e.g. benchmarking the prevention and treatment of pressure ulcers (Bankert *et al.*, 1996), which if ineffective may lead to a prolonged length of stay. Pain benchmarking may be seen as similarly motivated, as again inadequate pain management may lead to an increased length of stay. Pain management was indeed the first area considered by the Northwest Paediatric Benchmarking Group (Ellis, 1995) and by groups that have formed subsequently. Although benchmarking and the resultant development of practice are bound to have resource implications, such clinical practice benchmarking groups are clearly presented as focusing upon the continuous improvement of patient-centred care.

The Northwest Paediatric Benchmark Project (Ellis, 1995), using all of the previously listed available resources, identified through professional consensus eight factors in paediatric pain assessment and management that would

	KEY FACTORS	BENCHMARK STATEMENT
1.	Individualized pain assessment tools	Children/parents create their own pain assessment tool
2.	Pain assessed and recorded	Pain assessment is always undertaken and always recorded
3.	Pain control groups	Collaborative multidisciplinary paediatric pain control team
4.	Pain management protocols	Multidisciplinary protocols exist and are used for particular medical procedures and pain control management techniques
5.	Information	Verbal and reinforcing written information on pain control is given which the parents/child fully understand
6.	Documentation of planned care	Care is evaluated and the plan adapted
7.	Continuity of care	Plan for pain control starts on the first contact with the service and continues throughout the care episode (including on discharge from acute care setting)
8.	Partnership in planning	Care planned for pain control by child/carers and multidisciplinary team

Figure 13.1 Key factors in pain assessment and management identified by the Northwest Paediatric Benchmark Group as essential in ensuring that 'pain is at a level acceptable to the child and family' and benchmark statements of agreed best practice

support effective care delivery, with an overall outcome of 'Pain being at a level acceptable to the child and family' (see Figure 13.1).

These benchmark statements denote the identified or agreed best practice in the area. By placing these statements on the end of a continuum of practice and then identifying statements where current practice may exist along the continuum (see Figures 13.2 to 13.9), it is then possible for structured comparison to occur, i.e. benchmarking.

Practitioners in each area can score their practice upon the continuum and then, when the results have been collated, can identify where a higher score is being achieved and therefore seek help, with higher scorers not only sharing their developments but also assisting with action planning for development.

This structured comparison and sharing seeks to support all in achieving best practice. It allows recognition of examples of good practice, prevents complacency among those who claim that they 'do the best they can in the circumstances', supports practitioners' bids for better resourcing for their area if it is 'lagging behind', and allows effective networking to occur for the good of patient care. The factors highlight the development of best practice in three main areas.

Pain assessment tools

It is suggested that best practice in pain management can only be achieved where there is a means of assessing a patients' or clients' pain, and it is of value to consider where known practice areas would score upon the continuums shown in Figures 13.2 and 13.3.

No pain assessment tool is available	A pain assessment tool exists for some clients	Predetermined pain assessment tools exist	Patients/carers create their own pain assessment tool
0 2 4		6 8 10	

Figure 13.2 An example of a Benchmarking Continuum for Pain Assessment Tools (adapted from the Northwest Paediatric Benchmarking Groups Paediatric Pain Benchmark)

Pain is not formally assessed	Pain is assessed and recorded on an *ad hoc* basis	Pain assessment is always undertaken and always recorded
0 2	4 6	8 10

Figure 13.3 An example of a Benchmarking Continuum related to Pain Assessment and Recording (adapted from the Northwest Paediatric Benchmarking Groups Paediatric Pain Benchmark)

In order to respond correctly to a patient's or client's pain experience, and then to ascertain whether the response was effective, it is essential for best practice to assess the problem correctly. In many situations professional expectations of what pain a patient should be experiencing, and not the patient's actual experience, dictate the measures taken to relieve pain. Comparison with other patients undergoing the same operation is used, not the individualizing of care to be best practice for that patient, e.g. a postoperative patient who is prescribed a set number of doses of opiates before only being offered paracetamol. If it is accepted that individuals experience pain differently, then they must also be assessed individually. The assessment of patients who are developmentally mature and whose physical or mental state allows this may appear easy – a simple matter of questioning – but in fact many factors may influence the accuracy of this assessment. First the question has to be asked, and the way in which it is phrased may sway the answer given – for example, the use of closed and biased questioning of the form 'you're not in pain yet, are you?', the implication being that 'no' is the only likely and perhaps acceptable answer. Each time the question may be asked by a different carer, and indeed if no note is taken of the assessment the question may be frequently repeated, and there will be no record of reassessment that could suggest the efficacy of the pain-relieving methods being used.

A tool allows uniformity in assessment and record-keeping which, when consistently used (see Figure 13.3), will not only benefit the individual patient and carers, but will also provide valuable data for audit purposes. The value of tools appears to be unarguable, with many different tools in use, but again the issue of individuality may be raised as individual patients may have different ways of expressing themselves, e.g. patients who are unable for a variety of reasons to verbalize, or patients with special needs. Best practice may therefore be regarded as the existence (see Figure 13.2) and use (see Figure 13.3) of a tool that is actually individualized to that patient. For example, in paediatric oncology children are helped to design their own tools, drawing pictures that they feel express the different levels of pain, accompanied by words which they choose themselves, e.g. 'owie'.

However, for many areas it is accepted that this exercise, which may take some time, does not constitute an effective use of resources, e.g. if 28 day cases are to be admitted in 2 hours. Therefore, best practice in these areas may never reach the benchmark of best practice for all patients, but knowing what is best practice may assist professionals in striving to achieve the best they can in the context within which they are working. Indeed, if a special needs patient who is unable to use the pre-designed tool is admitted to a day-care area, it may be that time is well spent designing an individualized pain assessment tool.

Best practice in most areas requires the availability and consistent use of a pre-designed pain assessment tool. The vast number and variety of tools in use nationwide highlights the need for further research on the effectiveness of tools, but also sadly draws attention to the lack of sharing that occurs, with professionals everywhere using valuable time and resources to design and test yet another tool. In some hospitals it even appears that different professionals caring for the same patient insist on using separate tools.

Best practice must therefore not only be regarded as the existence of a pain assessment tool, individualized where necessary, but may also involve the sharing of that tool with others to prevent 'reinventing the wheel'.

Documentation/record-keeping and continuity

Patients experiencing pain are cared for by a vast number of people during any episode of care – not only by professionals but also by their families, friends, etc. It is therefore essential that, in order to achieve best practice in any area, care delivered and advice given are co-ordinated and consistent. This is dependent upon the establishment of good communication channels with professionals not just working side by side but also interacting (Sweet and Norman, 1995). This is especially important in the management of pain, as poor communication can lead to unnecessary and prolonged discomfort. The need for documented assessment has already been discussed, and it is also vital that planned care which meets the individual patients' needs is fully documented by all involved, so that the plan can be referred to at any time to allow consistency in delivery. For example, pre-emptive analgesia would not be given unless planned for, with carers instead waiting for pain to occur, or pharmaceutical methods might be used unnecessarily when massage had in fact been found to be effective. The sharing of earlier findings is essential, and evaluation must therefore be documented and plans updated (see Figure 13.3 and 13.4). The *Just for the Record* package (National Health Service Training Directorate, 1994) highlights the difficulties that all professionals seem to experience in keeping records. It is therefore important that as well as agreeing upon best practice, professionals also share the solutions that they have found concerning how to keep up-to-date, useful records.

In addition to records supporting professionals in best practice, meticulous record-keeping is also vital in view of the current litigious milieu in which health care decisions are made and care is delivered. It is no longer sufficient to claim as a professional that the care delivered was of a high standard; records kept may be examined in order to substantiate the claim, and may on a continuous basis be freely accessible to patients/clients and their carers. The need to share information therefore does not stop with the health professionals, but

Pain is not identified as a need/problem on the care plan	Pain is identified as a problem and care is planned	There is evidence of implementation of planned care	Care is evaluated and the plan adapted
0 2	4	6	8 10

Figure 13.4 An example of a Benchmarking Continuum related to documentation of planned care for pain assessment and management (adapted from the Northwest Paediatric Benchmarking Groups Paediatric Pain Benchmark)

No verbal pain control information given and no written information available	Verbal information about pain control not reinforced by written information	Written information on pain control given to reinforce verbal information but parents'/child's understanding not checked	Verbal and reinforcing written information on pain control is given which the parents/child fully understand
0 2 .4		6 8 10	

Figure 13.5 An example of a Benchmarking Continuum related to information on pain control (adapted from the Northwest Paediatric Benchmarking Groups Paediatric Pain Benchmark)

must include all those involved in care or likely to be involved in care in any setting (see Figures 13.5 and 13.6). Records that are truly patient-focused would therefore be completed by all individuals involved in care, and would be accessible to all, which includes being written in a language that can be understood by all of the parties involved (see Figure 13.5).

The practicalities of such a stance certainly raise many issues that, if solutions are to be found, would require sharing among those involved beyond the mere design of documentation. For professionals, combined education and training would be essential, to ensure that a common professional language exists (Walby and Greenwell, 1994), and indeed all patients and non-professionals involved would require education and guidance not only to understand entries but also to interpret them correctly. The problems are many, and indeed even joint assessment documentation demanded by the Greenhalgh research (Greenhalgh, 1994) addressing the reduction in junior doctors' hours, proved extremely difficult to implement (Sheffield Centre for Health and Related Research, 1994) with observations in practice suggesting that

No plan exists for the management of pain	Pain management plan only exists from when pain is a problem	Planning for pain management exists only for in-patient stay	Plan for pain control starts on the first contact with the service and continues throughout care episode (including on discharge from acute care setting)
0 2 4		6 8 10	

Figure 13.6 An example of a Benchmarking Continuum related to continuity of care in pain management (adapted from the Northwest Paediatric Benchmarking Groups Paediatric Pain Benchmark)

many professionals who claimed to be participating also maintained their own separate records.

Collaborative care planning is also now frequently cited as the way forward (Hewitson, 1992; Hornby, 1993; Kimball, 1993), with the focus seen as the patient and the plan aiming to formalize the co-ordination of all professionals' input, e.g. all professionals' management of pain appears within the one patient-focused plan. However, this could cause concern in two areas. First, the use of predetermined health-related group collaborative care pathways may fail to take into account the individual needs of the patients, and secondly, there may not be true collaboration in planning, with unequal recognition of the value of each professional's or carer's input.

Multidisciplinary collaboration

Best practice can only be achieved through true collaboration and sharing (Hornby, 1993) with an interdisciplinary team, members of which understand and value each other's input, and with the lead taken by the member who has a major contribution to make in ensuring that required outcomes are achieved for that patient, rather than being attributed the position of leader merely on the basis of membership of a particular profession (MacKay, 1993; Pillitteri and Ackerman, 1993). For example, in pain management many members of the multidisciplinary team may be involved (see Figure 13.7), and although the patient may most value the therapist's input, leadership responsibility may still appear to reside with the named medical practitioner, who visits fleetingly twice a week (Mallick, 1992). This does not constitute interdisciplinary working.

If care is to be patient-focused, all those involved in care should be involved in discussion, including the patient and carers (see Figure 13.8), and even if pre-determined care protocols (see figure 13.9) or care pathways have been identified, the patients must be involved in determining actual care delivery.

However, discussion between all professionals on principles of care and the identification of protocols of care that are guidelines for best practice is of value (Long, 1994) (see Figure 13.9). It allows all of those involved in care to share their particular knowledge and expertise (see Figures 13.7, 13.8 and 13.9), and agreement to be reached on what constitutes best practice. This can then

No pain control team	Uni-professional pain control teams	Collaborative multidisciplinary pain control team	Collaborative multidisciplinary pain control team (knowledgeable about care of specific client group)
0 2	4	6	8 10

Figure 13.7 An example of a Benchmarking Continuum for pain control groups (adapted from the Northwest Paediatric Benchmarking Groups Paediatric Pain Benchmark)

Uni-disciplinary plan for pain control	Plan for pain control only involves health care professionals	Care planned for pain control by patient/carers and multidisciplinary team

| 0 | 2 | 4 | 6 | 8 | 10 |

Figure 13.8   An example of a Benchmarking Continuum for partnership in planning (adapted from the Northwest Paediatric Benchmarking Groups Paediatric Pain Benchmark)

No pain management protocols exist	Ad hoc existence and use of protocols	Multidisciplinary protocols exist and are used for particular medical procedures and pain control management techniques

| 0 | 2 | 4 | 6 | 8 | 10 |

Figure 13.9   An example of a Benchmarking Continuum related to the existence of pain management protocols (adapted from the Northwest Paediatric Benchmarking Groups Paediatric Pain Benchmark)

support the structured development of personnel and the obtaining of resources to ensure that the care which is agreed upon as best practice can be delivered when required. However, difficulties arise in deciding whether protocols are merely guidance or dictate. For example, can they be adapted to patient need, or indeed can a practitioner fail to comply merely on the grounds of professional autonomy? If protocols are based on sound research and have been previously agreed upon, then explanation or indeed justification for transgression should be sought. Claiming professional autonomy as a non-negotiable right is not sufficient (Hugman, 1994; Parkin, 1995).

It is evident that, in considering factors involved in the process which supports achievement of the overall outcome of ensuring that 'pain is at a level acceptable to the patient', the benchmark statements set are not all concerned with achieving best practice in the care of particular patients, but refer to the organization and resourcing of care. This highlights the fact that achieving best practice is not merely a matter of actual patient–professional interaction and care delivery. To ensure effective communication and thus correct and consistent care, appropriate documentation has to be available (Figures 13.2, 13.5, and 13.9) and continuously kept (Figures 13.3, 13.4 and 13.6) and multidisciplinary working and partnership is essential (Figures 13.7, 13.8 and 13.9).

Comparison and sharing

Having set the benchmark for best practice in each factor, it is then of value to encourage practitioners to consider how near they are to achieving that best practice. Benchmarking is one method that can assist in structuring this deliberation by providing continuum statements against which to score (Ellis 1995). However,

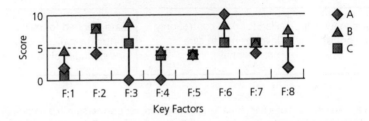

Figure 13.10 Example of a graph that allows comparison of the benchmark scores of hospitals A, B and C in the 8 key factor areas shown in Figure 13.1 (reproduced from the North West Paediatric Benchmarking Group)

the main value of benchmarking is that it allows comparison not only with best practice but also with others who have benchmarked their own practice.

Figure 13.10 shows a comparison line graph which would, for example, allow service A to compare its score in each factor, shown along the *x*-axis, with services B and C. In reality, service A would also need to know the structural and organizational background of services B and C in order to establish whether comparison was realistic. For example, service C may have access to many complementary therapists, whereas service A may be a small isolated service with access only to conventional medical services.

Having compared scores and accepted the reality of comparison, practitioners are then in a position to try to consider why there are differences in the scores achieved. This is where sharing becomes essential. Information may initially be available from the collated comments sent by participants to justify the chosen scores (see Figure 13.11).

In this example, service C is sharing with service A, who are members of their Paediatric Pain Control Group, and this can be immediately acted upon. Service A can send invitations to the individuals listed by service C, also acknowledging whether some attendants at hospital C are not available at hospital A. This may mean that service A will never score as high as service C. This highlights one of the dangers of comparison, which is that in some circumstances it may be demotivating to realize that a score may never be equalled. It is vital that this is not seen as a league table by participants – or

FACTOR SCORE	HOSPITAL	COMMENTS
9	C	Nurses ×2 per ward, paediatric pharmacist, paediatric psychologist, paediatric liaison anaesthetist, aromatherapist, play staff, theatre recovery, clinical audit
6	B	Pain control team hospital-wide = acute pain nurse and anaesthetist who collaborate with ward staff, parent, patient and doctor
0	A	Sister from paediatric ward on adult team

Figure 13.11 An example of a collated comments summary sheet referring to the benchmark continuum shown in Figure 13.8 (pain control groups) (reproduced from the North West Paediatric Benchmarking Group)

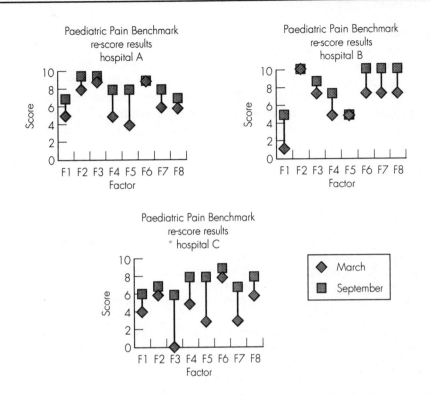

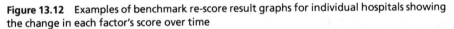

Figure 13.12 Examples of benchmark re-score result graphs for individual hospitals showing the change in each factor's score over time

indeed by their managers – but as a development support tool. It provides a structured means of identifying where to seek help with developments, and who would willingly share. A score on one factor may never be equalled or surpassed, but at least the participants are continuously striving to develop the service and to achieve best practice.

Re-scoring also motivates participants as, although on review the best practice benchmark may have developed further, it is the individual participants' development that is most important and encouraging (see Figure 13.12).

Figure 13.12 shows three examples of the pain re-score results of three paediatric services. In some factors – with the support of others and the sharing of initiatives and ideas – practice has developed, while in others the change is less evident. This may indicate that a decision was made to focus on certain key factors, e.g. the introduction of assessment tools, rather than to dilute effort across all of the factor areas. Overall, it is shown that practice has developed.

Conclusions

Benchmarking is only one way of structuring comparison and sharing in striving to achieve best practice, and it does rely on exceptionally good networking and openness. Research into effective management of a patient's pain is indeed essential, but it only becomes truly valuable if it brings about changes in practice. Practitioners, patients and carers need to use all available knowledge of what constitutes best practice in pain management, and to help each other by sharing what is happening in practice, so that all patients can expect to receive the best possible care. Professionals, and indeed all carers, must accept that comparison needs to be positively regarded as a motivator for change and as essential if care is to develop in a co-ordinated manner with efficient utilization of resources.

References

Action for Sick Children 1992: *Children and pain.* London: National Association for the Welfare of Children in Hospital Ltd.

Aspling, D.L. and Lagoe, R. 1996: Benchmarking for clinical pathways in hospitals: a summary of sources. *Nurse Economist* **14**, 92–7.

Atkins, S. and Murphy K. 1993: Reflection: a review of the literature. *Journal of Advanced Nursing* **18**, 1188–92.

Bankert, K., Daughtridge, S., Meehan M. and Colburn, L. 1996: The application of collaborative benchmarking to the prevention and treatment of pressure ulcers. *Advanced Wound Care* **9**, 21–9.

Bassett, C. 1992: The integration of research in the clinical setting: obstacles and solutions. A review of the literature. *Nursing Practice* **6**, 4–7.

Butterworth, T. and Faugier, J. 1992: *Clinical supervision and mentorship in nursing.* London: Chapman and Hall.

Carr-Hill, R.A. 1992: The measurement of patient satisfaction. *Journal of Public Health Medicine* **14**, 236–49.

Department of Health 1993: *Research for health.* London: Department of Health.

Diller, L. 1990: Fostering the interdisciplinary team, fostering research in a society in transition. *Archives of Physical Medical Rehabilitation* **71**, 275–8.

Ellis, J.M. 1995: Using benchmarking to improve practice. *Nursing Standard* **9**, 25–8.

Greenhalgh Report 1994: *The interface between junior doctors and nurses: a research study for the Department of Health.* Macclesfield: Greenhalgh and Company Ltd.

Hewitson, P. 1992: Collaborative care planning: a team approach to care. *International Journal of Health Care Quality Assurance* **5**, 12–16.

Hornby, S. 1993: *Collaborative care, interprofessional, interagency and interpersonal.* London: Blackwell Scientific Publications.

Hugman, R. 1994: *Power in caring professions.* Hong Kong: MacMillan Press Ltd.

Kimball, L. 1993: Collaborative care. *Journal of Health Care Quality in Promoting Excellence* **15**, 6–9.

Lam, E. 1994: Benchmarking best practice. *Nursing Times* **90**, 48–49, 51.

Lipsky, J.G. 1992: Commentary on how to steal the best ideas around. *Nursing Scan in Administration* **8**, 3.

London, J. 1993: On the right path: collaborative case management makes nurses partners in the care planning process. *Health Progress* **74**, 36–8.

Long, A. 1994: Guidelines, protocols and outcomes. *International Journal of Health Care Quality Assurance* **5**, 4–7.

MacKay, L. 1993: *Conflicts in care. Medicine and nursing.* London: Chapman and Hall.

McKeown, T. 1996: Benchmarks and performance indicators: two tools for evaluating organisational results and continuous quality improvement efforts. *Journal of Nursing Care Quality* **10**, 12–17.

Mallick, M. 1992: The role of the nurse on the consultants ward round. *Nursing Times* **88**, 49–51.

National Health Service Executive 1995: *Partnership in care.* London: Department of Health.

National Health Service Executive 1996: *Promoting clinical effectiveness.* London: Department of Health.

National Health Service Training Directorate 1994: *Just for the record.* Bristol: National Health Service Training Directorate.

Nolan, M. and Behi, R. 1995: Research in nursing – developing a conceptual approach. *British Journal of Nursing* **4**, 47–50.

Parkin, P.A.C. 1995: Nursing the future: a re-examination of the professionalisation thesis in the light of some recent developments. *Journal of Advanced Nursing* **21**, 561–7.

Pillitteri, A. and Ackerman, M. 1993: The doctor–nurse game – a comparison of 100 years – 1888–1990. *Nursing Outlook* **41**, 113–16.

Poulton, B.C. and West, M. 1993: Effective multidisciplinary teamwork in primary health care. *Journal of Advanced Nursing* **18**, 918–25.

Sheffield Centre for Health and Related Research 1994: *Reduction in junior doctors' hours: the nursing contribution.* London: Trent Regional Health Authority.

Sweet, S. J. and Norman, I. J. 1995: The nurse–doctor relationship: a selective literature review. *Journal of Advanced Nursing* **22**, 165–70.

Tolley, K.A. 1995: Theory from practice for practice: is this a reality? *Journal of Advanced Nursing* **21**, 184–90.

United Kingdom Central Council 1992: *Code of professional conduct.* London: United Kingdom Central Council.

Walby, S. and Greenwell, J. 1994: *Medicine and nursing: professions in a changing health service.* London: Sage.

Wilson, D. C. 1992: *A strategy for change: concepts and controversies in the management of change.* London: Routledge.

Useful contacts

Clinical Outcomes Group, National Health Service Executive, HCD-PHIB Room 408, Wellington House, 135–155 Waterloo Rd, London SE1 8UG

King's Fund, Promoting Action on Clinical Effectiveness, King's Fund Development Centre, 11–13 Cavendish Square, London W1M OAN

National Centre for Clinical Audit, BMA House, Tavistock Square, London WC1H 9JP

NHS Centre for Reviews and Dissemination, University of York, Heslington, York YO1 5DD

UK Cochrane Centre, Summertown Pavilion, Middle Way, Oxford OX2 7LG

The prevention of chronic pain

Richard G. Potter

Introduction

Acute pain would appear to be a simple concept familiar to all. It is the classic symptom that prompts people to consult health care professionals, who are expected to take a history of the problem, perform an examination and possibly organize some tests. A diagnosis is then made and a cure prescribed. This 'biomedical' model (Engel, 1977) of illness is entirely appropriate in many situations – a good example would be the diagnosis of an abscess which will be successfully treated either with antibiotics or by surgical drainage. Both clinician and patient are happy with the speedy and successful outcome. Frequently, however, in general medical practice this model may be applied in the absence of a firm diagnosis. Typically the problems are musculo-skeletal in nature and commonly they are spinal in origin. Over the first 4 weeks of such a pain problem this economical way of working is entirely justified by the need to exclude serious organic pathology and the knowledge that the natural history of the condition is favourable.

In contrast, chronic pain is a complex model (Tait *et al.*, 1989) comprising nociception (nerve fibre impulses), behavioural responses and cognitive factors (the sufferer's ideas about their illness). Such a model needs to be matched by an approach to care which has been termed 'biopsychosocial'. In some patients there may be a clear pathological diagnosis such as rheumatoid arthritis – the model holds no less true here and there is much evidence that psychosocial factors strongly influence such a patient's pain experience. However, many patients originally describe only minor trauma or an insidious onset of pain, and multiple investigations show no significant abnormalities. Clinical medicine has now matured so that we no longer automatically stigmatize such patients as malingerers or being prone to imaginary pains, but science is still struggling to identify the pathological basis of the disturbance, although we strongly suspect that it lies within the nervous system itself. We have, after all, accepted trigeminal neuralgia as a *bona fide* medical condition.

One of the great challenges for primary care is to gain a better understanding of why some patients with seemingly straightforward acute pain problems proceed to develop chronic pain and disability, despite the lack of a pathological diagnosis. Until such understanding is gained, we must amend our methods of pain management based on the evidence that we do have in order to reduce the incidence of chronic disability. The epidemic of chronic low back pain and disability over the past 10 years bears witness to the failure of medical management of these patients.

I intend to categorize pain according to its duration. I would define acute pain as that which is present for less than 4 weeks. Chronic pain has arbitrarily been defined as that which is present for longer than 6 months. I have introduced a third category, termed pre-chronic pain, which is pain that has been present for between 1 and 6 months. This label is intended to highlight a window of opportunity for the prevention of chronic pain.

Low back pain provides the paradigm for pain management because of its prevalence and its propensity for causing disability. The brisk biomedical approach is initially appropriate in a busy primary care setting especially when armed with the knowledge that 85 per cent of patients will have recovered within 6 weeks. However, there is a dramatic reduction in cure rate after 4 weeks, with 10 per cent of these patients still experiencing pain at 6 months.

Too frequently chronic care is practised as acute care repeated *ad nauseam*. A progressive shift from the biomedical to the biopsychosocial model of care should occur during the pre-chronic phase. Where a diagnosis cannot be made, a multidimensional formulation of the patient's problem will pave the way for a multidisciplinary approach to management. Aristotle described pain as 'an agony of the mind', a definition which was not bettered until 1986 when the International Association for the Study of Pain defined it as 'an unpleasant sensory and emotional experience associated with actual or potential tissue damage, or described in terms of such damage'. If we do not recognize the nature and danger of chronicity in the pre-chronic phase, repeated biomedical attempts at treatment are at risk of yielding only frustrated doctors, patients with disproportionate pain and disability, and wasted health care resources.

An epidemic of chronic pain and disability?

Despite the decline in heavy industry, the incidence of chronic low back pain has increased inexorably. This has major implications for the individuals involved, their families, and the costs to both employers and the state. Estimates suggest that the cost of back pain to the NHS is some £300 million annually, due to expenditure in both primary and secondary care (Table 14.1) (Moffat *et al.*, 1995). Between 1986 and 1992 sickness and invalidity benefit claims generally increased by 60 per cent, but for back pain the figure was 104 per cent (Moffat *et al.*, 1995). The vast majority of pain problems are managed in general practice. In an analysis of 1000 consecutive consultations in general practice, I established that 29.4 per cent were primarily for a pain problem of less than 3 months' duration. In total, 11.3 per cent of consultations involved a request for advice about a pain problem of duration over 3 months; the corresponding figure for pain of greater than 6 months' duration was 8.1 per cent (Potter, 1990). Figures for the prevalence of chronic pain in the region of 10 per

Table 14.1   Estimated annual health care demands for back pain (UK)

	Number of patients	
	1985 Office of Health Economics	1993 Clinical Standards Advisory Group
Surgical operations	11 000	24 000
In-patient treatment	63 000	100 000
Out-patient treatment	333 000	1 600 000
General practice consultations	22 200 000	3 700 000

cent are consistently found in both population studies and analyses of work-load in primary care. Of the 10 per cent of the population with chronic low back pain, perhaps 1 in 10 are disabled.

The term 'epidemic' seems to be justified and may help to galvanize us into action, although an explanation remains elusive. Increasing frequency of physical trauma or another organic cause are the most obvious possibilities, but there is no evidence of either. Indeed, our system of medicine is well prepared for such pathology, and we know that only 2 per cent of acute low back pain presentations are subsequently found to have a serious and specifically treatable lesion. The vast majority of these will be diagnosed during the early weeks of the problem. One of the primary concepts in the understanding and treatment of chronic pain is the patient's usage of passive coping strategies (e.g. bed rest, taking medication) and active coping strategies (e.g. gentle exercise, trying to distract oneself from the pain) (Jensen et al., 1991). An individual's behaviour in response to pain is governed by their 'locus of control'. This concept describes a person's perception of their problem either as one that they must solve themselves (internal locus) or one that must be solved by others (external locus) (Crisson and Keefe, 1988). If this phenomenon is a determinant of chronic pain behaviour, I am immediately tempted to speculate that it also governs the decision of a patient with an acute pain problem to consult or continue to consult a health care professional.

Consultation behaviour in general practice has long been studied. Over 30 years ago researchers pooled data from several studies in order to explore the relationship between the prevalence of illness and the utilization of health care services (see McWhinney, 1989). It was found that 75 per cent of an adult population reported an illness over the course of 1 month, but only 25 per cent consulted a doctor. Furthermore, it was demonstrated that for a given complaint, e.g. headache, pyrexia, or backache, there were wide variations in the likelihood of individuals consulting a doctor. Many factors appeared to influence the decision, including age, sex, socio-economic status, levels of anxiety and stress, and the state of interpersonal relationships.

Two concepts remain crucial in the consideration of consulting behaviour. In 1961, Mechanic (1961) defined 'illness behaviour' as 'the ways in which given symptoms may be differentially perceived, evaluated and acted (or not acted) upon by different kinds of persons'. The second concept is that of the 'sick role' described by Parsons (1951), in which the social dimensions of an illness were identified. The privileges of occupying the sick role include relief from financial responsibilities (i.e. going out to work) and being excused from interpersonal functions (e.g. being head of a household, childcare, sexual relationships, preparing meals). However, the role also has obligations, the most conspicuous of which is the continued search for a cure. As a primary care physician with an interest in chronic pain I suggest that the concepts and factors which determine consultation behaviour are identical to those which govern chronic pain behaviour. The acceptance of this hypothesis might provide insights into both the causes of the epidemic of chronic pain and the possible therapeutic manoeuvres which could be used to prevent the progression from acute to chronic pain.

The role of primary care

To paraphrase McWhinney (1989), the special skills of general practitioners and, by extension, all members of the primary health care team can be characterized as follows:

- the solution of undifferentiated clinical problems;
- preventive skills and risk factor identification;
- therapy based on multidimensional assessment;
- resource management skills.

A multidisciplinary team practising these skills at primary care level is potentially the ideal model to employ to tackle pain problems before the patient develops inappropriate chronic disability. In practice, however, this ideal has failed to emerge and the epidemic has proceeded apace. I perceive the reasons for this to be the workload pressures on primary care and a continued preference for biomedicine in both clinical practice and NHS administration. There are more optimistic signs, however, of which the 1994 Report of the Clinical Standards Advisory Group Committee on *Back Pain* is the clearest (Clinical Standards Advisory Group, 1994). Nevertheless, this document gives little consideration to cognitive factors, and implementation is likely to be haphazard.

An information booklet such as *The Back Book*[1] is an efficient medium through which to educate patients. This advice may well help 'willing disciples' regain function more quickly. However, I do not believe that this intervention alone would be sufficient to prevent a case of chronic pain.

It has taken the anaesthetists some 25 years to establish chronic pain as a discrete clinical entity rather than a symptom. This transformation has led to the development of broadly based therapeutic modalities for pain management. Like many other disciplines, pain specialists often feel that treatment would be more effective if patients were referred earlier. One way round this

[1]*The Back Book*, published in 1996 by the Stationery Office Ltd, St Crispins, Duke Street, Norwich NR3 1PD.

problem might be to employ the concept of pain management in primary care more widely. The following steps are required:

1. general acceptance that 'pain' may be the primary problem even in the first few weeks after onset;
2. investment of clinical time in a multidimensional assessment of the patient's problem;
3. effective teamwork with liaison to deliver a truly multidisciplinary therapeutic intervention.

The challenge is to incorporate such a system into the current workings of general practice (Potter, 1989). Interestingly, such a reorganization may not involve as many conflicting objectives as might at first appear. Step 3 could be achieved within a wide-ranging and forward-thinking review of the ways of working and responsibilities of primary health care team members.

Acute pain

When an individual first presents with an acute pain problem the imperative is the biomedical approach – a history of the pain, including its site, frequency, intensity, description, exacerbating and relieving factors and any associated symptoms. A past history of similar or other pain problems or other illnesses may suggest a cause for the current problem. A physical examination will give the patient confidence and may elicit diagnostic physical signs or important negative findings. Further investigations such as X-rays, blood tests, referral to a specialist or even hospital admission may be indicated. The whole process has generally been swift and focused and the questioning closed and doctor-centred. A specific diagnosis is made and curative treatment prescribed. Low back pain is rarely associated with serious underlying pathology such as malignancy or spinal cord compression, and these are usually diagnosed early. When no specific diagnosis is made, a knowledge of a favourable natural history of the complaint will be helpful in advising the patient.

In the management of a patient with a chronic pain problem, one important concept is a shift in the discussion from the intensity of the pain, with which the patient is frequently obsessed, to the activities that are performed and function that might be achieved. In the case of acute low back pain, doctors in the past were prone to advising excessive and prolonged rest. It is therefore not surprising that patients continue to feel that this is the correct treatment. We now know that 'early activation' after only 2–3 days of rest holds the best hope of preventing chronic pain and disability (Linton *et al.*, 1993). I suspect that busy doctors sometimes find it easier to collude with patients and agree to the more passive approaches to the control of pain, rather than to challenge the patient's ideas – the dangers are evident. I often advise patients that the only reason why I am prescribing painkillers is to facilitate their early mobilization. If little progress has been made 2 weeks after the onset of pain, physical treatment such as physiotherapy, osteopathy or chiropractic should be instituted if this has not already taken place. In the majority of cases steady improvement will occur, although further consultations may be useful to encourage complete resolution.

Pre-chronic pain

Failure of a pain problem, and typically of low back pain, to show sustained improvement after the first 4 weeks carries increasing risks of chronic pain and disability. Further efforts to exclude surgically treatable pathology such as a magnetic resonance imaging (MRI) scan may be justifiable, but there are risks. First, delays occur while waiting for tests or opinions, during which no progress is made. Secondly, the biomedical model of care is perpetuated whilst cognitive and behavioural factors may be intensifying. Thirdly, an abnormality may be found on investigation which is of little relevance to the pain but may be an expedient 'explanation' to give to the patient prior to discharging them from the orthopaedic clinic or finishing a consultation with the nihilistic advice to 'go away and live with it'.

A study of 98 MRI scans on healthy volunteers which demonstrated lumbar disc abnormalities in 64 per cent of cases, and the well-known lack of prognostic value of 'wear and tear' on lumbar spine X-ray both reveal a potential for the false attribution of symptoms to these findings (Jensen *et al.*, 1994). A pain patient's negative ideas about their problem will be compounded and their 'catastrophizing' about a dire prognosis will be intensified. Furthermore, the failure of modern medicine to cure the problem will be increasingly evident.

A shift in approach needs to be considered in order to redefine the problem in 'biopsychosocial' terms. One cue I have used is to look at the patient and consider not 'what is the cause of their *pain*' but 'what is the cause of their *distress*'. From this point more open questioning can flow, and an exploration of the person's mood, stresses, family and work situations, and ideas about their illness and its treatment can take place.

Our current research at Keele University (Potter *et al.*, unpublished results) suggests that three key factors have independent predictive value in the progression from pain of 4 to 12 weeks' duration over the subsequent 3 months:

- higher pain intensity on the None/Slight/Moderate/Severe verbal rating scale;
- low active coping strategies in the patient's own management of their pain;
- the presence of a past history of a pain problem of 3 months' duration or longer.

These three factors can all be determined or estimated at an ordinary consultation. The usage of coping strategies in particular can move the discussion on to levels of activity and reassurance that increasing function will not cause harm even if it is associated with a slight initial increase in symptoms. This approach can be facilitated by the use of patient information leaflets. Examination of the patient can be extended to include conscious observation of verbal (dramatic description), paraverbal (grunts and groans) and non-verbal (rubbing and grimacing) pain behaviours. Agreement may be reached on management even in the absence of a precise anatomical diagnosis, but the trust of the patient must be retained by explaining that although the cause of their pain is not understood, this does not imply that it is considered to be imaginary. In the absence of direct evidence that a patient is lying, the given description of the subjective experience of pain should always be accepted. Subsequent functional improvement will be accompanied by a reversal of the previous vicious circle of pain and disability.

The team members involved separately in this process are likely to be the doctor and physiotherapist, and possibly the occupational therapist. Failure to respond to the strategy in the standard primary care setting currently leaves the patient in a vacuum that is inevitably filled by further biomedical approaches, referrals to specialists and the consumption of resources with little prospect of appropriate therapy. Ultimately, possibly 2 or 3 years later, referral to a pain clinic may be made, although by this stage the prognosis will be poor.

Advanced pre-chronic pain management

For patients who are stalled in the vulnerable but potentially retrievable pre-chronic period, South Cheshire Health Authority piloted a pain management programme (Kavanagh, 1995; Potter *et al.*, 1996). The philosophy is identical to that of a chronic pain programme, but the objectives are more ambitious in terms of functional recovery and reduction in pain. This therapeutic intervention went well beyond even the Clinical Standards Advisory Group Report guidelines on low back pain, although spinal pain was present in all of our patients. The crucial ingredients were a fully integrated team approach and a concerted cognitive input to challenge the patients' invariably negative ideas about their illness, typically that 'hurt equals harm'.

Most candidates for the programme were waiting for a routine orthopaedic out-patient appointment and were either off work or, if they were not employed, were severely restricted in their daily functioning. The team consisted of a doctor (a general practitioner), nurse, occupational therapist, physiotherapist and cognitive behavioural therapist. The latter was intimately involved in devising the assessment and treatment of patients, but had little direct patient contact. Most of the patients assessed were suitable for the programme, but notable exclusions were those with serious organic pathology, hypochondriasis with little functional impairment, or poor intellectual function. Patients were treated in groups of 6 to 8 subjects in four half-day sessions in consecutive weeks, and were followed up 3 months later. The roles of each team member are set out in Table 14.2, but were by no means exclusive. Indeed, one of the strengths of the approach is that the same 'message' is given by all

Table 14.2 Roles of team members on Pre-Chronic Pain Management Programme

Physician	Clinical history and examination Review investigations and 'diagnosis' Challenge patients' ideas on illness Describe the concept of chronic pain
Nurse	Define patient's ideas on health Introduce usage of coping strategies Importance of sleep and relaxation Intimacy issues
Physiotherapist	Physical examination Education on spinal anatomy/posture Effects of rest and exercise Designing an exercise programme
Occupational therapist	Principles and practice of pacing and goal-setting Seating and stress positions Techniques of relaxation Everyday activities and functions
Psychologist	Underpinning of the input of all the other team members Illness behaviour and negative thoughts and feelings

of the team members. Initial results (Potter *et al.*, 1996) have suggested that 50 per cent of the patients made a full functional recovery, 37.5 per cent made a useful but incomplete recovery and 12.5 per cent of the patients showed a poor response.

The usage and evaluation of this type of therapeutic manoeuvre are in their infancy, but such an approach urgently needs development if modern medicine is to address the threat of the ongoing epidemic of chronic pain behaviour and disproportionate disability.

Summary and conclusions

Chronic pain has a prevalence in the region of 10 per cent and is associated with an epidemic of chronic disability. No physical factor can account for this epidemic, and I have suggested that a parallel can be drawn between consulting behaviour and increasing illness behaviour. Stresses in society (e.g. divorce, job insecurity) increase consultation behaviour, which can act as a safety valve offering the sanctuary of the sick role. A modest physical insult, typically to the lower back, results in disproportionate illness behaviour which in turn enhances and prolongs pain. Ten per cent of patients with 4 weeks of moderate or severe pain and marked disability will proceed to chronic pain (at 6 months) even in the absence of demonstrable organic pathology.

Chronic pain is a concept involving nociception and cognitive and behavioural dimensions, and is a condition with a poor prognosis. The challenge for primary care is to combat the epidemic by employing a multidimensional approach to care during the pre-chronic phase. General practice has the skills and potentially the structure to address this agenda. Much further development will be required if we are to escape the confines of biomedicine, which has so manifestly failed to address this problem.

References

Clinical Standards Advisory Group 1994: *Back pain. Report of the Clinical Standards Advisory Group Committee.* London: HMSO.

Crisson, J.E. and Keefe, F.J. 1988: The relationships of locus of control to pain coping strategies and psychological distress in chronic pain patients. *Pain* 35, 147–54.

Engel, G.L. 1977: The need for a new medical model: a challenge for biomedicine. *Science* 196, 129–35.

Jensen, M.C., Brant-Zawadzki, M.N., Obuchowski, N., Modic, M.T., Malkasian, D. and Ross, J.S. 1994: Magnetic resonance imaging of the lumbar spine in people without back pain. *New England Journal of Medicine* 331, 69–73.

Jensen, M.P., Turner, J.A., Romano, J.M. and Karoly, P. 1991: Coping with chronic pain: a critical review of the literature. *Pain* 47, 249–83.

Kavanagh, J. 1995: Management of chronic pain using the cognitive-behavioural approach. *British Journal of Therapy and Rehabilitation* 2, 413–18.

Linton, S.J., Hellsing, A.-L. and Anderson, D. 1993: A controlled study of the effects of an early intervention on acute musculoskeletal pain problems. *Pain* 54, 353–9.

McWhinney, I.R. 1989: *A textbook of family medicine.* New York: Oxford University Press.

Mechanic, D. 1961: The concept of ill behaviour. *Journal of Chronic Diseases* 15, 189–94.

Moffat, J.K., Richardson, G., Sheldon, T.A. and Maynard, A. 1995: *Back pain: its management and cost to society.* York: Centre for Health Economics, University of York.

Parsons, T. 1951: *The social system.* Glencoe, IL: The Free Press.

Potter, R.G. 1989: Chronic non-malignant pain: time to take on the challenge (editorial). *Journal of the Royal College of General Practitioners* 39, 486–7.

Potter, R.G. 1990: The frequency of presentation of pain in general practice: an analysis of 1000 consecutive consultations. *Journal of the Pain Society* 8, 112–16.

Potter, R.G., Chaddock, C., Crosby, A., Bird, G. and Wilde, V. 1996: *Report of the Pre-Chronic Pain Management Project to South Cheshire Health Authority.* Macclesfield: South Cheshire Health Authority.

Tait, R.C., Chibnall, J.T., Duckro, P.N. and Deshields, T.L. 1989: Stable factors in chronic pain. *Clinical Journal of Pain* 5, 323–8.

Child assent, consent and the refusal of painful procedures

Marilyn Persson and David Bunting

Introduction

Within this chapter the issues of assent and refusal of treatment as they relate to children, and the infliction of pain during medical procedures, will be examined. Many of the issues also have resonance within adult-oriented health care. Definitions of assent, consent and refusal will be proposed, and the resulting tensions that arise when children require painful procedures will be considered. As we practise in a tertiary Children's Hospital in New Zealand we shall reflect a South Pacific perspective, whilst acknowledging common issues with other centres around the world. Article 37 of the United Nations (UN) Convention on the Rights of the Child (1989) states that 'no child shall be subjected to torture or other cruel, inhuman or degrading treatment or punishment'.

If the child is denied a choice in the decision to administer a treatment that involves pain we may be guilty of breaking Article 37. Recognition of developmental and cognitive issues is important when considering children's ability to comprehend issues and to make an appropriate decision. The legal rights of children and their parents and the responsibilities of health care providers are all involved in muddying the waters when a decision is made that conflicts with the child's ability to give assent.

Definitions

Assent, as defined by the *Concise Oxford Dictionary* (Tompson, 1995), means 'to express agreement, to consent, mental or inward acceptance or agreement and to consent or sanction officially'. It derives from the Latin verb *'assentari'* meaning 'to think'. Porter states that:

> Assent is a term frequently used in the context of consent from minor children, who are not legally permitted to enter into a contract. Assent is

not a legal term, and has evolved from the ethical/moral perspective, which recognises the rights and responsibilities of children.

(Porter, 1985)

The Cumulative Index to Nursing and Allied Health Literature (CINAHL) lists only seven references to assent, and in the New Zealand setting the more commonly used expression of agreement is consent. However, the term of assent would appear to be a more appropriate concept to use for expressing agreement, in that assent implies that thought and decision-making are involved in the process. Informed consent is the usual name applied to this process.

Consent, as defined by the *Concise Oxford Dictionary* (Tompson, 1995), means to 'express willingness, to give permission or agree, a voluntary agreement, permission or compliance'. It is derived from the Latin verb *'consentire'* meaning 'to feel'. It has become commonplace that consent is required to be given before treatment is administered in the majority of medical procedures. There are exceptions where the patient may be unconscious or unable to make an informed choice. Legal avenues exist for clinicians to assume the responsibility if necessary. Where pain is expected to be part of this medical process, an explanation of the likely intensity and duration of the pain is necessary when gaining informed consent. Sanchez-Sweatman (1995) states that, in Canada: 'the question of whether a child can consent to medical treatment or whether consent should be sought from the child's parents or the courts is one frequently faced by nurses who work in paediatrics'.

A balance is required between the right of the child to be autonomous and the cognitive development required to comprehend these issues, which include the expected pain, the child's perception or interpretation of the pain, their resources to cope and adapt, and the likely effect of treatment upon the prognosis. Informed consent requires information, comprehension, intellectual competence and the absence of coercion.

Refusal, as defined by the *Concise Oxford Dictionary* (Tompson, 1995), is the 'act or an instance of refusing, the right or privilege of deciding to take or leave a thing before it is offered to others'. It is derived from the Latin verb *'recusare'* meaning 'to refuse'.

A central issue concerns how willing we are as health care providers to accept a child's refusal of a procedure that involves pain. Many of us may have heard the statement 'they will just have to get used to it', or something similar. Fowler states that:

> Self determination as an individual's exercise of the capacity to reform, revise and pursue personal plans for life does not know the boundaries of age. The paediatric population is a large aggregation that includes the very young and the almost adult.

(Fowler, 1988)

Because of the widely differing developmental level of understanding within this age range, the nature of the procedure and the age of the child become critical. A toddler who refuses a 'finger prick' for a blood test by crying and struggling is worlds apart from a teenager who refuses chemotherapy after giving a considered evaluation of their prognosis.

Tensions between consent and refusal

Tensions arise between assent, consent and refusal in a variety of clinical situations. If the child assents or consents to treatment that the adults think necessary, then problems do not usually occur. However, if the child refuses, there is a dilemma about whether their right to a decision should be upheld, or conversely whether it should be ignored and the procedure carried out regardless. Lansdown (1996) reports an additional twist to the consent–refusal debate. He states that 'American law in some states gives parents the right to consent to medical care for their dependent children but not the co-equal right to refuse care deemed medically necessary' (Lansdown, 1996, p.230).

It is important to bear in mind that consent/assent and refusal are rarely co-equal rights. The concept of 'best interests' also has relevance, since some decisions may be made in the best interests of the child even if this is contrary to their expressed wishes. However, as Rose points out, 'There is little discussion regarding what constitutes a "best interest" or how professionals know what it is' (Rose, 1997, p.74).

Charles-Edwards emphasizes that the 'best interests test' is 'an imperfect measurement but is the best available' (Charles-Edwards, 1995, p.65). Factors contributing to the consent–refusal dilemma include the age of the child or young person, their cognitive abilities and the developmental stage they have attained. There are no simple answers in relation to these issues. Thompson (1990) states that 'Developmental characteristics are somewhat relative in that individual differences of some children (e.g. abused, terminally ill, depressed or handicapped) may alter their ability to engage in a meaningful interaction meant to inform them and safeguard their rights'.

When children are young they are dependent on adults for the provision of all their life cares. Indeed, parents have a legal responsibility to make decisions about their child's medical care (Luke and Tyler, 1995). However, as children develop in maturity and in the range of their experiences, they begin to be more capable of making what could be considered reasonable decisions. The notion of 'reasonable' creates tensions of its own. This may reflect the perceived balance of risks and benefits (see Figure 15.1).

Issues arise when long-term illness is involved, as the child may move through different developmental stages and their ability to make decisions affecting their treatment may change. An example of this situation might be a child with cystic fibrosis, whose competence to make decisions involving treatment and painful procedures at 3 years of age will differ greatly from their decision-making skills at 14 years of age (Alderson, 1993; Atherton, 1994). However, there is a balance between parental responsibility and their right to decide and the child's autonomy (see Figure 15.2).

These decisions may be based on a variety of factors including prior experience, the understanding of both long- and short-term consequences, the child's view of the world, their trust and security with those giving the care, and the appropriateness of the explanation that they have received. If a balance is not achieved between these factors then the child may be misled or coerced and

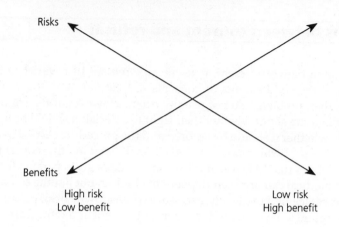

Risks

Benefits

High risk   Low risk
Low benefit   High benefit

Figure 15.1 Balance of risks and benefits (from Charles-Edwards, 1995). Reproduced with permission of Blackwell Science Ltd.

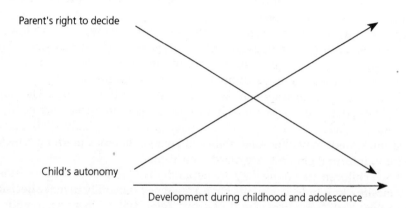

Parent's right to decide

Child's autonomy

Development during childhood and adolescence

Figure 15.2 Parent's and child's right of consent (from Charles-Edwards, 1995). Reproduced with permission of Blackwell Science Ltd.

their decision will not be based on an ethically valid interpretation. It is important to differentiate between a *general* capacity to understand and the *actual* capacity to understand a *particular* situation (Kennedy and Grubb, 1994). King and Cross state that:

> involvement must be appropriate to the level of capacity of the individual child. Intellectual capacity should be considered but also previous experience of the child's decision-making experience, the ability to consider consequences, level of impulsivity, misconceptions and their comfort with being given the responsibility of decision-making.
>
> (King and Cross, 1989)

Internationally there has been an increase in the debate on the child's rights. The Gillick v West Norfolk and Wisbech Area Health Authority (1985) case in the UK and the United Nations Convention on the Rights of the Child (1989) have been significant landmarks in this debate. In 1991 the Department of Health Report stated:

> The rights of children to give consent to treatment were reinforced by a judgement in the House of Lords in 1985 [the Gillick case] which stated that 'the parental right to determine whether or not their minor child below the age of 16 years will have medical treatment terminates if and when the child achieves sufficient understanding and intelligence to enable him or her to fully understand what is proposed.
>
> (Department of Health, 1991)

A decision has to be made by the health professional as to whether the child is competent to consent to medical treatment if he or she is under the age of 16 years. The questions arise as to how this assessment is made, by whom, and what criteria health professionals use. Children mature at different speeds. This is acknowledged by McHale (1996) and is undisputed. Some children of a certain age may be capable of making a decision regarding painful medical treatment, whereas another child of the same age or older may not. McHale (1996) also suggests that the assessment of competence is proportional to the type of decision in each individual case. For example, a child may be able to make an informed treatment decision for a minor procedure but be unable to make a similar decision with regard to other more major treatment (Atherton, 1994).

Children are individuals, and hence should be treated as such. Age in years cannot always be a factor determining whether the child is consulted about his or her wish for treatment. More emphasis should be placed on the child's cognitive ability. This then raises the concern that a child who has been assessed by the health professional as competent to make an informed decision about their treatment, considers the options and refuses!

Legal issues

Cases in law have demonstrated that the assent/refusal to treatment made by the child is respected only when they agree with what the health professional and the parent believe is an appropriate decision. McDowell (1996) states that 'the law in New Zealand as to when a child has the right to consent or refuse consent to their own medical treatment is confused and fragmented'.

The clarity of the legal situation of consent appears to differ widely between countries and even between states. Elliston (1996) highlights the difference between English and Scottish law. They both have set ways to determine whether a child is to be regarded as competent, but the court may overrule this decision in England, whereas in Scotland a child who is considered competent may indeed have their decision respected. In the USA the Presidents' Commission (1982) recognizes the ability of an older child to be self-determining. Each province in Canada also has laws that address competence differently. It is necessary for practitioners to be aware of these legal differences and to consider the lack of clear and consistent legal guidelines as they relate to their own practice.

Painful procedures are only one aspect of treatment, but they can be crucial to the success or failure of that treatment. From a child's perspective, the pain may be the most significant issue. In a practical sense, refusal of consent to a painful procedure may be the first step that a child or young person takes in a decision about their overall treatment. If the child is considered competent to make these seemingly small decisions, then a consensus needs to be reached involving the child, his or her parents and the clinical team as to how overall decisions about treatment are to be made.

At times, when there is conflict, even the parental decisions can be overruled. This occurs when the health professional uses legal avenues to enforce treatment. Thus power can be seen to be transitory, with no single person wielding it consistently. Historically, children were seen as vulnerable and in need of adult protection. This is in contrast to the modern view that children have the right to decide on the matters that affect them most directly (Children Act, 1992). However, although this view is widely proposed, difficulties remain in the implementation of these valued principles. Atherton suggests that:

> our own personal belief system may be influenced by the stance we take between these two points. The position that we take on these contrasting views not only affects what rights we believe the child has, but also how hard we are prepared to protect those rights.
>
> (Atherton, 1994)

Strategies

A number of key questions appear to be significant in considering assent and refusal (see Table 15.1). These questions compel professionals to consider what is deemed reasonable in the process of gaining the child's assent to a painful procedure.

Previous bad experiences can result in children developing generalized anxiety about their health care, as well as extreme distress in response to specific procedures (Jay *et al.*, 1983). Psychological preparation for children and their parents prior to medical procedures is imperative (Patterson and Ware, 1988; Smith *et al.*, 1989, Douglas, 1993). A basic approach would involve giving the child understandable information about the impending procedure at a cognitively appropriate level (Douglas, 1993; Medforth, 1995). This needs to occur in a psychologically supportive environment in which the attitudes of staff display trust and respect for the children's decisions (Alderson, 1991). Psychological preparation using a doll to 'play out' the procedure and a book

Table 15.1   Questions of significance in terms of assent and refusal

- How much should the child know?
- Who is best qualified to make the final decision? (child, parents, physicians or courts)
- What is the decision based on? (research, experience, anecdote, or trial and error)
- When is a child old enough to have his or her decision respected?
- Is this decision only to be respected if it complies with what we as the health team believe is in the best interests of the child?

of photographs illustrating what would happen were found to have beneficial effects on children undergoing lumbar puncture for chemotherapy (Månsson et al., 1993).

The role that paediatric nurses, pain nurses, play specialists and colleagues have in preparing the child for the painful procedure is vital in assisting the child during this difficult time. Preparation for the procedure should involve teaching the child, as well as the parents, strategies for coping with the procedure ahead. Strategies such as relaxation, breathing, distraction, positive self-talking, hypnosis and creative imagery and other non-pharmacological techniques can be readily taught to the child and parents and used during the procedure (Kuttner, 1989; Broome et al., 1992; Broome, 1994; Carter, 1994; Pederson and Harbaugh, 1995). The teaching of these techniques helps the child to gain a sense of competence, control and age-appropriate independence.

McGrath and deVeber (1986) demonstrated that a supportive presence helped children to deal with repeated lumbar punctures. Involving parents in a support role during the procedure helps the child to cope with the painful aspects (Dolgin and Phipps, 1989). Visintainer and Wolfer (1975) found that children coped better when their parents were present. However, caution is needed, and Jay et al. (1983) have reported a 'positive correlation between parental anxiety and the distress children experience with medical procedures'.

It is important to remember that parental presence may actually increase manifestation of the child's distress (Blount et al., 1990; Manne et al., 1992; Dahlquist et al., 1994, 1995). Pharmacological interventions should be used in conjunction with these supportive strategies for painful procedures. Preparations such as topical local anaesthetics, e.g. EMLA® cream, should be an integrated part of procedures such as venipuncture (Alder, 1990; Anderson et al., 1993). It is important that the appropriate medication is used – one which will effectively reduce the pain during a procedure and not simply sedate the child. Using an inhalation analgesic such as Entonox for the child who is able to hold the mask him- or herself is effective as it not only gives the child the control over their pain management during the procedure, but it also combines the technique of focusing the child on their breathing and relaxation. Following appropriate teaching and explanation to both child and parent, the use of analgesic agents can provide adequate pain relief during short pain-evoking procedures. Other pharmacological agents can also be used effectively. Strategies such as timing the peak effect of the analgesic medication in conjunction with the painful procedure should be planned when using analgesic agents. In some cases general anaesthesia may be the most appropriate and sensitive option.

How well the initial procedure is managed will influence subsequent medical procedures and the child's willingness to assent to future painful procedures. When a child copes successfully with a procedure, his or her confidence is increased. Care should be taken with each painful procedure to manage it most effectively. The procedure should not be treated in isolation, but rather in the context of subsequent events that the child may have to encounter and endure.

If a negative experience occurs, then it is crucial that there is an opportunity for the child to talk about what happened to them. Being able to express their anger and fears is vital if improved strategies for any future procedures are to be instigated. Sugarman (1990) states that 'pain increases anxiety and that pain can be minimised through prediction, prevention, awareness and acknowledgement of pain'.

In the 1990s children are being taught to respect their bodies, to know about what is 'good' and 'bad' touching, and that they have the power to refuse adult touching with which they are uncomfortable. It seems contradictory that the control of their body should be relinquished when they are receiving health care. Pearce (1994) suggests that an important role of nurses is in the prevention of the 'erosion of a child's right to self-determination and autonomy'. Nurses are able to achieve this by involving the child in decisions that affect them. The nurse is often the person who is most able to provide age-appropriate information and explain treatment implications clearly. This helps the child to develop an informed opinion about his or her treatment. A nurse is likely to be the professional who spends the most time with a child in hospital and is in a unique position to help the child with this process. An essential part of the development of trust by the child and their family is honesty. As health professionals we must be prepared to be honest with children when we explain procedures. The extra time spent in preparation and explanation may reduce the likelihood of further problems with painful procedures. It is better to say 'this will hurt, but we can help you with some ways to be able to cope with the pain', rather than for the child to be misled.

New Zealand perspective

The situation in New Zealand is in many ways comparable with that in other countries. The legal situation is unclear, with the Courts enforcing treatment against a child and his or her parents' wishes on more than one occasion in recent years. The consensus among those working in children's health is that the rights of the child are becoming increasingly recognized and considered.

Unfortunately, the use of restraint for the imposition of treatment against a child's wishes does still occur. However, by using a considered approach that includes appropriate explanation to the child and consultation with the parents, children can be given a sense of choice and some power over the circumstances of the procedure.

These strategies, which are frequently employed in clinical practice in New Zealand, help to reduce the occurrence of refusal and gain the child's assent to the procedure. However, it needs to be acknowledged that this does not fully enshrine a child's rights, and it relies on the 'good will' of the practitioners involved. The comment has been made in discussing this issue with a number of practitioners in New Zealand that if a refusal occurs it is most likely to be because of fear or anxiety about the likely pain, and that if adequate preparation is given, then the experience for the child is greatly improved.

If negotiation is possible, then those involved can help the child to make a decision that is appropriate and that can minimize the pain and reduce the likely incidence of similar problems in the future. LeBel-Schwartz (1990) has commented that the 'interpretation of a painful stimulus is influenced by physical, cognitive, emotional and social factors'. If we are able through our practice to have some influence on each of these factors when we care for a child, then the overall outcomes can be more positive. It is the nature of the health care system that, when presented with a life-threatening event, action must be taken. In these circumstances consideration of assent or refusal may be difficult or even impossible. If precipitous action has been taken then the child and family need to be followed up so that they gain a better understanding of these intense experiences. In this way post-traumatic stress may be reduced.

Awareness of the cultural background of the child and how this affects their ability to express their own views must be paramount. Consideration of whether they would feel comfortable saying 'no' to a health professional, and how their culture may view pain, is necessary in order to facilitate appropriate responses to their pain and management of the issues of assent and consent.

The health system in New Zealand is predominantly government funded. The government was a signatory to the Treaty of Waitangi (1840) along with the Maori who are New Zealand's Tangata Whenua (first people). This Treaty, signed in 1840, enshrined in law certain Maori rights. In recent years greater commitment has been shown to honouring the treaty, and part of this has resulted in increased consideration of Maori attitudes to health. Most hospitals now have Maori health workers on their staff who work from a Maori health perspective and are able to provide a service that can help to bridge this cultural gap.

Conclusions

In conclusion, the right of the child to make a decision either to assent to or refuse a painful procedure is a right that has gained more prominence in recent years (Department of Health, 1991). A balance needs to be struck between the rights of the child, the wishes of the parents, the urgency or necessity of the procedure and the clinicians' need to provide treatment that adheres to the relevant ethical and legal systems. Currently, it would appear from the literature that most countries have adopted a conservative approach which values the views of parents and clinicians over those of the child. This situation may be in the process of changing, and we need to be prepared for the impact that this will have on our practice. Obviously the developmental and cognitive level of the child must be taken into consideration.

In the future we believe that it will become necessary to look at the issue from the child's perspective and for their views to act as a guide to our intervention. The situation that currently exists in New Zealand is that age in years is the factor which determines whether the child's or young person's wishes are upheld. At present there is no clear precedent to guide the way. We must each evaluate our own perspectives and our beliefs about children's rights. As health professionals working with children we must uphold their rights, especially when they are associated with painful procedures. Children are often unaware of their right to pain relief, and rely on others to relieve their pain and protect them from harm. We must therefore maintain our role as advocates of the child's right to make decisions. Elliston (1996) challenges the law to 'protect the decision-making of competent persons, not the competent person themselves'.

References

Alder, S. 1990: Taking children at their word. *Professional Nurse* 5, 398–402.

Alderson, P. 1991: Children's consent to surgery. *Paediatric Nursing* 3, 10–13.

Alderson, P. 1993: *Children's consent to surgery.* Buckingham: Open University Press.

Anderson, C.T.M., Zeltzer, L.K. and Fanurik, D. 1993: Procedural pain. In Schechter, N.L., Berde, C.B. and Yaster, M. (eds) *Pain in infants, children and adolescents.* Baltimore, MD: Williams and Wilkins, 435–58.

Atherton, T. 1994: The rights of the child in health care. In Lindsay, B. (ed.) *The child and family. Contemporary nursing issues in child health care.* London: Ballière Tindall, 3–21.

Blount, R.L., Sturges, J.W. and Powers, S.W. 1990: Analysis of child and adult behavioral variations by phase of medical procedure. *Behavior Therapy* 21, 3–48

Broome, M.E. 1994: *Parents in pain.* Paper presented at Collaboration in Care Conference, 10–12 November 1994, Jersey, Channel Islands.

Broome, M.E., Lillis, P.P., McGahee, T.W. and Bates, T. 1992: The use of distraction and imagery with children during painful procedures. *Oncology Nursing Forum* 19, 499–502.

Carter, B. 1994: *Child and infant pain: principles of nursing care and management.* London: Chapman and Hall.

Charles-Edwards, I. 1995: Moral, ethical and legal perspectives. In Carter, B. and Dearmun, A.K. (eds.) *Child health care nursing: concepts, principles and practice.* Oxford: Blackwell Science, 61–75.

Dahlquist, L.M., Power, T.G., Cox, C.N. and Fernbach, D.J. 1994: Parenting and child distress during cancer procedures. A multidimensional assessment. *Children's Health Care* 23, 149–66.

Dahlquist, L.M., Power, T.G. and Carlson, L. 1995: Physician and parent behavior during invasive pediatric cancer procedures: relationships to child behavioral distress. *Journal of Pediatric Psychology* 20, 477–90.

Department of Health 1991: *Welfare of children and young people in hospital.* London: HMSO.

Dolgin, M.J. and Phipps, S. 1989: Pediatric pain: the parents' role. *Pediatrician* 16, 103–9.

Douglas, J. 1993: *Psychology and nursing children.* London: Bristish Psychological Society Books, in conjunction with Macmillan.

Elliston, S. 1996: If you know what's good for you: refusal of consent to medical treatment by children. In McLean, S. (ed.), *Contemporary issues in law, medicine and ethics.* Darmouth: Aldershot, 29–56.

Fowler, M. 1988: Paediatric informed consent. *Heart and Lung* 17, 584–5.

Gillick v West Norfolk and Wisbech Area Health Authority 1985: All ER 402.

Jay, S.M., Ozlins, M., Elliott, C.H. and Caldwell, S. 1983: Assessment of children's distress during painful medical procedures. *Health Psychology* 2, 133.

Kennedy, I. and Grubb, A. 1994: *Medical law: text with materials,* 2nd edn. London: Butterworths.

King, N.M.P. and Cross, A.W. 1989: Children as decision-makers: guidelines for paediatricians. *Paediatrics* **115**, 10–16.

Kuttner, L. 1989: Management of young children's acute pain and anxiety during invasive medical procedures. *Pediatrician* **16**, 39–44.

Lansdown, R. 1996: *Children in hospital. A guide for family and carers*. Oxford: Oxford University Press.

LeBel-Schwartz, A. 1990: Pain management in children. In Jellinek, M. and Herzog, D. (eds), *Psychiatric aspects of general hospital paediatrics*. Chicago: Year Book Publishers, 98–113.

Luke, S. and Tyler, J. 1995: Children: parental responsibility. *British Journal of Nursing* **4**, 847.

McDowell, M. 1996: *Medical treatment and children: assessing the scope of a child's capacity to consent or refuse to consent. Parental authority and the exercise of freedom of religion*. Unpublished thesis, Univesity of Auckland, Auckland.

McGrath, P. A. and de Veber, L.L. 1986: Helping children cope with painful procedures. *American Journal of Nursing* **86**, 1278–90.

McHale, J. 1996: Consent to treatment and the child patient. *Health Care Risk Report* June, 14–16.

Manne, S.L., Bakeman, R., Jacobsen, P.B., Gorfinkle, K., Bernstein, D. and Redd, W.H. 1992: Adult–child interaction during invasive medical procedures. *Health Psychology* **11**, 241–9.

Månsson, M.E., Björkhem, G. and Wiebe, T. 1993: The effect of preparation for lumbar puncture on children undergoing chemotherapy. *Oncology Nursing Forum* **20**, 39–45.

Medforth, N. 1995: Strategies to reduce children's perception of pain. *Nursing Times* **91**, 34–5.

Patterson, K.L. and Ware, L.L. 1988: Coping skills for children undergoing pain medical procedures. *Issues in Comprehensive Pediatric Nursing* **11**, 113–43.

Pearce, G. 1994: Sensitive choices. *Nursing Times* **90**, 35–6.

Pederson, C. and Harbaugh, B.L. 1995: Nurses' use of nonpharmacologic techniques with hospitalized children. *Issues in Comprehensive Pediatric Nursing* **18**, 91–109.

Porter, J. 1985: Regulatory considerations when children are involved as subjects in research. *Journal of School Health* **55**, 175–8.

President's Commission for the Study of Ethical Problems in Medicine and Biomedical and Behavioural Research 1982: *Deciding to forego life–sustaining treatment*. Washington, DC: US Government Printing Office.

Rose, P. 1997: Best interests versus autonomy: a model for advocacy in child health care. *Journal of Child Health Care* **1**, 74–7.

Sanchez-Sweatman, L. 1995: Children and consent to treatment. *Canadian Nursing Journal* **91**, 57–9.

Smith, K.E., Ackerson, J.D. and Blotcky, A.D. 1989: Reducing distress during invasive medical procedures: relating behavioral interventions to preferred coping style in pediatric cancer patients. *Journal of Pediatric Psychology* **14**, 405–19.

Sugarman, M. 1990: Caring for children in hospitals. In Jellinek, M. and Herzog, D. (eds), *Psychiatric aspects of general hospital paediatrics*. Chicago: Year Book Publishers, 28–40.

Thompson, R. 1990: Vulnerability in research: a developmental perspective on research risk. *Child Development* **61**, 1–16.

Tompson, D. (ed.) 1995: *Concise Oxford Dictionary*. Oxford: Clarendon Press.

Visintainer, M. and Wolfer, J. 1975: Psychological preparation for surgical paediatric patients. The effects on children and parents' stress response and adjustment. *Paediatrics* **56**, 189–202.

Children and their experience of pain

Bernadette Carter

Pain hurts – stupid!

(Jonathan, aged 7 years)

Introduction

Children experience pain as part of everyday life – as part of the rough-and-tumble of growing up. This sort of pain often hurts for a while and then is largely forgotten. A kiss, a cuddle, the right sort of attention, a hanky to wipe up the tears, a suitably large sticking plaster and the chance to tell their friends all about it are often all that is necessary to manage the experience. The majority of painful episodes in childhood occur outside the health care arena. Pain is usually managed within the child's usual environment of family and school. Pain generally becomes the concern of health care professionals only when it is severe enough for the family to seek help, or when the health care professionals are involved in instigating the pain in some way. Whilst everyday hurts are important to the child, it is the 'bigger' pains that this chapter will focus upon. This focus is a relatively recent phenomenon.

Jerrett (1985) identified a real problem when she highlighted the dearth of research focusing on children in the mid-1980s: 'In the vast research on pain, few studies have been done on children, yet their experiences are as of great concern as those of adults' (Jerrett, 1985, p.83).

This was also noted by Beyer and Byers (1985), who highlighted the limited state of knowledge about children's pain. However, little over a decade later the research desert is starting to bloom and the situation is much improved. There has been a surge of interest in children's pain among researchers and practitioners (Gillies, 1993). On the surface it would seem that tremendous progress has been made, and indeed in some ways it has. Yet children's pain is still largely a hidden problem (Cleeland, 1993). There are many areas of children's pain that have not been addressed, either because a problem has not been identified or because the issue is inherently 'tricky' to tackle. Pain research in adults is acknowledged to be difficult and these difficulties are compounded in young children. Communication problems between adults and children lie at the root of some, but not all, of these difficulties. Anand and Craig (1996) acknowledge that issues such as 'self-report' are incompatible with the current International Association for the Study of Pain (IASP) definition of pain (Merskey and Bogduk, 1994). They credit the existing definition as having provided the stimulus for 'seminal advances' in many areas of pain research. However, they analyse the tensions inherent within some of the assumptions upon which the definition is based, and they suggest that these tensions may force the definition to be reconsidered. Their discussion also highlights the progress that has been made in thinking about children's pain, with children's pain now firmly established in professional thinking.

Within this chapter I shall focus on some of the factors which influence the way in which children experience pain (specifically the child-centred charac- teristics) and the coping strategies that children employ to cope with pain. The importance of the family will act as a thread running through the chapter. This discussion will be set in the context of historical attitudes and beliefs about children's pain, as well as current beliefs, values and thinking. I shall draw on both acute and chronic pain literature where appropriate, although much of the early work focused on acute, often procedural, pain. I shall be focusing on children under 12 years of age.

Historical attitudes towards children's pain

A summary of historical attitudes appears to read as a long, 'bloody' and misguided mishandling of children's pain. Historically their pain was ignored. Schechter (1989) summarized the reasons for under-treatment within four categories (see Table 16.1), these being 'incorrect assumptions about pain and its management; personal and societal attitudes about pain; the complexity of pain assessment in children; and inadequacies in research and training' (Schechter, 1989, p.784).

The recent focus on children's pain has resulted both from a deeper pro- fessional commitment and from awareness of pain in general, but is also reflective of changing social concerns. Everson-Bates (1988), writing around the time of the emergence of the first substantial output of children's pain research papers, stated that 'societal concern for individual children and their rights is a recent phenomenon' (Everson-Bates, 1988, p.234).

It is sometimes hard to recall that only a few decades ago the dominant belief was that children did not experience or remember pain in the same way that adults do. This dismissive and casual attitude resulted in widespread mismanagement of children's pain. Children received little if any analgesia for many painful situations, including postoperative and intra-operative pain, and pain whilst receiving intensive therapy. Swafford and Allen (1968), in a study of postoperative medication, noted that of 60 postoperative children, only two individuals received any analgesia. Their explanation shows how far removed thinking was from any real appreciation of what a child was experiencing:

Pediatric patients seldom need medication for relief of pain, they tolerate pain well. The child will say he does not feel well or that he is uncomfortable or that he wants his parents but often he will not relate this unhappiness to pain.

(Swafford and Allen, 1968, p.133)

This quote must haunt the authors, although any indignation we express about the apparent lack of insight is only possible due to research produced since the Swafford and Allen study. Subsequent research refutes their analysis and supports a more informed and sophisticated understanding of children's pain. Indeed, scrutiny of their article suggests an interest in children's pain management within the limits of collective concern about the risks of narcotics. Swafford and Allen's statement also serves to reflect the pain myths that abounded at that time (see Table 16.2). Pain was not a priority, at least not for many professionals – who continued to see it merely as a side-effect of illness or intervention, and as something which could legitimately be ignored. Children had no perceived right to pain management, and professionals had no perceived duty to manage their pain.

Refutation of these myths came through the work of a relatively small number of professionals who were committed to trying to understand children and their pain, and to pushing for improved practice and more research. The

Table 16.1 Explanations for undertreatment

Incorrect assumptions	Attitudes	Complexity of pain assessment	Research and training inadequacy
There is a correct amount of pain for a given injury	Pain is necessary because of its religious implications	Pain is difficult to assess in children because they often cannot or will not tell us, in ways we can understand, the extent of their discomfort	*Research* Research is limited by inadequate assessment techniques
Children's nervous systems are too immature to experience pain	Pain is necessary because it is character-building		Research is complicated by ethical constraints
Children metabolize opioids differently	The use of analgesics is evidence of a weak character	There is no single universally accepted, well-standardized measure of pain assessment in children	*Training* There are few sources of information regarding pain mangement in children
Children have no memory of pain	Some families have attitudes which denigrate the open discussion of pain and its treatment	Inadequate assessment techniques foster undertreatment because PRN dosing is based on the patient's report of need for analgesics	Faculty discomfort with pain management transmits a lack of concern for this problem to trainers
Children become easily addicted to narcotics	Physicians and nurses tend to have attitudes about pain in children minimizing their role as causers of pain	Inadequate assessment techniques complicate research on pain and its management	There is limited information on pain management in the medical school curriculum

Source: Schechter, N.L. 1989: The undertreatment of pain in children: an overview. *Pediatric Clinics of North America* **36**, 781–94. Reproduced with permission of W.B. Saunders Company

tragedy of their efforts was that, despite the developing body of knowledge, practice itself was slow to change. Knowing that children *did* experience pain, *could* report their pain and *were* frightened of injections had only a small initial impact on practice. Today, however, practice is more active in utilizing research findings, and with the advent of pain teams and clinical nurse specialists

Table 16.2 Misconceptions and evidence about pain in children and infants (from Carter, 1994; developed from Burr, 1987, and Whaley and Wong, 1989)

Misconception/fallacy	Facts/evidence
Neonates/infants cannot remember pain	Neonates may be able to remember pain and this may lead to long term sequelae (Fitzgerald and Anand, 1993)
Neonates/infants are incapable of experiencing pain due to immaturity of the central nervous system	Volpe (1981) demonstrated that complete myelination is not required for pain perception. Neonates exhibit behavioural, physiological and hormonal responses to pain (Anand *et al.*, 1985; Owens and Todt, 1984; Franck, 1986)
Neonates cannot cognitively appreciate pain	Booker (1987) proposes that the neonate may be able to perceive pain at the cortical level
Children and infants experience less pain than adults	Younger children may perceive a greater intensity of pain than older children (Fowler-Kerry and Ramsay-Lander, 1987)
Infant's and children's behaviour accurately reflects their pain	Sleeping children (Hawley, 1984) and children who are playing/active (Eland, 1985) may be experiencing pain but coping with it (McCaffery, 1979; Eland, 1985)
Children cannot describe and/or locate their pain	Children as young as 3 years have used self-report tools (Beyer and Wells, 1989) and can locate their pain (Eland and Anderson, 1977)
Children do not want to be involved in their pain management	Eland (1981) showed that a level of autonomy increased a child's feelings of control
The use of opioids causes respiratory depression and addiction	There is no greater risk for children and adolescents in terms of addiction (Porter and Jick, 1980). Dilworth and MacKellar (1987) showed no incidences of addiction in postoperative children. 'Fear of creating opioid addiction should never be a reason for withholding opioid analgesics from anyone who needs them for pain relief' (McCaffery and Wong, 1993, p. 305). The risk of respiratory depression is no greater in children than in adults, providing the dose is appropriate
Children will be truthful about their pain	Children will often withdraw when coping with pain and may not admit to their pain. Fear of what will happen next may prevent them from disclosing the truth (Mather and Mackie, 1983)
Injections do not hurt	Eland (1981) reported that children described the injection as the 'worst hurt'. Mather and Mackie (1983) state that children fear injections more than anything else in hospital

children's pain is being managed more appropriately than before (Lloyd-Thomas and Howard, 1994). The situation is still by no means perfect (Royal College of Surgeons and College of Anaesthetists, 1990; Consumers' Association, 1995) but, thankfully, it represents a vast improvement on conditions 10 to 20 years ago. Problems persist as a result of the real and intrinsic difficulties of children's pain, but also because of deficits in some professionals' attitudes and education (McIlvaine, 1989).

Children's experience of pain

It is difficult, if not impossible, for an adult (regardless of how well meaning or well informed) to write accurately about a child's experience of pain. Even the best research is an adult representation of children's experiences – an interpretation of what adults believe children are saying. (Autobiography may come close, but even that is affected by the lens of hindsight.) Children's conceptualizations of illness and pain are often very different to those of adults. Whilst we cannot experience their pain, it is essential that we do appreciate their anxieties, concerns, responses and coping strategies. It is only by doing this that we can hope to mediate their pain experience. It is essential to remember that children are individuals, and that generalizations based on research findings need to be used with caution. Pain is unique not only to the child experiencing it, but also in relation to all of their previous experiences of pain (Carter, 1994).

There is consensus in the literature that many factors are involved in the child's experience of pain, including the child's vulnerability, their cognitive development, and their family, as well as physiological, psychological, social, cultural and contextual factors. A number of models have been proposed which provide frameworks for understanding the interplay of these factors – their nature and diversity provides a clue to the complexity of the experience of pain. McGrath's (1989) model of the situational, behavioural and emotional factors demonstrates the relationship between these key factors and the child's experience (see Figure 16.1). The mutual interplay of these elements can be managed as a fundamental way of mediating the intensity and quality of the child's experience. Each factor within the model is supported by research evidence. By utilizing this knowledge, professionals can provide different interventions, e.g. to modify the child's fears and expectations about a painful procedure and the type of support being offered to them. This model provides a strong and respected framework for understanding, and although other models have been proposed, such as those of Stevens et al. (1987) and Covelman et al. (1990), it is McGrath's model which is returned to time and time again.

An attractive aspect of the model proposed by Covelman et al. (1990) (see Figure 16.2) is the focus on the family, which is recognized as being of immense importance to the child's experiences of acute and especially chronic pain. The model of Covelman et al. places emphasis on the social ecology of the child and

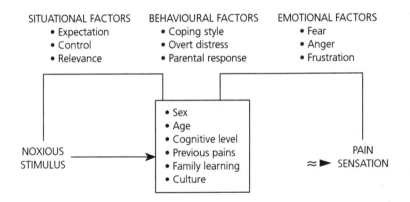

SITUATIONAL FACTORS
 • Expectation
 • Control
 • Relevance

BEHAVIOURAL FACTORS
 • Coping style
 • Overt distress
 • Parental response

EMOTIONAL FACTORS
 • Fear
 • Anger
 • Frustration

 • Sex
 • Age
 • Cognitive level
 • Previous pains
 • Family learning
 • Culture

NOXIOUS
STIMULUS

PAIN
≈ ► SENSATION

Figure 16.1 A model of the situational, behavioural and emotional factors that affect a child's pain (reproduced with permission of Elsevier Science, Inc. from McGrath, 1989). © 1998 by the US Cancer Pain Relief Committee

the role of the family's transactional patterns. The child's attributes are seen as 'contributory to the pain experience, but are modulated by a complex circular transactional system between the child and his or her environment' (Covelman et al., 1990, p.227).

Covelman et al. particularly stress the therapeutic opportunities inherent in using this transactional approach, which they found encouraged them to extend their 'focus to include not just the child–environment interactions but the ongoing transactional pattern between the child–family and the medical system' (Covelman et al., 1990, p.227).

For me, this model's strength lies in the identification of the vulnerability of the child to both acute ('one-off') pains *and* chronic ongoing or repeated pains. This vulnerability is physical, psychological and social, and should lie at the heart of efforts to appreciate the child's experience of pain. I believe that this model has much to offer in terms of the consideration of chronic pain and the effect that this has on the family. However, a significant drawback to the acceptance of this model is that it has developed from a model for psycho-somatic illness in children (Minuchin et al., 1975). Some people may have reservations about accommodating this aspect in their approach to children's pain, somatic or otherwise.

Varni's (1995) model is being utilized in practice as a means of structuring prevention and intervention strategies for children who are experiencing chronic pain. Within this model, Varni et al. (1996) (see Figure 16.3) postulate 'a number of factors that may influence pediatric pain perception and associated functional status outcome parameters in an effort to identify potentially modifiable constellations of factors be targeted for biobehavioral treatment' (Varni et al., 1996, p.155).

This model provides a framework that is congruent with my own experi-ences of working with children with chronic pain. The model itself is acknowl-edged as being complex, but this reflects the complexity and dynamic and integrative nature of pain.

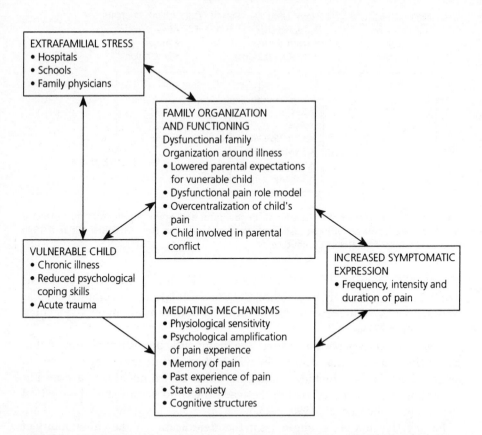

Figure 16.2 Open systems model of dysfunctional adaptation to pediatric pain (reproduced with permission from Covelman *et al.*, 1990). Reproduced with permission of Lippincott-Raven Publishers

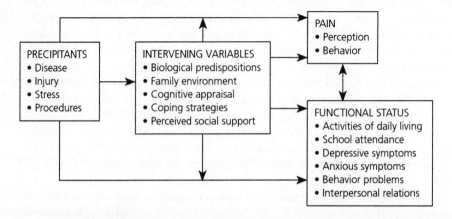

Figure 16.3 Biobehavioral model of pediatric pain (from Varni *et al.*, 1996). © Williams & Wilkins (reproduced with permission)

Children's personal characteristics and their effect on the experience of pain

One of the most obvious differences between adults and children is their age and level of cognitive development. Both of these are crucial factors in determining their understanding of pain and their ability to communicate and share their experiences (Gaffney and Dunne, 1986). Children's descriptions of their pain reflect their cognitive level (Haslam, 1969; Swanwick, 1990; McCready *et al.*, 1991). Research into children's understanding of pain has developed from and alongside research into children's conceptualizations of general health and illness issues (e.g. Perrin and Gerrity, 1981; Green and Bird, 1986; Perrin *et al.*, 1991; Kury and Rodrigue, 1995; Crisp *et al.*, 1996; Rushforth, 1997). Many of these studies are based on a cognitive development approach arising from a Piagetian stance. Gillies (1995), whilst warning that children are individuals, provides an excellent overview of the way in which children's perceptions and reactions to pain can be associated with Piaget's stages of development (see Table 16.3).

However, a more questioning stance is now being adopted towards Piaget, with some authors considering a different approach (Eiser, 1989; Rushforth, 1997). Whilst recognizing that there is a developmental trend in understanding, there is the assumption that children's development is more flexible. Rather than compartmentalizing children into different age categories to indicate their likely cognitive development, Carey (1985) identifies a theory based on the notion of 'novice to expert shift', whereby children move from novice to expert as their knowledge and understanding increase. This approach does not impose the limits to understanding that are traditionally associated with Piagetian theory, and it emphasizes the need for children to be assessed and treated as individuals – an issue that is fundamental when considering pain. The background studies on children's conceptualizations about illness and those which have focused on children's understanding of pain emphasize that, whilst age is an important factor, it is a poor indicator unless it is linked to an assessment of cognitive development/level. Even young children are generally able to provide relatively sophisticated descriptions of their pain, and to locate their pain spatially. Early research suggested that children under the age of 7 years were unable to report pain accurately (McBride, 1977). However, the child's ability to report pain, based on their own experiences and using their own vocabulary, is now accepted. McGrath, reporting on a study of children's experiences of pain, states that 'Although the language they use, the ingenuity of their pain descriptors, and the quality and diversity of their pains are different, it is clear that all these children understand the concept of pain and the multidimensional nature of pain experiences' (McGrath, 1993, p.42).

Jerrett and Evans' (1986) study of the pain vocabulary of school-aged children identified a wide range of pain descriptors used by children that reflect their own previous experiences (not necessarily just painful ones) and their own view of the world. Children used sensory, affective and evaluative words, and there were some differences between older and younger children. Descriptors included buzzing, banging, unhappy, sad, bad, awful and terrible. Other studies include those by Savedra *et al.* (1981), who demonstrated the differences between hospitalized and non-hospitalized children, the hospitalized children using more words related to fear and anxiety. Again a range of descriptors was identified. Gaffney and Dunne's (1987) study supported their hypothesis that children frequently interpret pain as a result of a transgression or careless behaviour. The notion of pain as punishment is one that occurs fairly consistently in the illness literature.

In a study I recently undertook (which was not specifically focused on language), the children who were chronic pain veterans 'admitted' to using 'medical words' to describe their pain to doctors and nurses, and using different words to describe it to friends and family. They felt that using medical words 'got the point across in a way they [professionals] could understand' (Carter, 1997, and in press) – a case of children accommodating adult inadequacies! Children not only use single words to describe their pain, but they also draw on imagery to explain their pain. These descriptions often evoke

Table 16.3 Recognition of pain, by Piaget's stages of development. Developed from Beales (1986), Gaffney and Dunne (1986), Mills (1989), Swanwick (1990), McCready *et al.* (1991) and Gillies (1995)

Infants	0–2 years	Babies of 1 month perceive localized pain (by withdrawal of the limb); pain is not understood; from 6 months they can recall painful experiences; verbal reports of pain and location may occur at about 18 months; security develops with consistency
Preoperational stage	2–7 years	Pain is physical and is present on the surface of the body, i.e. everything is taken at face value; pain may be interpreted as punishment; pain cannot be related to positive future outcomes; cannot reason beyond the present; do not understand how treatment, e.g. analgesics, helps pain; a concrete object is needed for reassurance
Concrete operations	7–12 years	Cause and effect begin to be understood, e.g. reason for immunization; treatment which appears unrelated to illness is accepted; begin to perceive psychological pain; begin to question, but do not necessarily understand what is happening, rather than taking everything at face value
Formed logical operations	12–18 years	Begin to think abstractly, understanding cause and effect; logical reasoning develops; will accept that organs can malfunction; may hide or deny pain to avoid appearing 'weak'; psychological factors may be understood as contributing to disease; understand that short-term discomfort may lead to long-term cure; may worry constantly if knowledge is incomplete

powerful images and provide substantial clues about how the experience feels for the child. Ross and Ross provide a boy's description of his headache: 'Like there's this big monster in there, see, and he's growing like crazy and there's no room and he's pulling the two sides of my head apart he's getting so big' (Ross and Ross, 1984, p.189).

This is a graphic description that goes well beyond merely identifying that he has a headache. An 11-year-old child in my recent study described his chronic back pain to me as follows:

> deep inside . . . normally two sorts of pain to it but I always have one pain and that's more of a just stabbing pain . . . sometimes constant . . . but it can get worse just twitching . . . and I get spasms. . . . When I get stabbing pain I can, can sort of be paralysed for a couple of seconds . . . sort of not be able to move . . . maybe not because I can't but because I don't want to because it makes it worse.
>
> (Carter, 1997)

Interestingly, in the same study the children said that they did not talk much about their pain because mostly people (and they *were* including health professionals in this group) got bored and were not interested.

Simple visual/graphic scales have been developed as a means of overcoming some of the difficulties associated with children's linguistic development. These provide a structured method of attempting to determine the intensity of children's pain. Used appropriately, these can provide reliable information about intensity scores, but they yield little information about the quality of a child's pain experience.

Gender has been explored as a factor that influences pain experience. Some differences have been identified in studies on children by Savedra *et al.* (1982) and Ross and Ross (1984), and in studies on infants by Grunau and Craig (1987) and Carter (1995). However, these studies do not provide sufficient evidence that gender itself has a significant impact. It would seem that pain is influenced by social and cultural issues. Gillies (1991), for example, found that male nurses and doctors expected girls to hide their pain more than boys, and that female doctors and nurses and the mothers believed that boys would hide their pain more than girls (Gillies, 1991, 1995). McGrath proposes that 'Most likely, boys and girls are equally sensitive to pain but differ in their response to pain. Familial, cultural and societal expectations may gradually shape different pain behaviors for boys and girls' (McGrath, 1993, p.43).

Previous experience of pain

It is generally accepted that early experiences of pain provide the basis for increasing sophistication of understanding about pain. Children relate a current pain experience to previous experience(s). Children's responses develop as they learn more about pain and extend their understanding about its quality, intensity, cause(s), emotional consequences, and so on. The perception of pain is not a learned response (Anand and Craig, 1996), but experience of pain is modified by previous exposure to painful situations. An early animal study by Melzack and Scott (1957) demonstrated significant behavioural changes in young dogs as a result of repeated exposure to pain.

Worrying evidence is now being produced which suggests that the same is true outside the animal model, and that early and substantial exposure to pain during the neonatal period can have a major impact on the way in which pain is perceived during childhood. Certainly research that I undertook, exploring preterm babies' responses to painful stimuli, provided evidence that the way in which individual babies responded (physiologically and behaviourally) to painful stimuli changed during their period of hospitalization (Carter, 1995). Studies by Grunau *et al.* (1994) and Gunnar *et al.* (1995) have demonstrated the impact that early exposure to pain can have on children. These neonatal follow-up studies are intriguing and really break new ground – the implications for neonatal practice could be immense.

More established evidence surrounds children's experience of repeated procedural pain, as well as the more 'everyday' pains that are part of growing up. McGrath's (1990) study of pain experiences in children demonstrated the diversity of ways in which children hurt themselves and experience pain, including broken bones, headaches, falling over, falling off bikes, tummy pains, and bites from various pets and insects. These experiences provide the context for children's subsequent pains. Unlike many procedural pains, especially repeat procedural pain, the everyday injuries are largely unexpected and accidental, and generally heal quickly. Whilst there is obviously an emotional and psychological component which should not be underestimated, the context is different to the emotional turmoil that may result from, for example, the child dreading a medical procedure or yet another admission for treatment.

The importance of family and culture

In the early years the family is often the prime focus for learning for the child. Children learn about pain from their family in the same way that they learn about other things. The family provides the means of enculturation with respect to pain (Turk *et al.*, 1983; Mathews *et al.*, 1993). The child learns from their family the means of expressing pain, what is 'acceptable' as pain behaviour, and how to cope with their pain. They also learn how to evaluate the meaning and importance of their pain. Children model their pain responses both on how they see their parents and siblings handling their pain, and on their parents' expectations of them. As the child grows, develops and starts to move away from the family, they use other models (teachers, friends and hero-figures) on which to base their pain behaviour and responses. They also access models through books, the television and other resources. Studies have shown that birth order can exert an effect on children's experience of pain. Vernon (1974) found that first-born children showed a greater sensitivity to pain than later-born children. It is possible that this results from parents being extra-protective towards their-first born child, but less so towards their second and subsequent children.

Another area of interest within the family-based literature is the degree to which children whose parents experience chronic pain are affected. Adult-focused research by Payne and Norfleet (1986) suggests a greater likelihood of pain patients belonging to families that appear to have a higher incidence of pain or illness than of belonging to families that do not. A study by Edwards *et al.* found 'the strong association between the number of pain models in an individual's family and his/her current reports of pain' (Edwards *et al.*, 1985, p.382).

The notions of reinforcement, secondary gains, inappropriate coping and an external locus of control could all contribute to increased pain reporting. It is interesting to note that many of these studies identify the methodological difficulties inherent in researching such a complex issue. Dura and Beck (1988) demonstrated that children in families where the mother had chronic pain experienced significantly more self-reported depressive symptoms compared to children in control families where the mothers did not have pain. Studies on the effects on the family of a chronically ill parent would suggest that family members are less well adjusted and develop poorer coping styles (Armistead *et al.*, 1995; Kotchick *et al.*, 1996). Robinson *et al.* (1990), in a matched study of children suffering from recurrent abdominal pain (RAP), concluded that children who experienced RAP were more likely than the controls to come from families where 'recurrent painful illness (particularly migraine) is a parental feature' (p.180). They also identified that expression of symptoms could often be triggered by adverse life events. However, they stressed that they could not 'apportion the relative magnitude of modelling vs. genetic endowment in the parental contribution to its aetiology' (p.180). Roy *et al.*, in a study which explored the impact of parental chronic pain on children, concluded that 'the influence of parental chronic pain on the psychosocial well-being of their children is not self-evident. ...The notion that parents with chronic pain endanger the well being of their children should be viewed with caution' (Roy *et al.*, 1994, p.25).

There does not seem to be a strong consensus of opinion as yet, and more studies are obviously needed. Thus, whilst the family is a strong means of pain enculturation, it would appear that even where there is a significant pain model within the family, children do not necessarily develop disturbed pain expression or response.

Culture again provides a model for learning about pain, but it is dangerously oversimplistic to suggest that culture overrides the individual response to, expression and experience of pain. There have been few cultural studies of children, and often these studies would appear to be considering ethnic rather than cultural differences. Abu-Saad's (1984) research considered Arab-American, Chinese-American and Latin-American children, but found very few cross-cultural differences between the types of pain reported. However, it is possible that these children – regardless of their parents' country or area of origin – were predominantly culturally American. Other studies have not provided definitive evidence of cultural differences, although it is widely assumed that they do exist. Importantly, Bernstein and Pachter state:

It is not clear exactly what it is about culture and ethnicity among *children* that we should be aware of or study with respect to pain. Consequently, there is no well-accepted model for grouping cultures or ethnic groups. No formula, therefore, factors the importance of culture in the assessment of pain and effectiveness of its management in children.

(Bernstein and Pachter, 1993, p.119)

Banoub-Baddour and Laryea (1991) emphasize the need for culturally sensitive care for children experiencing pain.

Coping with pain

Literature on how children cope with pain has arisen from two major areas – first, from literature related to hospitalization and how children deal with admission(s) (Saylor *et al.*, 1987; Spirito *et al.*, 1994; Lansdown, 1996), and secondly, from studies that addressed how adults cope with stressful situations. The models that underpin stress research tend to be adopted when researching coping. One difficulty that is encountered when addressing the 'coping' literature is the diversity of terminology that is utilized. Smith *et al.* (1989) identified this as an issue in the opening remarks of their paper, and usefully provided a summary: 'Although nomenclature differs among investigators, coping style has commonly been conceptualized as a tendency to repress, minimize, or avoid information on one extreme to a more sensitized awareness, vigilant, or active information-seeking style on the other' (Smith *et al.*, 1989, p.406).

This point is emphasized by Branson and Craig (1988), who provide an excellent summary considering the lack of integration of research findings which they propose 'may impede progress in the investigation of children's coping' (p.409).

Coping is closely linked to the notion of stress. Stress is only a meaningful concept when it is applied to an individual – what will stress one child will not be seen to be stressful by another child. Stress, like pain, is individually perceived. Almost regardless of approach, models related to stress and coping appear to divide people into one of two groups, namely those who cope, seek information and have a strong internal locus of control, and those who do not cope, avoid information, have an external locus of control, and catastrophize situations. This is useful in so far as it allows children who do not cope well to be identified. However, there is a risk involved in labelling a child as a non-coper or a catastrophizer, as it has rather negative connotations. Children may also either use spontaneous coping strategies (self-coping) or draw on learned coping strategies. A number of theoretical frameworks have been developed to examine children's coping strategies and pain.

Lazarus (1966) divided the coping process into two modes, namely direct action coping and intrapsychic/cognitive coping. Direct action coping involves physically preparing for the stressful event, whereas cognitive coping is directed towards preparing the mind for the event. Cognitive coping is the coping strategy most frequently utilized by children with pain, and includes distraction, imagery and mental preparation, e.g. rehearsing the event (Brown *et al.*, 1986). Ellerton *et al.* (1994) provide a theoretical model reflecting Lazarus' model of stress and coping in which coping behaviour is dependent on three major areas, namely the context of the situation, the resources (basically personal characteristics) available to the child, and the child's own appraisal of the situation. They propose that the outcomes of 'effective and ineffective coping are manifested in somatic health, social function and morale' (Ellerton *et al.*, 1994, p.74).

Peterson *et al.* (1990), drawing on concepts from the transactional coping model, highlight the fact that coping consists of three discrete stages – appraisal, encounter and recovery. Importantly, they note that a child's coping behaviours may be different within each stage. The way in which a specific stressor may be responded to may also differ at each stage. They acknowledge that, since this model suggests so many different responses are possible within each stage, there is little chance of predicting the response and thus being able to mediate it. However, they emphasize that 'in reality most individuals produce one of a small number of responses to appraisal of, encounter with and recovery from a stressor' (Peterson *et al.*, 1990, p.199).

It is important, however, to assess coping styles so that appropriate behavioural and other interventions can be instigated. Bachanas and Blount (1996) report using the Behavioral Approach-Avoidance and Distress Scale (BAADS) as a method of assessing coping style in children undergoing immunizations. The BAADS was originally developed by Hubert *et al.* (1988). It consists of two subscales, namely, the Approach-Avoidance scale (indexed children's coping style during a stressful painful procedure or event) and a Distress subscale (which indexes crying, agitation and other implicated factors). Bachanas and Blount (1996) suggest that some difficulties inherent within the BAADS limit its clinical application, as the Approach-Avoidance subscale potentially 'measures the quantity rather than type of coping'. Within their discussion, Bachanas and Blount (1996) highlight the complexity of classifying and measuring coping styles.

Appraisal of the stressor (such as a painful procedure) is an important component of the coping response. Appraisal can be modified by good preparation of the child through age/cognitive level-appropriate information-giving, play therapy, relaxation and other strategies, which all allow the child to 'meet' the painful stressor in a prepared manner. Children who had actively sought information as an appraisal coping strategy showed reduced levels of anxiety and higher pain tolerance (Siegel and Smith, 1989). This finding is also supported by studies by Peterson and Toler (1986) and Hubert *et al.* (1988), in which information-seeking behaviour resulted in better coping than was observed in children who used information avoidance behaviour.

Information-giving is a fundamental part of preparing a child to cope with a painful procedure, although the timing of the information would appear to be important (Melamed *et al.*, 1983). Smith *et al.* (1989) found that children who were told that they would be given detailed information during the procedure (lumbar puncture or bone marrow aspiration) had higher anticipatory heart rates than children who were not told this prior to the event. They further suggest that the value of information-giving may depend on whether the children have already had experience of the procedure. They postulate that provision of information to repressor children (those who normally cope by avoiding information) may actually enhance their internal locus of control, enhance their coping and reduce their experience of pain. Månsson et al. (1993), in a study examining the effects of a preparation programme for children undergoing lumbar puncture during chemotherapy, found that prepared children were more able to express their feelings and anxiety. The preparation had many beneficial effects on children's co-operation in stressful situations.

Children can utilize a vast range of spontaneous and learned strategies. Siegel and Smith (1989) identified the categories of coping strategies (see Table 16.4). Studies have been undertaken to consider the effectiveness of these strategies as intervention, e.g. self-talk (Patterson and Ware, 1988; Carter, 1997), imagery and distraction (Kuttner, 1989; Fowler-Kerry and Ramsay-Lander, 1990; Doody et al., 1991; Broome et al., 1992; Manne et al., 1992), relaxation (May, 1992), hypnotherapy (Zelter and LeBaron, 1982; Kuttner, 1988; Olness, 1989; Valente, 1991), deep breathing, making decisions about aspects of their care, and holding their parents (Hester and Barcus, 1986). Medforth (1995) reports the value of distraction via bubble blowing and imagery as helpful for children who have difficulty coping with painful procedures. Spontaneous coping strategies in children are probably a vastly underestimated resource which could be tapped to the child's advantage.

A number of the studies that have considered coping styles and pain have focused on procedural pain (Field et al., 1988; Smith et al., 1989; Collier and MacKinlay, 1993; and Ellerton et al., 1994). A number of investigations have focused on the efficacy of measures intended to reduce anxiety by enhancing coping strategies and thus reducing pain (Zelter and LeBaron, 1982; Jay et al., 1985; Katz et al., 1987). Spirito et al. (1994) identify children as either active copers or avoidant copers: 'certain children ("active" copers) seek out information about a stressor to master the stress. These active approaches can be either cognitive or behavioral. Avoidant copers block information about the stressor or behave in ways to avoid the stressor' (p.314).

An issue that is consistently identified within the literature is the relevance of the age of the child and their ability to use spontaneous coping strategies. Put simply, older children generally have a wider repertoire of coping skills to draw upon than their younger counterparts. Ellerton et al. (1994) found that young children appeared to lack the personal resources for effective or adaptive coping, and were dependent on supportive input from their parents and from staff to help them develop and utilize good coping skills. They also reported that there was an increase in the number of coping strategies used when children appraised a situation as being painful. However, Peterson et al. (1990) warn that the relationship between age and coping is rather ambiguous due to some of the methodological weaknesses and limitations of the available studies. Indeed the ambiguity between chronological age and coping skills would be supported by the difficulties of linking age and understanding/conceptualization as discussed earlier. A better guide may be to assess children individually in relation to linking cognitive level and coping.

The individuality of children's styles of coping with painful procedures was determined by Broome *et al.* (1990), who further stated that:

> Assumptions about the meaning of any behaviors, should be validated with the child, and his/her perception periodically assessed. To be most effective in reducing the child's perception of pain during procedures, interventions need to incorporate each child's individual meanings and coping styles.
>
> (Broome *et al.*, 1990, p.366)

The importance of attending to individuality of coping style is demonstrated by a study by Fanurik *et al.* (1993), which showed that mismatched interventions actually reduced coping abilities. Hester (1989) reports a study (Hester and Barcus, 1986) in which children described their own comforting strategies and what other people could do to help them feel more comfortable. The strategies proposed by the children reflected their age/cognitive level and previous experience, and examples included holding teddy, crying, calling for their parents, trying to control it, and getting mad with it.

One of the key factors influencing a child's experience of pain is their family. Young children experience the world through their family who (ideally) provide protection and support. Despite the identification of the importance of the family, there is still relatively little research on the impact of children's pain either on the family or on parental perceptions of their children's pain. Indeed, there has been a historical reluctance by some health care professionals to allow parents to be present during procedures, the explanation often being that the parents will become distressed and upset the child, and thus make his or her pain worse. Whilst there may be a small grain of truth in this, it does rather reflect health professionals' own anxieties about being observed. Gonzales *et al.* (1989) found, in their study of young children undergoing injections, that not allowing parents to be present during the procedure was 'an unjustified practice' (p.461). Carter (1995) emphasizes that parents play a vital role in helping to interpret children's symptoms, since they have a wealth of experience about how their child generally copes with pain. Children themselves, in a study by Ross and Ross (1984), stated overwhelmingly that the 'thing that helped most' during a painful procedure was the presence of their parents.

The need for parental/family support is evident in a number of studies (Tesler *et al.*, 1981; Watt-Watson *et al.* 1990; Ellerton *et al.*, 1994; Ferrell *et al.*, 1994; Spirito *et al.*, 1994; Carter, unpublished results). Cohesive family styles were associated with children with sickle cell disease using active coping styles for pain management (Kliewer and Lewis, 1995). However, Ellerton *et al.* (1994) reported that even though young children needed the support of their parents in order to enhance their coping skills, health care professionals displayed few supportive actions towards the parents. Considering the interplay between parental anxiety and children's anxiety and increased pain, this is an area that needs closer attention.

Table 16.4 Categories of coping strategies (from Siegel and Smith, 1989)

Category	Definition of coping strategy
Distraction	
External	Indicates that he or she does something to divert his or her attention away from the procedure by focusing on some aspect of the immediate environment (e.g. looking at a picture on the wall, counting floor tiles)
Internal	Indicates that he or she does something to divert his or her attention away from the procedure by focusing on some part of the body or sensation unrelated to the procedure (e.g. concentrates on heart beating)
Imagery	Indicates that he or she thinks about or imagines some pleasant event, activity or situation to divert attention away from the procedure (e.g. thinks about playing an electronic game, imagines self at school, thinks about being at a party)
Reinterprets sensations	Indicates an attempt to reinterpret or alter by some cognitive process (other than by distraction) the sensory stimulation produced by the procedure (e.g. thinks about it as being cool or as pressure rather than as hurting, burning or stinging)
Fantasy	Imagines he or she is some imaginary character who does not feel pain (e.g. Superman) or pretends that some magical event is happening (e.g. waving a magic wand) to make the pain disappear
Mental rehearsal	Indicates some attempt to prepare for the experience by mentally planning how he or she will confront it
Information-seeking	
Relevant	Indicates an attempt to ask questions or gather information that is related to the medical procedure
Irrelevant	Indicates an attempt to ask questions or gather information that is unrelated to the medical procedure
Positive self-statements	Indicates thinking about positive aspects of the procedure; reassures self that he or she can tolerate the procedure; thinks about how he or she had handled previous procedures successfully; makes self-reinforcing statements for doing well during the procedure; thinks about the experience (e.g. 'the doctor is doing this to help me', 'it doesn't hurt so bad, I can get through this OK')
Negative self-statements	Indicates thinking about distressing aspects of the current procedure and problems in tolerating it (e.g. thinks about how much it was hurting and wanting it to stop)
Catastrophizing thoughts	Indicates thinking about distressing or bad things that might happen or that have occurred in the past (e.g. thinks about the last time it really hurt)
Affective expression	Indicates that he or she thought about or actually displayed some affective response (e.g. cried, yelled, got angry) as a means of tension or stress reduction

Affective inhibition	Indicates an attempt to reduce emotional distress by specifically controlling or inhibiting feelings such as trying not to cry or yell
Relaxation	Indicates that he or she engaged in some activity or thought about something with the specific intent of relaxing or making self feel calm
Seeking help/emotional support	Indicates that he or she thought about asking or actually asked someone for help, comfort, sympathy or emotional support, such as asking the nurse to hold his or her hand, or thought about mother being in the room, to call for help or comfort if needed
Physical activity	Indicates that he or she attempts to place a part of the body in a certain position (e.g. holds arm rigid) or that he or she engages in a particular physical activity (e.g. holds breath, massages arm) for the specific purpose of reducing discomfort
Seeks active termination of procedure	Engages in any activity or thinks about engaging in an activity with the specific purpose of immediately terminating the procedure (e.g. escaping from the room, pushing the doctor away, verbalizing that he or she wants the procedure stopped)
Passive acceptance	Indicates some decision that presumes that nothing could be done to change the situation or to make it better or less stressful in some way
No strategy reported	After sufficient prompting from the examiner, the child indicates that he or she did not engage in any activity or did not think about anything

Beales (1986) demonstrated that anxious parents could communicate their anxiety and distress to the child and thus create an anxiety–pain cycle. Alexander et al. (1986) found that the child's pain was a family stressor, with parents and siblings experiencing feelings of helplessness, anger, guilt and depression. Jay et al. (1983) and Vardaro (1978) demonstrated a positive correlation between parental anxiety and the distress that children exhibited during painful procedures. Some studies have addressed the comparative level of accuracy, in terms of assessing pain intensity, between nurses and parents (Manne et al., 1992; Dalquist et al., 1995). These types of studies dominate the parent-focused pain literature, but they do not specifically address the parents' subjective experience of their children's pain.

In a study (Carter, unpublished results) exploring the effect on their family of a child experiencing chronic pain, the devastation was evident. In this study emotional consequences, as well as changes in the family dynamics, were notable. The child's parents expressed feelings of frustration, despair, anger and hopelessness. They noted that this emotional turmoil changed the family in subtle and dramatic ways. One mother wrote in her 'research' diary, 'You have to live with previously unknown TENSION!!!!'. Life was described as 'not being a real existence any more' by another mother, who summed up the changes the family experienced as a result of her child's chronic pain as follows: 'you're made to feel a bit of a freak and your child's a freak and your family's a freak. And it's really not'.

It is obviously problematic for the family, and yet there is often little support provided to help the family to cope – not only with their own feelings but to provide more effective support for their child's pain. Miles and Carter (1982) reported on parents who were encouraged to be involved and to stay and support their child during painful procedures. However, they urge that parents need to be provided with information and skills (such as relaxation and distraction techniques) prior to the procedure. The need to provide parents with information about pain is also emphasized by Bauchner (1991) and Bauchner *et al.* (1989, 1991). Bauchner *et al.* (1991) suggest that parents can be allies, but that they themselves need care, support and advice about how to help their child (Dearmun, 1993; Broome, 1994). Dolgin and Phipps emphasize the importance of the parents' role:

> incorporating the parent into the treatment process is of utmost importance. The parents' role as the child's provider and protector is most compromised in conditions of crisis, such as the child in pain. . . .Involving the parent in the child's care serves not only to restore the parental role, but also to reinforce the alliance between physician and parent as partners in meeting the child's medical needs.
>
> (Dolgin and Phipps, 1989, p.108)

Conclusions

It is impossible for us, as adults, to enter the world of a child and fully appreciate what pain feels like to them. Trying to remember our own childhood encounters of pain may make us feel as if we have come a step closer – but it is only the child who really knows what it feels like to face yet another injection, another phase of surgery, or another day of struggling with recurrent pain. Yet even though it is difficult for us to appreciate their experience, we cannot dismiss it. Children are vulnerable, and their experiences of pain are *all too real* to them. Children, given the opportunity, can be articulate about their pain and can provide many clues about how a painful experience has affected them. However, adults are not always good at listening to children. It is easy to dismiss a child's description of pain because it does not fit easily into our expectation of their experience. Thus children often have to cope not only with their pain but with adults' attitudes as well. If we do stop and listen to what children are saying, we can help to ease the pain for them. What may seem like a bizarre story about 'bad rabbits eating my ears' was actually a pretty good description by a young child of bad earache. Such images do not just give us insight into something of the child's experience, but they also provide us with a way in to help them to cope with their pain. Children's imaginations and their creativity mean that stories, imagery and distraction can work (those bad ear-eating rabbits were finally sorted out by having their ears tied to big, blue balloons which made them float away!).

Children's pain is important, and we cannot afford to ignore it. It affects both children and their families. Many of the factors that influence a child's pain can be modified, although this takes real commitment on the part of professionals. It means that we have to believe and respect children in terms of their reports of pain and the way in which they cope. We need to respect the crucial role the family has to play by helping parents to support their children. Whilst we might not be able to protect the child from painful experiences altogether, we need to ensure that they know that we care and that we are doing our best to understand.

References

Abu-Saad, H. 1984: Cultural group indicators of pain in children. *Maternal Child Nursing Journal* 13, 187–96.

Alexander, D., White, M. and Powell, G. 1986: Anxiety of non-rooming-in parents of hospitalized children. *Child Health Care* 15, 14–20.

Anand, K.J.S. and Craig, K.D. 1996: New perspectives on the definition of pain. *Pain* 67, 3–6.

Anand, K.J.S., Brown, M.J., Causson, R.C. *et al.* 1985: Can the human neonate mount an endocrine/metabolic reponse to surgery? *Journal of Pediatric Surgery* 20, 41–8.

Armistead, L., Klein, K. and Forehand, R. 1995: Parental physical illness and child functioning. *Clinical Psychology Review* 15, 409–22.

Bachanas, P.J. and Blount, R.L. 1996: The Behavioral Approach-Avoidance and Distress Scale: an investigation of reliability and validity during painful medical procedures. *Journal of Pediatric Psychology* 21, 671-81.

Banoub-Baddour, S. and Laryea, M. 1991: Children in pain: a culturally sensitive perspective for child care professionals. *Journal of Child and Youth Care* 6, 19–24.

Bauchner, H. 1991: Procedures, pain and parents. *Pediatrics* 87, 563–5.

Bauchner, H., Vinci, R. and Waring, C. 1989: Pediatric procedures: do parents want to watch? *Pediatrics* 84, 907–9.

Bauchner, H., Waring, C. and Vinci, R. 1991: Parental presence during procedures in an emergency room: result from 50 observations. *Pediatrics* 87, 544–8.

Beales, J.G. 1986: Cognitive development and the experience of pain. *Nursing* 3, 408-10.

Bernstein, B.A. and Pachter, L.M. 1993: Cultural considerations in children's pain. In Schechter, N.L., Berde, C.B. and Yaster, M. (eds), *Pain in infants, children and adolescents.* Baltimore, MD: Williams and Wilkins, 122–33.

Beyer, J.E. and Byers, M.L. 1985: Knowledge of pediatric pain: the state of the art. *Children's Health Care* 13, 150-59.

Beyer, J.G. and Wells, N. 1989: The assessment of pain in children. *Pediatric Clinics of North America* 36, 837-54.

Booker, P.D. 1987: Postoperative analgesia for neonates. *Anaesthesia* 42, 343-5.

Branson, S.M. and Craig, K.D. 1988: Children's spontaneous strategies for coping with pain: a review of the literature. *Canadian Journal of Behavioural Science* 20, 402-12.

Broome, M. 1994: *Parents in pain. Paper presented at Collaboration in Care Conference,* 10-12 November 1994, Jersey, Channel Islands.

Broome, M.E., Bates, T.A., Lillis, P.P.Y. and Wilson McGahee, T. 1990: Children's medical fears, coping behaviors, and pain perceptions during a lumbar puncture. *Oncology Nursing Forum* 17, 361-7.

Broome, M.E., Lillis, P.P.Y., Wilson McGahee, T. and Bates, T.A. 1992: The use of distraction and imagery with children during painful procedures. *Oncology Nursing Forum* 19, 499–502.

Brown, J.M., O'Keefe, J., Sanders, S.H. and Baker, B. 1986: Developmental changes in children's cognition to stressful and painful situations. *Journal of Pediatric Psychology* 11, 343-57.

Burr, S. 1987: Pain in childhood. *Nursing* 24, 890–6.

Carey, S. 1985: *Conceptual change in childhood*. Boston, MA: MIT Press.

Carter, B. 1994: *Child and infant pain. Principles of nursing care and management.* London: Stanley Thornes.

Carter, B. 1995: Pantomines of pain, distress, repose and lability. Unpublished doctoral thesis. Manchester: Manchester Metropolitan University.

Carter, B. 1997: The experience of living with chronic pain. An exploratory study. *International Children's Nursing Conference. Evidence-Based Practice*, Jersey, 28–30 November.

Cleeland, C.S. 1993: Treating pain in children: can there be a global perspective? In Schechter, N.L., Berde, C.B. and Yaster, M. (eds), *Pain in infants, children and adolescents*. Baltimore, MD: Williams and Wilkins, 649–53.

Collier, J. and Mackinlay, D. 1993: Play at work. *Play Preparation Guidelines for the Multidisciplinary Team* 1, 123–5.

Consumers' Association 1995: Managing acute pain in children. *Drug and Therapeutics Bulletin* 33, 41–4.

Covelman, K., Scott, S., Buchanan, B. and Rosman, B. 1990: Pediatric pain control: a family systems model. *Advances in Pain Research Therapy* 15, 225–36.

Crisp, J., Ungerer, J.A. and Goodnow, J.J. 1996: The impact of experience in children's understanding of illness. *Journal of Pediatric Psychology* 21, 57–72.

Dalquist, L.M., Power, T.G. and Carlson, L. 1995: Physician and parent behavior during invasive pediatric cancer procedures: relationships to child behavioral distress. *Journal of Pediatric Psychology* 20, 477–90.

Dearmun, A. 1993: Towards a partnership in pain management. *Paediatric Nursing* 5, 8-10.

Dilworth, N.M. and MacKellar, A. 1987: Pain relief for the pediatric surgical patient. *Journal of Pediatric Surgery* 22, 264–6.

Dolgin, M.J. and Phipps, S. 1989: Pediatric pain: the parents' role. *Pediatrician* 16, 103–9.

Doody, S.B., Smith, C. and Webb, J. 1991: Nonpharmacologic interventions for pain management. *Critical Care Nursing Clinics of North America* 3, 69–75.

Dura, J.R. and Beck, S.J. 1988: A comparison of family functioning when mothers have chronic pain. *Pain* 35, 79–89.

Edwards, P.W., Zeichner, A., Kuczmierczyk, A.R. and Boczkowski, J. 1985: Familial pain models: the relationship between family history of pain and current pain experience. *Pain* 21, 379–84.

Eiser, C. 1989: Children's concepts of illness: towards an alternative to the stage approach. *Psychology and Health* 3, 93-101.

Eland, J. 1981: Minimizing pain associated with prekindergarten intramuscular injections. *Issues in Comprehensive Pediatric Nursing* 5, 361–72.

Eland, J. 1985: The child who is hurting. *Seminars in Oncology Nursing* 1, 116–22.

Eland, J.M. and Anderson, J.E. 1977: The experience of pain in children. In Jacox, A. (ed.) *Pain: a sourcebook for nurses and health professionals*. Boston, MA: Little, Brown and Co., 453–73.

Ellerton, M.L., Ritchie, J.A. and Caty, S. 1994: Factors influencing young children's coping behaviors during stressful healthcare encounters. *Maternal-Child Nursing Journal* 22, 74–82.

Everson-Bates, S. 1988: Research involving children: ethical concerns and dilemmas. *Journal of Pediatric Health Care* **2**, 234–9.

Fanurik, D., Zeltzer, L.K., Roberts, M.C. and Blount, R.L. 1993: The relationship between children's coping styles and psychological interventions for cold pressor pain. *Pain* **53**, 213–22.

Ferrell, B.R., Rhiner, M., Shapiro, B. and Dierkes, M. 1994: The experience of pediatric cancer pain. Part 1. Impact of pain on the family. *Journal of Pediatric Nursing* **9**, 368–79.

Field, T., Alpert, B., Vega-Lahr, N., Goldstein, S. and Perry, S. 1988: Hospitalization stress in children: sensitizer and repressor coping styles. *Health Psychology* **7**, 433–46.

Fitzgerald, M. and Anand, K.J.S. 1993: Developmental neuroanatomy and neurophysiology of pain. In Schechter, N.L., Berde, C.B. and Yaster, M. (eds), *Pain in infants, children, and adolescents*. Baltimore, MD: Williams and Wilkins, 11–31.

Fowler-Kerry, S. and Ramsay-Lander, J. 1987: Management of injection pain in children. *Pain* **30**, 169–75.

Fowler-Kerry, S. and Ramsay-Lander, J. 1990: Utilizing cognitive strategies to relieve pain in young children. *Advances in Pain Research Therapy* **15**, 247–53.

Gaffney, A. and Dunn, E.A. 1986: Developmental aspects of childrens' definitions of pain. *Pain* **26**, 105–17.

Gaffney, A. and Dunne, E.A. 1987: Children's understanding of the causality of pain. *Pain* **29**, 91–104.

Gillies, M.L. 1991: A study of postoperative pain in children and adolescents. *Health Bulletin* **52**, 193–6.

Gillies, M.L. 1993: Post-operative pain in children: a review of the literature. *Journal of Clinical Nursing* **2**, 5–10.

Gillies, M.L. 1995: Pain management. In Carter, B. and Dearmun, A.K. (eds), *Child health care nursing: concepts, theory and practice*. Oxford: Blackwell Science, 193–221.

Gonzales, J.C., Routh, D.K., Saab, P.G. *et al.* 1989: Effect of parent presence on children's reactions to injections: behavioral, physical and subjective aspects. *Journal of Pediatric Psychology* **14**, 449–62.

Green, K.E. and Bird, J.E. 1986: The structure of children's beliefs about health and illness. *Journal of School Health* **56**, 325–8.

Grunau, R.V.E. and Craig, K.D. 1987: Pain expression in neonates: facial action and crying. *Pain* **28**, 395–410.

Grunau, R.V.E., Whitfield, M.F., Petrie, J. and Fryer, E.L., 1994: Early pain experience, child temperament and family characteristics as precursors of somatization: a prospective study of preterm and fullterm children. *Pain* **56**, 353–9.

Gunnar, M.R., Porter, F.L., Wolf, C.M., Rigatuso, S. and Larson, M.C. 1995: Neonatal stress reactivity: predictions to later emotional temperament. *Child Development* **66**, 1–13.

Haslam, D. 1969: Age and perception of pain. *Psychonomic Science* **15**, 86.

Hawley, D.D. 1984: Postoperative pain in children: misconceptions, descriptions and interventions. *Pediatric Nursing* **10**, 20–3.

Hester, N.O. 1989: Comforting the child in pain. In Funk, S.G., Tornquist, E.M., Champange, M.T., Copp, L.A. and Wiese, R.A. (eds), *Key aspects of comfort: management of pain, fatigue and nausea*. New York: Springer Publishing Co. Inc., 290–317.

Hester, N. and Barcus, C. 1986: Assessment and management of pain in children. *Pediatrics: Nursing Update* **1**, 3.

Hubert, N.C., Jay, S.M., Saltoun, M. and Hayes, M. 1988: Approach-avoidance and distress in children undergoing preparation for painful medical procedures. *Journal of Clinical Child Pyschology* **17**, 194–202.

Jay, S.M., Ozolins, M., Elliott, C.H. and Caldwell, S. 1983: Assessment of children's distress during painful medical procedures. *Health Psychology* **2**, 133–47.

Jay, S.M., Elliott, C.H., Ozlins, M., Olson, R.A. and Pruitt, S.D. 1985: Behavioral management of children's distress during painful medical procedures. *Behavioral Research Therapy* **23**, 513–20.

Jerrett, M.D. 1985: Children and their pain experience. *Children's Health Care* **14**, 83–9.

Jerrett, M. and Evans, K. 1986: Children's pain vocabulary. *Journal of Advanced Nursing* **11**, 403–8.

Katz, E.R., Kellerman, J. and Ellenberg, L. 1987: Hypnosis in the reduction of acute pain and distress in children with cancer. *Journal of Pediatric Psychology* **12**, 379–94.

Kliewer, W. and Lewis, H. 1995: Family influences on coping processes in children and adolescents with sickle cell disease. *Journal of Pediatric Psychology* **20**, 511–25.

Kotchick, B.A., Forehand, R., Armistead, L., Klein, K., Wierson, M. 1996: Coping with illness: interrelationships across family members and predictors of psychological adjustment. *Journal of Family Psychology* **10**, 358–70.

Kury, S.P. and Rodrigue, J.R., 1995: Concepts of illness causality in a pediatric sample: relationship to illness duration, frequency of hospitalization, and degree of life threat. *Clinical Pediatrics* **34**, 178–82.

Kuttner, L. 1988: Favourite stories: a hypnotic pain-reduction technique for children in acute pain. *American Journal of Clinical Hypnosis* **30**, 289–95.

Kuttner, L. 1989: Management of young children's acute pain and anxiety during invasive medical procedures. *Pediatrician* **16**, 39–44.

Lansdown, R. 1996: *Children in hospital. A guide for family and carers.* Oxford: Oxford Medical Press.

Lazarus, R.S. 1966: *Psychological stress and the coping process.* New York: McGraw-Hill.

Lloyd-Thomas, A.R. and Howard, R.F. 1994: A pain service for children. *Paediatric Anaesthesiology* **4**, 3–15.

McBride, M. 1977: Can you tell me where it hurts? *Pediatric Nursing* **3**, 7–8.

McCaffery, M. 1979: *Nursing management of the child in pain.* New York: JB Lippincott.

McCaffery, M. and Wong, D.L. 1993: Nursing interventions for pain control in children. In Schechter, N.L., Berde, C.B. and Yaster, M. (eds), *Pain in infants, children and adolescents.* Baltimore, MD: Williams and Wilkins, 295–316.

McCready, M., MacDavitt, K. and O'Sullivan, K.K. 1991: Children and pain: easing the hurt. *Orthopaedic Nursing* **10**, 33–42.

McGrath, P.A. 1989: Evaluating a child's pain. *Journal of Pain and Symptom Management* **4**, 198–214.

McGrath, P.A. 1990: *Pain in children: nature, assessment and treatment.* New York: Guilford Publications.

McGrath, P.A. 1993: Inducing pain in children: a controversial issue. *Pain* **52**, 255–7.

McIlvaine, W.B. 1989: Perioperative pain management in children: a review. *Journal of Pain and Symptom Management* **4**, 215–29.

Manne, S.L., Jacobsen, P.B. and Redd, W.H. 1992: Assessment of acute pediatric pain: do child self-report and parent ratings measure the same phenomenon? *Pain* **48**, 45–52.

Månsson, M.E., Björkhem, G. and Wiebe, T. 1993: The effect of preparation for lumbar puncture on children undergoing chemotherapy. *Oncology Nursing Forum* **20**, 39–45.

Mather, L. and Mackie, J. 1983: The incidence of post-operative pain in children. *Pain* **15**, 271–82.

Mathews, J.R., McGrath, P.J. and Pigeon, H. 1993: Assessment and measurement of pain in children. In Schechter, N.L., Berde, C.B. and Yaster, M. (eds), *Pain in infants, children and adolescents*. Baltimore, MD: Williams and Wilkins, 97–111.

May, L. 1992: Reducing pain and anxiety in children. *Nursing Standard* **6**, 25–8.

Medforth, N. 1995: Strategies to reduce children's perception of pain. *Nursing Times* **91**, 34–5.

Melamed, B., Dearborn, M. and Hermecz, D. 1983: Necessary considerations for surgery preparation: age and previous experience. *Psychosomatic Medicine* **45**, 517.

Melzack, R. and Scott, T.H. 1957: The effects of early experience on the response to pain. *Journal of Comparative and Physiological Psychology* **50**, 155–61.

Merskey, H. and Bogduk, N. 1994: *Classification of chronic pain*, 2nd edn. Seattle: IASP Task Force on Taxonomy, IASP Press.

Miles, M. and Carter, M. 1982: Sources of parental stress in pediatric intensive care units. *Children's Health Care* **11**, 65–9.

Mills, N.M. 1989: Pain behaviour in infants and toddlers. *Journal of Pain and Symptom Management* **4**, 184–90.

Minuchin, S., Baker, L. and Rosman, B. (1975) *Psychosomatic families: anorexia nervosa in context*. Cambridge, MA: Harvard Press.

Olness, K. 1989: Hypnotherapy: a cyberphysiologic strategy in pain management. *Pediatric Clinics of North America* **36**, 873–84.

Owens, M.E. and Todt, E.H. 1984: Pain in infancy: neonatal reaction to heel lance. *Pain* **20**, 77–86.

Patterson, K.L. and Ware, L.L. 1988: Coping skills for children undergoing painful medical procedures. *Issues in Comprehensive Pediatric Nursing* **11**, 113–43.

Payne, B. and Norfleet, M.A. 1986: Chronic pain and the family: a review. *Pain* **26**, 1–22.

Perrin, E.C. and Gerrity, P.S. 1981: There's a demon in your belly: children's understanding of illness. *Pediatrics* **67**, 841–9.

Perrin, E.C., Sayer, A.G. and Willett, J.B. 1991: Sticks and stones may break my bones. . .reasoning about illness causality and body functioning in children who have a chronic illness. *Pediatrics* **88**, 608–19.

Peterson, L. and Toler, S.M. 1986: An information-seeking disposition in child surgery patients. *Health Psychology* **5**, 343–58.

Peterson, L., Harbeck, C., Chaney, J., Farmer, J. and Muir Thomas, A. 1990: Children's coping with medical procedures: a conceptual overview and integration. *Behavioral Assessment* **12**, 197–212.

Porter, J. and Jick, H. 1980: Addiction rare in patients treated with narcotics. *New England Journal of Medicine* **302**, 123.

Robinson, J.O., Alverez, J.H. and Dodge, J.A. 1990: Life events and family history in children with recurrent abdominal pain. *Journal of Psychosomatic Research* **34**, 171–81.

Ross, D.M. and Ross, S.A. 1984: Childhood pain; the school aged child's viewpoint. *Pain* **20**, 179–91.

Roy, R., Thomas, M., Mogilevsky, I. and Cook, A. 1994: Influence of parental chronic pain on children: preliminary observations. *Headache Quarterly, Current Treatment and Research* **5**, 20–6.

Royal College of Surgeons of England and College of Anaesthetists 1990: *Report of the Working Party on Pain after Surgery*. London: Royal College of Surgeons of England.

Rushforth, H. 1996: Nurses' knowledge of how children view health and illness. *Paediatric Nursing* **8**, 23–7.

Savedra, M., Tesler, M., Ward, J., Wegner, C. and Gibbons, P. 1981: Description of the pain experience: a study of school-aged children. *Issues in Comprehensive Pediatric Nursing* 5, 373–80.

Savedra, M., Gibbons, P.T., Tesler, M.D., Ward, J.A. and Wegner, C. 1982: How do children describe pain? A tentative assessment. *Pain* 14, 95–104.

Saylor, C., Pallmeyer, T., Finch, A.J., Eason, L., Trieber, F. and Folger, C. 1987: Predictors of psychological distress in hospitalized pediatric patients. *Journal of the American Academy of Child and Adolescent Psychiatry* 26, 232–6.

Schechter, N.L. 1989: The undertreatment of pain in children: an overview. *Pediatric Clinics of North America* 36, 781–94.

Schechter, N.L., Berde, C.B. and Yaster, M. 1993: Pain in infants, children, and adolescents: an overview. In Schechter, N.L., Berde, C.B. and Yaster, M. (eds), *Pain in infants, children and adolescents*. Baltimore, MD: Williams and Wilkins, 3–10.

Siegel, L.J. and Smith, K.E. 1989: Children's strategies for coping with pain. *Pediatrician* 16, 110–18.

Smith, K.E., Ackerson, J.D. and Blotcky, A.D. 1989: Reducing distress during invasive medical procedures: relating behavioral interventions to preferred coping style in pediatric cancer patients. *Journal of Pediatric Psychology* 14, 405–19.

Spirito, A., Stark, L.J. and Tyc, V.L. 1994: Stressors and coping strategies described during hospitalization by chronically ill children. *Journal of Clinical Child Psychology* 23, 314–22.

Stevens, B., Hunsberger, M. and Browne, G. 1987: Pain in children; theoretical, research and practice dilemmas. *Journal of Pediatric Nursing* 2, 154–66.

Swafford, L.I. and Allen, D. 1968: Pain relief in the pediatric patient. *Medical Clinics of North America* 52, 131–6.

Swanwick, M. 1990: Knowledge and health. *Paediatric Nursing* 2, 18–20.

Tesler, M. D., Wegner, C., Savedra, M., Gibbons, P.T. and Ward, J.A. 1981: Coping strategies of children in pain. *Pediatric Nursing* 5, 351–9.

Turk, D.C., Meichenbaum, D. and Genest, M. 1983: *Pain and behavioural medicine: a cognitive-behavioural perspective*. New York: Guilford.

Valente, S.M. 1991: Using hypnosis with children for pain management. *Oncology Nursing Forum* 18, 699–704.

Vardaro, J.A. 1978: Preadmission anxiety and mother–child relationships. *Journal of the Association for the Care of the Child in Hospital* 8, 8–15.

Varni, J.W. 1995: Pediatric pain: a decade's biobehavioral perspective. *Behavioral Therapy* 18, 65–70.

Varni, J.W., Rapoff, M.A., Waldron, S.A., Gragg, R.A., Bernstein B.H. and Lindsley, C.B. 1996: Chronic pain and emotional distress in children and adolescents. *Developmental and Behavioral Pediatrics* 17, 154–61.

Vernon, D.T.A. 1974: Modeling and birth order in responses to painful stimuli. *Journal of Research in Social Psychology* 29, 794–9.

Volpe, J. 1981: *Neurology of the newborn*. Philadelphia, PA: Saunders.

Watt-Watson, J.H., Evernden, C. and Lawson, C. 1990: Parents' perceptions of their child's acute pain experience. *Journal of Pediatric Nursing* 5, 344–9.

Whaley, L. F. and Wong, D. L. 1989: *Essentials of pediatric nursing*, 3rd edn. St Louis, MO: Mosby.

Zelter, L. and LeBaron, S. 1982: Hypnosis and nonhypnotic teaching for reduction of pain and anxiety during painful procedures in children and adolescents with cancer. *Journal of Pediatrics* 101, 1032–5.

Young people and acute pain

Marjorie L. Gillies

Introduction

Young people are defined in different ways, but a generally accepted age group is 10–19 years (Department of Health, 1995). They are different from either adults or children in that they have specific age-related needs which include growing independence, an increasing need for privacy and a desire to comply with peer pressures (Coleman, 1980). Young people use the health service less than children and adults, but a significant number do receive care (Taylor and Müller, 1995). In general, the health care needs of young people are often not met in terms of their age-related needs, and recommendations for altering the practice of health professionals caring for this group have not been implemented (Gillies and Parry-Jones, 1992). Young people are usually nursed with children or adults, and hence the approach to their care is dictated by the group with which they are nursed, e.g. those in paediatric wards may be treated as though they are children. In a similar context, the management of acute pain in children and adults remains inadequate, despite recent increasing clinical and research attention (Royal College of Surgeons and College of Anaesthetists, 1990; McGrath, 1995; Romsing *et al.*, 1996). It is reasonable, therefore, to assume that the management of young people's pain will not be different.

Acute pain has been chosen as the focus for this chapter because, although young people can experience chronic or recurrent pain, the acute form is more common. Young people commonly experience acute pain as a result of trauma or, in hospitals, from surgical or medical procedures. The way in which they deal with pain may vary according to their past experience of pain, the cause of their suffering, their maturity, their emotional well-being or the attitudes of their carers. Each of these will be addressed, giving examples from a research study that has recently been completed (Gillies *et al.*, in preparation[1]). An overview of the recognition and management of pain in young people will follow, and consideration will be given to implications for practice. However, the first section will consider young people as a specific group because an understanding of adolescence is central to this chapter.

Young people

Young people are referred to using a variety of terms, such as teenagers, adolescents, or children. Regardless of which term is preferred, there is broad agreement, at World Health Organization level, that although young people are no longer children, they have not yet reached adulthood (Paxman and Zuckerman, 1987). To offer a definition of young people is difficult because the maturational process occurs at different times in different individuals and in different cultures, but a generally accepted age group is 10–19 years (Department of Health, 1995).

Young people differ from adults and children because they have specific physiological, psychological and social needs (Coleman, 1980). The physical development that occurs in puberty and the accompanying growth spurt are changes which require psychological adjustment and, for some young people, cause anxiety, e.g. concern about the rate of change in comparison with peers (Coleman, 1980): body image is therefore important. Nevertheless, it is crucial to recognize that adolescence is not always, or even usually, a difficult period for young people (Brannen *et al.*, 1994; Hobsbaum, 1995). Cognitive development is less obvious than the physiological changes, but is just as salient. Children already have the ability to think and, to some extent, to reason, but in young people these abilities develop further, allowing, for example, contradiction of adults to take place, while problem-solving becomes easier. Changes in self-image also occur as a result of the physical and cognitive development, but also because of the diminishing dependent role of the child and the emerging independent role which leads to adulthood. Relationships with parents change as a result, as young people become less dependent on them, while friendships and relationships with peers (of both sexes) become increasingly important.

In the UK health care system, the concept that adolescents may differ both from children and from adults, and therefore require separate care to meet their needs, is sometimes viewed controversially. The opinions of health professionals vary widely as to whether young people should be nursed with children or adults or in separate adolescent units, which are rare in the UK. In general, the health care needs of young people have not been met in terms of their developmental stage, and recommendations for altering the practice of health professionals caring for this group are seldom implemented (Gillies and Parry-Jones, 1992). Examples of important issues are as follows:

- the age at which young people can legally consent to or refuse treatment;
- the need for privacy at a stage when easily embarrassed;
- consideration of the dependence–independence continuum and the effect of hospitalization on this; and
- the need for peer company, particularly in an otherwise unfamiliar environment (Gillies, 1992).

Young people are perceived in different ways by adults, some of whom enjoy contact with them, are aware of their needs and can communicate effectively with them – some think that 'adolescents have a different outlook on life' (from adults and children) (Gillies *et al.*, in preparation[1]). However, other adults have difficulty in developing or maintaining relationships with young people. One contributory factor could be the label which some adults give young people, e.g. that of being rebellious and disobedient, when in fact they are asserting themselves in their quest for independence (Hadfield, 1967). Comments such as 'I don't believe in adolescence' are still heard.

The fact that health professions have not taken account of the issues deemed necessary for the effective care of young people is likely to impinge on more specific needs, such as the experience of pain. For example, the need for acute pain services, including those for children, was reported in 1990 (Royal College of Surgeons and College of Anaesthetists, 1990) but no consideration was given to young people. In practice, specialist pain posts have been created and pain relief is now receiving higher priority than ever before, but there is growing evidence that postoperative pain in young people could be managed more effectively (Tyler, 1990; Horimoto *et al.*, 1996; Gillies *et al.*, 1997; Gillies *et al.*, in preparation[1]).

Acute pain

The causes of pain are many and complex, particularly if recurrent and chronic pain are included. This chapter addresses only acute pain, which is often a sign that something is wrong and is usually the result of trauma, surgery or medical procedures, e.g. lumbar puncture. Acute pain is often intense and may last for days or weeks (Schechter *et al.*, 1993). Its recognition is complicated in young people by various influences, as it is in children and adults. These include the cause and type of pain, culture, environment, emotion, physiological factors, past experience of pain and development. In principle, these are the same for young people as they are for children, and are described elsewhere (Gillies, 1995). However, there are factors specific to young people, e.g. communication difficulties, gender differences, the effects of and past experience of pain, maturational stage and emotional well-being, which should be considered.

Communication has to be effective for pain to be assessed, relieved and the effect evaluated. Difficulties in communication are known to exist between adults – including health professionals – and young people (Gillies, 1992). Adults who feel uncomfortable with young people will not be as effective in their verbal and non-verbal communication as those who enjoy the company of the younger group and recognize their needs. In addition, the confidence of young patients in their carers is necessary if they are to confide their fears. Where pain is concerned, health professionals' interpretation of their young patient's behaviour, i.e. non-verbal communication, has been shown to be unreliable (Vetter and Heiner, 1996).

Gender differences and similarities in reaction to pain have been reported in the literature (Lander *et al.*, 1990; Fowler-Kerry and Lander, 1991; Erickson, 1992). Fowler-Kerry and Lander (1991) examined 90 males and 90 females aged 5–17 years following venepuncture and found many similarities between the sexes, but males tended to underestimate and females tended to over-estimate the level of pain, despite similar pain scores. On the other hand, Erickson (1992) argued that males and females have similar pain thresholds, but that their pain-related behaviour often differs, with males displaying a macho image while females are expected to be less tolerant of pain. However, this is to some extent dependent on culture and upbringing (Facett et al., 1994). Preliminary findings (Gillies et al., in preparation[1]) indicate that most health professionals support the view that differences exist, with adolescent males often displaying a macho image, neither admitting to pain nor acknowledging a need for analgesics, while females are more likely to voice complaints about pain. Although nurses and doctors commonly believe that young people deny the presence of pain, most young people, regardless of sex, will admit to pain. Allowing young people the option of admitting to pain by talking about the fact that they will not lose face is helpful, as it offers the patient control, rather than an out-of-control feeling created by unrelieved pain.

The perception of pain increases if the young person is afraid, worried or tired, and in addition to altering mood, pain may also change behaviour and self-esteem. Young people are more likely to report pain than children, but are less likely to display pain-related behaviour such as crying. Displays of pain behaviour in the presence of others and quiet behaviour when alone may be misinterpreted by health professionals as meaning that the pain is less severe than it really is (Erickson, 1992). This may contribute to health professionals not believing the complaints. If asked, most young people will describe their pain, e.g. as 'stabbing pain' or 'booming in and out', and the majority have the cognitive skills to use pain measures. Almost all young people will be able to localize the site of their pain.

Memory for painful experiences is reported from 6 months of age (Schechter et al., 1993). It is therefore likely that by the time young people are teenagers they will have had numerous experiences involving pain of varying severity. Examples of painful experiences most frequently cited by young people include fractured bones, previous surgery, muscular or ligament injuries and earache (Gillies et al., in preparation[1]). Some such episodes, experienced as children or in the teenage years, may cause immense distress, the memory of which might influence pain perception in the future.

Maturational stage is difficult to measure because it is an ongoing process through which individuals pass at their own pace. However, attempts have been made to measure it, e.g. by rating self-image in 12 different areas and as a whole, to give a measure of psychological adjustment to adolescence, using the Offer Self-Image Questionnaire – Revised (Offer et al., 1992; Siefen et al., 1996). Although not without recent criticism (Abella et al., 1994), the measure is useful. Very few studies have been conducted to investigate the effect of psychological adjustment to adolescence on the clinical needs or care of young people. Nevertheless, research is important when considering the health care needs of this group, and the experience of pain in particular. Evidence support-ing this view was obtained recently by Gillies et al. (in preparation[1]), who suggest that young people who are poorly adjusted psychologically to their stage of development in adolescence are more likely to experience higher levels of pain than their well-adjusted peers. Furthermore, the presence of anxiety was related to dissatisfaction with body image. Similar findings have been reported by Brown and Moerenhout (1991) in relation to dental treatment, but more research is required in this area.

Emotional state, particularly anxiety, is known to be linked with pain perception. Anxiety arises because of worry, e.g. about a situation or an impending event. The importance of considering emotional state and acute pain in young people following burns has been described by Favaloro (1988), who argues that nurses need to know about adolescent behaviour, and in particular emotional control, so that the young victims can be helped to cope with their pain.

Preoperative preparation, i.e. the provision of information, can play a major role in the reduction of postoperative anxiety and related pain. The principal areas that worry young people in relation to surgery are the anaesthetic, pain and injections. Fear of the unknown causes emotional upset. However, if details about what is to happen are given and taken on board, then the reality may be less upsetting than originally anticipated. Health professionals usually give some information to patients, but the provision of detailed information may be less common practice. Moreover, information may be given but not received – it may be misunderstood and not clarified, or not heard. In other words, the information has to be desired. There are a few young people who simply do not want to know, and their wishes have to be respected.

Support for the link between pain and anxiety in young people has been found by Gillies *et al.* (in preparation[1]), who suggest that pain severity is directly linked to clinical anxiety and depression. Individuals with such symptoms are more likely to experience moderate or severe pain postoperatively than young people who do not display such clinical symptoms. Although depression has been linked less often than anxiety to acute pain, its inclusion raises an interesting point. It is not unusual to observe patients who have undergone surgery feeling 'low' afterwards, but it could be said to be unusual for health professionals to consider that this feeling might be serious enough to warrant further intervention, possibly involving more effective pain relief and reassurance. However, the unfortunate label of 'troublemakers/attention-seekers' that is sometimes attached to young people, and concerns voiced by health professionals about drug dependency, may contribute to infrequent administration of strong analgesics. The outcome for such patients is likely to be more pain, and feeling worse, both physically and mentally, than they might have done had they received effective analgesia.

Parents should not be forgotten. Despite the fact that many young people are becoming increasingly independent of their parents, the latter still wish to be involved in what is happening to their child. The amount of information given to parents varies depending on where the young person is nursed. In a paediatric setting, parental involvement is maximized, and this includes minute detail about what is happening. On the other hand, in an adult setting there is less involvement of relatives. Young people are neither adults nor children and, although the desires of parents should be listened to, the rights of the young person need to be considered as well. A compromise should be negotiated between the young person, his or her parents and the health professionals in order to keep all parties satisfied, thereby reducing parental anxiety which could be transferred to the young person, with the possibility of increasing pain perception.

The attitudes of health professionals to young people vary, and can have a negative or positive influence on the care which is received. Preconceived ideas about the severity of pain, such as: *'postoperative pain is not all that severe'* and *'not in the same league as labour or renal colic'*, that may be held by health professionals make accurate assessment of the existence and severity of pain subjective and difficult. On the other hand, acknowledgement that any pain is as severe or unpleasant as the patient says it is will result in a greater likelihood of appropriate assessment and consequent pain relief. The administration of analgesics is also influenced by attitudes such as *'adolescents clock-watch for drugs'*.

It is not difficult to see why analgesics, especially strong ones, are not administered often or regularly when beliefs such as this exist. In the absence of evidence that young people receive effective pain relief or 'clock-watch' for pain-relieving drugs, their right to high-quality care, including pain relief, should be respected. The lack of sensitivity towards a particularly vulnerable group may enhance their negative experience of hospitalization and surgery, not forgetting continuing inadequately relieved pain. The influence on health care of professionals with positive attitudes to young people can be demonstrated in the clear understanding that some of them display. For example, a grasp of the importance of preoperative information and its possible effect on the experience of some young people is explained by one health professional as *'guilt associated with feeling pain if (adolescents are) not pre-warned'*.

Accurate pain assessment is crucial if pain relief is to be effective. Most health professionals believe that they are able to assess a young person's pain adequately but this contradicts the views of many young people (Gillies *et al.*, in preparation[1]). The usual but unreliable methods of assessing young people's pain include reliance on verbal and non-verbal communication, measurement of clinical signs, e.g. blood pressure, and observation of behaviour. A few formalized methods of measuring young people's pain exist, but they are infrequently used. Those that are more commonly used are visual analogue, numerical or word-graphic rating scales (see Figure 17.1).

The Adolescent Pediatric Pain Tool (APPT) is a self-completion pain measure, designed specifically to assess postoperative pain (location, intensity and descriptions) in patients aged 8–17 years (see Figure 17.2). It is simple to use, not time-consuming, has been validated in the USA and is relatively inexpensive (Savedra *et al.*, 1990). To the author's knowledge the APPT has been used only twice in the UK (Savedra, 1996, personal communication; Gillies *et al.*, 1997; Gillies *et al.*, in preparation[1]).

The McGill Pain Questionnaire, which is well known and on which the APPT is based, is more suitable for the assessment of recurrent or chronic pain, and is not described here (Melzack, 1975).

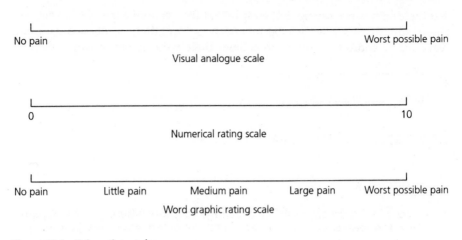

Figure 17.1   Pain rating scales

Pain management

The management of young people's pain follows similar principles to those recommended for other age groups. Analgesics prescribed for young people are varied, often with a number of drugs of differing strengths and times of action being prescribed at any one time. The choice about whether and when to administer the drug lies with the health professional. When faced with a choice of administering an opiate or a non-opiate, many nurses will select non-opiates, while few will opt for the opiate, with potentially serious implications for pain relief. Fear that pain may not be adequately treated contributes to anxiety (Erickson, 1992), which in turn raises pain perception. One young person once told the author that the worst (postoperative) pain was *'dead sore but nurse didn't give me anything 'cos I'd be sick, so I just took it (the pain) for a while and went back to sleep'*. The problem of effectively relieving postoperative pain can be complicated by unpleasant side-effects such as nausea and vomiting. Kart *et al.* (1996) have identified the importance of alleviating such problems while still adequately relieving the pain.

The method of analgesic administration can be important. Oral analgesic administration is often the route of choice, but can in itself be problematic. Some people, regardless of age, have difficulty in swallowing tablets. This possibility is catered for in children, who may be given an alternative liquid medicine, but adults are often expected to swallow tablets. Young people are often treated like adults and so are given tablets. This sometimes results in refusal to take pain relief, and failure to explain or question the reason for the refusal may lead to continuing unrelieved pain. An alternative route is injections – never a popular choice! Although many young people fear injections, they (unlike children) will often accept one if pain relief is going to follow (Erickson, 1992). However, there is a small number of young people who will always refuse injections, preferring to suffer their pain. This does not mean that their pain is not severe, but simply that they cannot cope with injections. These individuals are likely to be anxious because of their unrelieved pain, and every effort should be made to relieve their pain in other ways. Patient-

CODE _____

DATE _____

ADOLESCENT PEDIATRIC PAIN TOOL (APPT)

INSTRUCTIONS:

1. **Colour in the areas on these drawings to show where you have pain. Make the marks as big or as small as the place where the pain is.**

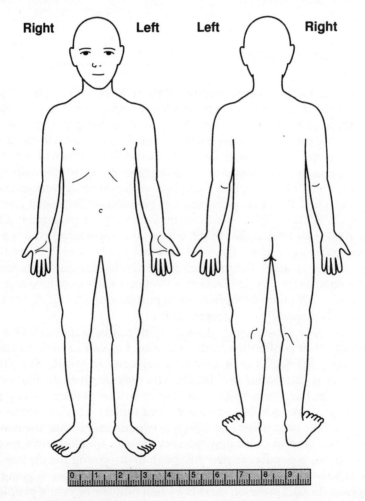

Figure 17.2 Continued on next page

2. **Place a straight, up and down mark on this line to show how much pain you have.**

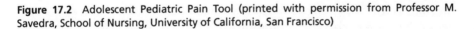

No pain	Little pain	Medium pain	Large pain	Worst possible pain

3. **Point to or circle as many of these words that describe your pain.**

1	5	10	15
annoying	blistering	awful	off and on
bad	burning	deadly	once in a while
horrible	hot	dying	sneaks up
miserable	**6**	killing	sometimes
terrible	cramping	**11**	steady
uncomfortable	crushing	crying	
2	like a pinch	frightening	If you like,
aching	pinching	screaming	you may add
hurting	pressure	terrifying	other words:
like an ache	**7**	**12**	
like a hurt	itching	dizzy	_____
sore	like a scratch	sickening	
3	like a sting	suffocating	_____
beating	scratching	**13**	
hitting	stinging	never goes away	_____
pounding	**8**	uncontrollable	
punching	shocking	**14**	
throbbing	shooting	always	
4	splitting	comes and goes	
biting	**9**	comes on all of	
cutting	numb	a sudden	
like a pin	stiff	constant	
like a sharp knife	swollen	continuous	
pin like	tight	forever	
sharp			
stabbing			

For office use only.

BSA: _____
IS: _____

#S(2-9) _____ /37 = _____ %
#A(10-12) _____ /11 = _____ %
#E(1,13) _____ /8 = _____ %
#S(14,15) _____ /11 = _____ %
#S(2-9) _____ /67 = _____ %

Figure 17.2 Adolescent Pediatric Pain Tool (printed with permission from Professor M. Savedra, School of Nursing, University of California, San Francisco)

controlled analgesia, used routinely for adults and children, has been recommended and used for young people (Tyler, 1990; Gaukroger, 1993).

Analgesics are more often refused by young people than by children. Reasons for this include the belief that the pain is not severe enough to warrant analgesics, the belief that swallowing would be painful, concern about dependency and possibly concern that admitting to pain is not 'adult' behaviour, thereby putting the credibility of their macho image in doubt. On the other hand, misunderstandings can influence behaviour: '(he) wanted to be aware of where the pain was so (he) didn't do anything to hurt it'. Specific information about how pain can be relieved, the methods of achieving this and the benefits of effective analgesia would have prevented this mistaken belief. Dealing with unexpected pain can be difficult for a young person who does not want to be seen to be 'weak', yet who wishes to remain in control.

The reasons for failure to give analgesics include side-effects, dependency, and over- or under-dosage. Dependency on drugs given for acute pain in hospital is rarely reported, but this possibility cannot be excluded completely. Therefore, it is important that health professionals do not allow their personal concerns about drug dependency to cloud their judgement about analgesic administration. However, it is also important to acknowledge that there will be a few young people presenting for health care who already have an existing drug or substance dependency. For this reason, health professionals working with young people should have a basic knowledge of how to identify those at risk of drug abuse. This includes poor school performance, social isolation apart from drug-using friends, and rebelliousness (McKenzie and Kipke, 1992), and it has implications for admission procedures.

Non-pharmacological methods of relieving pain include the use of heat or cold and physiotherapy and, less commonly, transcutaneous electrical nerve stimulation (TENS), acupuncture and aromatherapy. The latter are rarely used with young people, possibly because specific training is required for some and, although a number of health professionals hold the relevant qualifications, there is little provision made for the use of such practices within the health care system. Distraction as a means of pain relief is perceived sceptically by many health professionals, but many parents believe that it is useful, and young people actively use it as a means of coping with pain (Gillies *et al.*, in preparation[1]). Guided imagery has been used successfully in the reduction of anxiety and pain postoperatively in adults who have undergone major surgery (Tusek *et al.*, 1997), but to the author's knowledge it has not been attempted with young people.

Implications for clinical practice

It is true to say that some of what is written in this chapter could be applied to adults and children, as well as to young people. However, it is important that, just as developmental stage needs to be taken into consideration for children, the same is true for young people. They should be recognized as a group with needs that differ from those of adults or children. When caring for young people with acute pain, the aim of effectively relieving that pain will be enhanced by taking into account their past experience of pain, emotional state, psychological adjustment to adolescence and gender, and by using formal pain measures and giving analgesic drugs regularly. Ensuring that communication skills are effective and being aware of the possible need for a change in attitudes will also have a beneficial effect. By following these suggestions, the relief of acute pain in young people will be enhanced, and in addition their overall recovery is likely to benefit.

Endnote

1. This research examined the postoperative pain experience of young people, in addition to assessment of their emotional state and their psychological adjustment to adolescence. The research will be available shortly in several papers that are currently being prepared for publication. For further information please contact Marjorie Gillies, Department of Child and Adolescent Psychiatry, University of Glasgow, Caledonia House, Royal Hospital for Sick Children, Glasgow G3 8SJ, UK.

References

Abella, A., Knauer, D., Palacio Espasa, F. and Cramer, B. 1994: A self-evaluation questionnaire for adolescents: the Offer Self-Image Questionnaire: usefulness and limits in clinical evaluation. *Neuropsychiatrie de l'Enfance et de l'Adolescence* **42**, 681–92.

Brannen, J., Dodd, K., Oakley, A. and Storey, P. 1994: *Young people, health and family life*. Buckingham: Open University Press.

Brown, D. and Moerenhout, R. 1991: The pain experience and psychological adjustment to orthodontic treatment of preadolescents, adolescents and adults. *American Journal of Orthodontic and Dentofacial Orthopedics* **100**, 349–56.

Coleman, J. 1980: *The nature of adolescence*. London: Methuen.

Department of Health 1995: *Child health in the community: a guide to good practice*. Consultation draft. London: Department of Health.

Erickson, C. 1992: Assessment and management of pain. In Friedman, S., Fisher, M. and Schonberg, S. (eds), *Comprehensive adolescent health care*. St Louis: Quality Medical Publishing, Inc., 108–18.

Facett, J., Gordon, N. and Levine, J. 1994: Differences in postoperative pain severity among four ethnic groups. *Journal of Pain and Symptom Management* **9**, 383–9.

Favaloro, R. 1988: Adolescent development and implications for pain management. *Pediatric Nursing* **14**, 27–9.

Fowler-Kerry, S. and Lander, J. 1991: Assessment of sex differences in children's and adolescents' self-reported pain from venepuncture. *Journal of Pediatric Psychology* **16**, 783–93.

Gaukroger, P. 1993: Patient-controlled analgesia in children. In Schechter, N., Berde, C. and Yaster, M. (eds), *Pain in infants, children and adolescents*. London: Williams and Wilkins, 203–11.

Gillies, M. 1992: Teenage traumas. *Nursing Times* **88**, 26–9.

Gillies, M. 1995: Pain management. In Carter, B. and Dearmun, A.K. (eds), *Child health care and development. Concepts, theory and practice*. Oxford: Blackwell Science, 193–221.

Gillies, M. and Parry-Jones, W. 1992: Suitability of the paediatric setting for hospitalised adolescents. *Archives of Disease in Childhood* **67**, 1506–19.

Gillies, M., Parry-Jones, W. and Smith, L. 1997: Postoperative pain in adolescents: a pilot study. *Journal of Clinical Nursing* **6**, 77–8.

Hadfield, J. 1967: *Childhood and adolescence*. Harmondsworth: Penguin.

Hobsbaum, A. 1995: Children's development. In Carter, B. and Dearmun, A.K. (eds), *Child health care and development. Concepts, theory and practice*. Oxford: Blackwell Science, 130–56.

Horimoto, Y., Yoshioka, H., Suzuki, A., Fujino, S. and Takano, T. 1996: What do adolescents desire for the postoperative pain relief? A speculation from an interview with a patient. *Japanese Journal of Anaesthesiology* **45**, 1160–63.

Kart, T., Van der Laan, K., Crombach, J. *et al.* 1996: Postoperative pain management in children has been improved but can be further optimised. *European Journal of Pediatric Surgery* **6**, 259–64.

Lander, J., Fowler-Kerry, S. and Hill, A. 1990: Comparison of pain perceptions among males and females. *Canadian Journal of Nursing Research* **2**, 39–49.

McGrath, P.J. 1995: Annotation: aspects of pain in children and adolescents. *Journal of Child Psychology and Psychiatry* **36**, 717–30.

McKenzie, R. and Kipke, M. 1992: Substance use and abuse. In Friedman, S., Fisher, M. and Schonberg, S. (eds), *Comprehensive adolescent health care*. St Louis: Quality Medical Publishing, Inc., 765–86.

Melzack, R. 1975: The McGill Pain Questionnaire: major properties and scoring methods. *Pain* **1**, 277–99.

Offer, D., Ostrov, E., Howard, K. and Dolan, S. 1992: *Offer Self-Image Questionnaire, Revised*. Los Angeles, CA: Western Psychological Services.

Paxman, P. and Zuckerman, R. 1987: *Laws and policies affecting adolescent health*. Geneva: World Health Organization.

Romsing, J., Sonnergaard, J., Hertel, S. and Rasmussen, M. 1996: Postoperative pain in children: comparison between ratings of children and nurses. *Journal of Pain and Symptom Management* **11**, 42–6.

Royal College of Surgeons and College of Anaesthetists 1990: *Commission on the provision of surgical services. Report of the Working Party on Pain After Surgery*. London: Royal College of Surgeons and College of Anaesthetists.

Savedra, M., Tesler, M., Holzemer, W. and Ward, J. 1990: *Adolescent Pediatric Pain Tool (APPT): user's manual*: San Francisco, CA: University of California, School of Nursing.

Schechter, N., Berde, C. and Yaster, M. 1993: Pain in infants, children and adolescents: an overview. In Schechter, N., Berde, C. and Yaster, M. (eds), *Pain in infants, children and adolescents*. London: Williams and Wilkins, 3–9.

Siefen, G., Kirkcaldy, B., Athanasou, J. and Peponis, M. 1996: The self-image of Greek, Greek-migrant and German adolescents. *Social Psychiatry and Psychiatric Epidemiology* **31**, 241–7.

Taylor, J. and Müller, D. 1995: *Nursing adolescents. Research and psychological perspectives*. Oxford: Blackwell Science.

Tusek, D., Church Strong, S., Grass, J. and Fazio, V. 1997: A significant advance in the care of patients undergoing elective colorectal surgery. *Diseases of the Colon and Rectum* **40**, 172–8.

Tyler, D. 1990: Patient-controlled analgesia in adolescents. *Journal of Adolescent Health Care* **11**, 154–8.

Vetter, T. and Heiner, E. 1996: Discordance between patient self-reported visual analogue scale pain scores and observed pain-related behavior in older children after surgery. *Journal of Clinical Anaesthesia* **8**, 371–5.

Pain in later life

Trevor M. Corran and Beatrice Melita

Introduction

Findings from surveys, clinical and experimental studies demonstrate the high prevalence of persistent and chronic pain during the later years of life. Harkins (1988) has previously addressed the myth that older people feel pain differently to younger individuals because of age *per se*. Over the last decade there has been increasing evidence refuting the notion that pain is invariably a consequence of ageing. Physical pathology or psychological factors underlie the reporting of pain. It is Harkins' (1996) contention that earlier research evidence did not support the notion that older people, through stoicism or physiological insensitivity, experience less pain. He emphasizes that older people are as much subject to the ravages of pain as younger people. Indeed, many factors point to an increased vulnerability to the impact of pain. A line of argument which is being advanced in very recent publications indicates that the older person in pain may 'be confronted with a predicament that threatens to overwhelm him or her' and 'yet many are able to draw upon reserves and strategies that ameliorate the situation. For others chronic pain is a torment that has both physical and emotional dimensions' (Farrell *et al.*, 1996a, p.81).

This section focuses on the dimensions of pain. The multidimensionality of pain was a concept originally addressed by Melzack and Wall in their now well-known 'gate control theory of pain' (Melzack and Casey, 1968). The multidimensionality of pain is summarized as consisting of the sensory-discriminative, affective-motivational and cognitive-interpretive dimensions. The interaction of age and other variables with these dimensions will be the focus of this chapter. It is argued here that age brings specific health problems, a fact that is clearly demonstrated in a recent review by Gibson and Helme (1995). They point out that less than 25 per cent of individuals remain disability free by the age of 70 years, and less than 15 per cent by the age of 80 years (Gibson and Helme, 1995). Recent evidence suggests the existence of a complex relationship between age, disease and pain (Harkins, 1996). According to Harkins, 'It is likely that chronic pain represents a major source of morbidity, reduced quality of life, and contributes to mortality in the old' (Harkins, 1996, p.456).

Melding (1991) decried the lack of attention paid to the research and treatment of pain in the elderly. It has taken a considerable amount of time for the significance of pain in the elderly to be recognized, and its relevance becomes clearer with epidemiological evidence. There has been room for optimism in cent years as a greater emphasis is being given to researching the older ulation, and an increasing number of publications focusing on the issue of pain in older people have been produced. Helme and Gibson (1996) investigated the volume of research through a Medline review, using the key words 'pain' and 'elderly' or 'aged'. The review revealed 848 references from 1975 to 1979. Fifteen years, later between 1990 and 1994, the number had more than doubled to 1876. It is a timely change, as they believe that it mirrors the increasing number of older people in the world. Using a cut-off point of '65 years for ageing', the elderly population in 1992 was 342 million, and was increasing by one million each month.

Two subgroups of old people are not specifically addressed in this chapter, namely older women and cancer patients. Women are extremely vulnerable to diseases of old age, due to their higher survival rates and higher prevalence of medical problems. Given the relationship between pain and disease, there is a high likelihood that a significant proportion of older women are living with chronic pain (Roberto, 1994). Not only has there been a paucity of research on older people in the past, but even less attention has been given to gender differences. This is an area that will need significantly more investigation in the future.

Only a very small number of cancer patients are referred to pain clinics, and it is from such clinics that much of the research and understanding of chronic pain are obtained. All (1994) reported that 60 to 85 per cent of individuals with advanced cancer have either severe or chronic pain. Non-pharmacological strategies have been suggested as being useful. However, other specialist centres have more specifically addressed the needs of cancer patients.

The distinction between younger and older people is further delineated in order to provide additional insights into the experience of pain in later life. Despite a gradual increase in the amount of research on chronic pain in older people, a smaller group is still being neglected in the investigations, namely those regarded as the 'frail old' or the 'old old'. The 'young old' are considered to be those aged between 60 and 70 years, and the 'old old' are 75 years of age or older (World Health Organization, 1963). More recently, the 'oldest old', over 85 years of age, have been ascribed their own specific features (Suzman et al., 1992). The term 'frail' is taken to indicate the decreased reserve in various organ systems that develops with advanced age (Farrell et al., 1996a). Epidemiological studies of pain acknowledge the further differentiation of older people by focusing on two main populations, namely those in the community and the 'oldest old', who are predominantly represented in nursing homes. This chapter will explore the differences and similarities between younger and older people's experience of pain across the dimensions established by the gate control theory of pain.

Prevalence of pain in the community

Farrell et al. (1996a) provide a summary of epidemiological studies which, despite some variation in absolute prevalence rates, indicates that pain in older people is a common experience. Helme and Allen (1992) report the results of a survey of medication use in the community in Australia, where it was found that 47 per cent of individuals, with a mean age of 79 years, suffered from a condition which caused them pain. This is consistent with the often cited Canadian study (Crook *et al.*, 1984), which found that by the age of 80 years, 40 per cent of individuals were reporting the presence of chronic pain. Gibson and Helme (1995) comment on the high quality of recent epidemiological investigations which focus on a narrower population of individuals aged 65 years and over. These studies add important information to our understanding of the prevalence of pain in older people because of tailored sampling methods designed specifically to recruit older individuals. The high number of older adults sampled, and the more comprehensive representation of the 'old' elderly, have identified higher rates of pain at 60 to 80 per cent.

With better research methods, an important trend has been identified. Roy and Thomas (1987) reported a decrease in the prevalence of pain in older people the 'oldest old', aged 80 to 89 years, of 64 per cent, compared to 81 per cent for the younger elderly, aged 64 to 69 years. This finding is discussed by Farrell *et al.* (1996a), who suggest that factors contributing to these differences may include survivorship, increased rates of institutionalization and psychological and physiological changes in pain perception and reporting.

Qualitative factors in the measurement of pain further demonstrate the significance of pain in older people. Helme and Allen's (1992) Australian study indicated that, of those subjects who acknowledged having pain, 13 per cent reported 'strong', 'severe' or 'excruciating' pain. The majority reported 'just noticeable' pain (33 per cent), followed by reports of 'moderate' and 'mild pain' of 26 per cent and 16 per cent, respectively. Pain interfering with life 'nearly always' was reported by 22 per cent. In summary, it is evident that pain has to be regarded as an important factor in the experience of older people in the general community.

Nursing home populations

As many older people live in assisted accommodation rather than in the community, epidemiological research of pain prevalence in nursing-home settings also deserves separate consideration. A comprehensive study by Parmelee *et al.* (1993) of 758 residents living in a large multi-level care facility found that the overall prevalence of 'bothersome pain' in the previous few weeks was 79.9 per cent. Interestingly, a study by Roy and Thomas (1986), which surveyed 97 people living in a nursing home and 35 individuals attending an elderly day-hospital programme, found that 83 per cent of subjects reported having current pain-related problems which were attributed to musculoskeletal disorders of the back, joints and muscles. Whilst the reported intensity of pain was low, 93 per cent of those with pain had been suffering for more than 12 months, and one-third reported pain of duration longer than 10 years. A similar study of 97 nursing-home residents, conducted by Ferrell *et al.* (1990), found that 71 per cent suffered from at least one pain complaint. The majority of residents reported recurrent intermittent pain, and one-third indicated the presence of constant pain.

The significance of pain prevalence in the 'oldest old' is reinforced by Sengstaken and King (1993), who estimate that 43 per cent of all individuals who were 65 years old in 1990 will enter nursing homes at some time before they die. The complications created by the interaction of ageing variables with pain indicate the importance of understanding pain in the 'old old'. For instance, another aspect of pain prevalence in the 'oldest old' in nursing-home populations was the very strong association between pain and depression, which indicated a significant need for depression to be aggressively treated. Stein and Ferrell (1996) also refer to additional difficulties and problems presented by non-communicative patients with pain. These people require frequent assessments to evaluate current pain and discomfort. Indeed, the investigation of pain in dementia confronts us all with situations that demand examination of the very nature of the pain experience. The pain clinic, which has for so long focused predominantly on younger adults, can play a significant role in investigating the clinical experience of pain of all older people.

The pain clinic population

The nature of the population that attends multidisciplinary pain clinics is relevant. Melding (1991) notes that ageing brings about changes in psychological and social functioning, and there is some additional support for the notion that social dysfunction is an indicator for a multidisciplinary pain clinic referral. Kwentus et al. (1985) pointed out that multidisciplinary pain clinics should be suitable for older people, particularly as non-pharmacological treatment is often superior to pain medication. Nevertheless, older people represent only 7 to 10 per cent of pain clinic patients and, due to their comparatively lower numbers in pain clinics, older patients have been under-represented in research studies and treatment programmes.

The 'oldest old' are unlikely to be able to attend pain clinics – the primary source of study of clinical pain – and those who are included in pain clinic studies are likely to be the mobile 'young old'. There is evidence to suggest that younger patients attending pain clinics differ from the general population (Crook et al., 1989) in that they have higher levels of mood disturbance associated with chronic pain.

In order to address these problems, two multidisciplinary pain clinics for the elderly were established in Melbourne. The first of these was opened over a decade ago (Helme et al., 1989). Data collected from the second pain clinic for the elderly in Melbourne support a similar conclusion to that of Crook et al. (1989), indicating significantly higher levels of depression in the pain clinic population. Helme et al. (1989) report that arthritis was the most common diagnosis in the pain clinic, followed by post-herpetic neuralgia and patients presenting with emotional and functional symptoms of sufficient severity to meet the criteria of a somataform pain disorder (American Psychiatric Association, 1994).

Dementia and pain

Previous epidemiological surveys ignored the impact of dementia in pain prevalence estimates. As with other aspects of pain in older people, Parmelee (1996) notes the paucity of research into pain and dementia and the relationship between the two. Surveys have failed to screen older people for cognitive impairment and its relevance to understanding prevalence rates is critical, because people with cognitive impairment have a tendency to report lower levels of pain (Farrell *et al.*, 1996b). Some discussion of the relevance of this dimension within the general population of older people is therefore necessary.

The review by Farrell *et al.* (1996b) of the relevant literature reveals conflicting reports on the relationships between pain variables and cognitive impairment. Parmelee (1996) argues that the evidence tends to support an equal risk of pain in all older people, but that those with dementia are less likely to complain for a number of reasons. Dementia and its consequent problems, such as impaired formal operational thinking, leads to the formation of less sophisticated concepts of illness and pain. This may lead to miscommunication about the pain, resulting in the underlying pathology being masked by behavioural disturbances. Due to difficulties in assessing the cognitively impaired, problems associated with chronic pain in older people are likely to be compounded. In nursing homes, 75 per cent of residents are estimated to be cognitively impaired, and 25 per cent of older people in more independent congregate apartments have been identified as cognitively impaired. Similar rates were found by Jorm and Henderson (1993). The combined chronic pain and dementia prevalence data suggest that a significant problem exists in this population group. In fact, one study reported that 66 per cent of cognitively impaired people present with chronic pain (Sengstaken and King, 1993).

Parmelee (1996) tentatively concluded that there was an association between cognitive impairment and decreased propensity to report pain. Farrell *et al.* (1996b) also noted that there is less reporting of pain by cognitively impaired people, and even less by those who are significantly cognitively impaired. It is not yet clear whether this data represents a diminution in the experience of pain or a deterioration in recall and communication of symptoms. Complaints of all types of symptoms diminish as a function of cognitive impairment and, concomitantly, pain complaints would also decrease (McCormick *et al.*, 1994). Farrell *et al.* (1996b) suggest that there are various reasons for the reduced capacity to report pain, and it is also possible that less pain is experienced as a function of the disease. However, Parmelee (1996) indicates that even when health status is controlled, cognitive impairment continues to be associated with a bias against the reporting of pain.

Acute and clinical pain

In general, acute pain serves a protective role, drawing attention to actual or potential tissue damage and protecting those tissues from further damage (Gibson *et al.*, 1994). Helme and Gibson (1996) consider that pain resolves spontaneously with the natural history of an injury or illness following appropriate intervention. Health status may restrict treatment options, but treatment will be focused on the symptomatic presentation of the injury or illness in order to limit suffering (Gibson *et al.*, 1994). Findings from epidemiological studies indicate a distinct difference in the prevalence of acute pain compared to chronic pain. The distinction between chronic and acute pain is often made on a temporal basis – pain which has existed for more than 6 months is considered to be chronic. In addition, a further distinction is sometimes made between sub-acute pain, of 3 to 6 months' duration, and acute pain, which can be of less than 3 months' duration. Harkins (1996) suggests adopting the definition proposed by Bonica (1990) for chronic pain. Pain is considered to be chronic when it extends beyond the normal time for healing or is associated with a chronic pathological process which causes the pain to be continuous, or to recur at intervals over months or years.

Prevalence rates of 5 per cent for acute pain are consistent across all age groups (Crook *et al.*, 1984). Kwentus *et al.* (1985) reviewed differences in the presentation of acute pain between the younger and older patients and found that the reporting of pain for some acute conditions differs according to age. For example, pain associated with myocardial infarction was reported by people of advanced age to be less painful. Gibson and Helme (1995) point to similar evidence with regard to abdominal pain. However, as Harkins (1996) comments, pain associated with musculoskeletal and other cardiovascular disorders increases with age. Overall, the research infers a relative absence or low levels of pain in the presentation of some disease states in elderly adults.

Perception of severe and persistent pain

Gibson and Helme (1995) summarize pain as a complex perceptual experience that incorporates sensory, emotional and cognitive components. The context in which noxious information is processed, the cognitive beliefs of the individual, and the meanings attributed to the presence of noxious sensation are recognized as important factors in shaping the overall experience of pain (Melzack, 1973).

It is well recognized that sensory changes occur with 'normal ageing'. Harkins' (1988) review of the evidence considers age-related changes in the skin senses in conjunction with physiological changes in other body systems, and demonstrates that decreases in acuity occur across the senses. It follows that changes in pain perception should also occur. However, at the time of publication of Harkins' paper, research had noted little difference in experimental pain perception between younger and older people. Similarly, Ferrell (1991) indicated that there was little evidence regarding differences in pain perception. Sorkin *et al.* (1990) went even further in concluding that the similarities between younger and older people were greater than the differences.

More recent experimental evidence indicates that the sensory discriminative dimension is affected by age, and suggests that the increase in pain threshold is due to physiological and neurological changes (Helme and Gibson, 1996). Gibson and Helme's (1995) comprehensive review of physiological, psychological, laboratory and clinical studies, points to morphological, physiological and functional changes which occur in nociceptive pathways with advancing age. In particular, they found that age-related changes in stimulation are likely to be significant but few systematic studies have addressed this issue. There was no conclusive evidence of changes in the density of structure of nerve endings, while electrophysical studies indicated slower central processing of information from stimuli and reduced cortical activity.

Parmelee (1994) considers that age differences are not necessarily due to differences in sensory experience, but are more likely to be related to the person's labelling of a stimulus as painful. Indeed, as stimuli are processed, interpreted and ascribed meaning, more complex cognitive structures come into play such that differences in presentation and report occur (Helme and Gibson, 1996).

A study of age differences in clinical pain in 297 patients ranging in age from 18 to over 90 years was recently conducted by Corran *et al.* (1994). It involved a series of tests which attempted to synthesize and describe the patient's problem. In essence the tests describe the pain, its cause, and the person's mood state, behaviour and interaction with the environment. The results indicated no apparent age-related differences in pain when assessed by sensory or affective descriptors or measures of depressed mood. However, some differences in anxiety level, impact of pain and coping styles were found. Helme and Gibson (1996) conclude from this study that the description of pain across age groups was very similar, even though the causes of pain were different.

Price (1988) discusses the way in which a painful stimulus is given meaning. He presents an heuristic model which considers the parallel activation of sensory-discriminative functions, physiological arousal and pain-related motor responses. According to Price, emotional states are dependent on sequential processing of cognitive processes. As a result of these processes, unremitting pain is in some instances associated with significant mood disturbance and functional impairment. However, in the majority of cases, pain is most probably tolerated with minimal negative emotional and physical impact. Factors that distinguish patients along this clinical spectrum have been the subject of considerable speculation and investigation (Farrell *et al.*, 1996a) but, as usual, research has focused on younger populations.

Age-related differences in pain perception are probably mediated by alterations in the peripheral and central nervous system pain pathways, and by the individual's adoption of a more cautious or stoical approach in reporting the presence of pain (Gibson *et al.*, 1994). The reasons for this approach are derived from survey evidence which suggests that it could be partly due to the older person's expectation that they will experience pain with increasing age (Gibson and Helme, 1995). These factors tend to reduce the impact of mild aches and pain, because the elderly are more likely to attribute mild aches to ageing. A review of the evidence indicates the existence of subtle differences between younger and older people in coping with pain, degree of disability and psychological impact (Gibson and Helme, 1995). However, more severe pain is attributed to illness equally across the age groups and indicates that, when strong pain is felt, the old will suffer – in their own way – as much as the young. These findings are consistent with experimental evidence which has shown that, once the supra-threshold level of the painful stimuli is reached, the severity of pain is reported equally by the different age groups (Helme and Gibson, 1996).

Contemporary explanations of the nexus between pain, mood disturbance and disability commonly adopt a cognitive-behavioural model. This model has been shown to be applicable to older people when it is adapted for treatment of the various conditions (Manetto and McPherson, 1996). However, the benefits of behavioural cognitive strategies in pain management in the elderly are still unclear. Positive outcomes have been achieved at multidisciplinary pain clinics (Middaugh et al., 1988; Hornsby et al., 1991) where cognitive-behavioural programmes are an integral component of treatment. Figure 18.1 sets out a model for chronic pain which integrates the mode of processing of information, as suggested by Price (1988), the relationship with general belief systems, and specific cognitions implicated in the aetiology of affective states (e.g. Beck, 1976; Ellis, 1979) associated with chronic pain. The model demonstrates how a painful stimulus, such as that derived from an arthritic joint, is interpreted as painful. Cognitive factors will mediate between the emotional/ behavioural response and the painful event. If the stimulus is persistent or chronic, changes in thoughts and beliefs about the pain will continue to be modified until the beliefs of some people become extremely maladaptive, and significant suffering will then be experienced.

The role of cognitive and behavioural variables in the experience of chronic pain in the elderly is considered to explain, in part, the relationship between pain and disability (Farrell et al., 1996a). Research on the role of cognitive constructs in pain and their impact on older people has been limited, but some useful information has been obtained to date. Keefe and Williams (1990) reported no age differences in coping strategies, although there was a trend for older adults to use 'praying and hoping' more frequently than their younger counterparts. This trend was confirmed in a study of a much larger sample of older people with chronic pain. It also identified increased use of strategies such as 'praying and hoping', but less use of 'ignoring of pain' strategies, among older people (Corran et al., 1994). Subtle differences emerged in the efficacy of the strategies employed by older people to ameliorate their experience of pain and depression. Whereas younger subjects employed ignoring of pain to good effect, older subjects obtained most benefit from the use of self-coping statements. In a more recent study it was suggested that cognitive-behavioural factors are of relatively less importance for older people in mediating the relationship between pain and depression (Turk et al., 1995). This result may require replication before a conclusion which diminishes the role of cognitive factors in the experience of chronic pain in older people can be drawn.

In summary, age-related differences in psychological factors may contribute to altered pain perception and reporting of pain in older people. Changes in expectations and misattribution are likely to alter the cognitive import and fundamental meaning of mild pain symptoms in the elderly. A response bias due to 'stoicism' or 'cautiousness' by the older person in labelling a noxious sensation as painful will result in under-reporting of pain, particularly for faint or mild pain sensations (Gibson and Helme, 1995). The vast majority of studies report a modest increase in pain threshold by older people in comparison to the young. Anecdotal evidence regarding the relationship between pain and pathology, as noted by Gibson and Helme (1995), leads to inappropriate stereotyping and ageist attitudes. It is therefore important, and worth emphasizing, that when an older person does report pain, it should be considered in

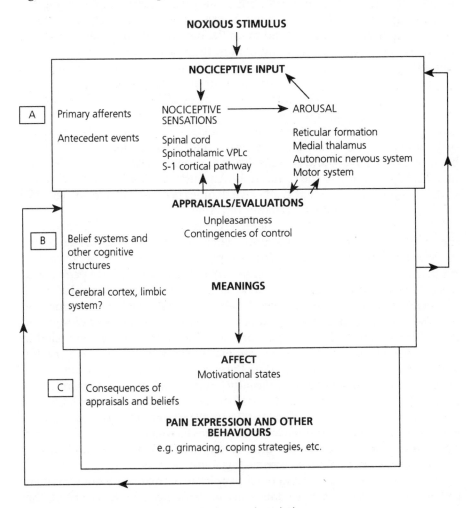

Figure 18.1   A model of chronic pain biology and psychology

exactly the same way as when a young adult reports pain (Gibson and Helme, 1995).

Age differences in the prevalence and presentation of clinical pain

There is increasing evidence to support the view that some age differences exist for specific subgroups of people and disorders. The prevalence of pain in older people in some circumstances is difficult to delineate due to a number of methodological problems in conducting research (Gibson and Helme, 1995). Epidemiology of the prevalence of pain varies according to the questions asked. Persistent pain is extremely common in community-dwelling older people (Gibson and Helme, 1995), but acute pain remains stable, at approximately 5 per cent of the population, across all age groups. The prevalence figures for persistent pain depend upon the time frame sampled through the questions (e.g. 'have you had any pain in the last 2 weeks, 6 months, or 12 months?') and the temporal definition of chronic pain used in the research (pain for longer than 3 months, 6 months, or 'persistent' pain).

A study of physical and mental functioning of 2792 older people (mean age 75 years) living in the community in south-west France reported that 68.3 per cent suffered from persistent joint pain (Bauberger-Gateau et al., 1992), whereas other studies (Crook et al., 1984; Anderson and Worm-Pederson, 1987; Brattberg et al., 1989) have found persistent pain prevalence rates of 25 to 50 per cent of older people living in the community. An Australian survey of medical use in the community, found that 47 per cent of older people with a mean age of 79 years reported suffering pain (Helme and Allen, 1992).

Other consistent trends have emerged. The prevalence of articular joint pain (i.e. involving the knee or hip) is more than double in older adults (aged over 65 years) compared to young adult samples. Conversely, the prevalence of headache shows a progressive decrease with increasing age after a peak prevalence at 45-50 years of age. Gibson and Helme (1995) also report a reduction in the frequency of facial/dental pain and abdominal/stomach pain during ageing. The prevalence of chest pain appears to peak during late middle age and then decrease during the later part of the life span. In a study conducted in Iowa by Mobily et al. (1994), joint pain was found to be most prevalent, followed by leg pain and back pain. With the exception of leg pain, the prevalence of other pain was found to be significantly lower in subjects over 85 years of age compared to adults aged 65 to 74 years. The findings with regard to back pain are more equivocal. Some studies report a small but significant increase in back pain with advancing age, whereas other studies have shown the reverse trend. The reasons for such disparate findings are not entirely clear, and further studies are needed in order to resolve this issue.

In general, it seems likely that older people are particularly prone to pain in certain body sites, such as the joints, legs, arms and neck. However, headache, abdominal pain, chest pain, facial pain and visceral pain appear to peak in late middle age (45–55 years) but decrease with advancing age, whilst age-specific rates for back pain remain equivocal and require further investigation. The collective results of studies indicate that chronic pain rates peak in older people by the age of 65 years, but reported pain declines in the 'old old' and the 'oldest old' (Roy and Thomas, 1987; Mobily *et al.* 1994; Gibson and Helme, 1995).

Helme and Gibson (1996) conclude that specific neurological factors may contribute significantly to the differences in prevalence associated with specific types of pain. It is clear from the vast majority of studies that pain in older people is a significant problem, and it can be concluded that pain is more prevalent among older people when compared to young and middle-aged people. This is largely due to the consequences of degenerative and spine diseases, together with leg and foot disorders. However, in the extremes of old age, the trend changes and even decreases in specific disorders (Helme and Gibson, 1996). Findings which indicate decreasing pain with increasing age after 65 years are attributed to reduced survivorship or increased rates of institutionalization of the 'oldest' adults. An alternative view suggests that the 'oldest old' accept pain more readily and therefore fail to endorse questions pertaining to the presence of 'bothersome pain' or of being 'often troubled by pain'. Other factors concerning age-related physiological changes which may lead to some mild pain symptoms in the 'oldest old' for specific disorders have been discussed above. However, Harkins (1996) contends that the notion of an age-related decrease in the prevalence of pain perception remains controversial. Irrespective of the exact reasons, it would appear that the 'older old' (85 years or older) living in the community, report significantly less pain than older adults in the previous decades of life.

Problems which could occur as a result of difficulties in identification of pain in the 'oldest old' have been emphasized by Ferrell (1991). She reported that only 15 per cent of patients in pain had received medication during the previous 24 hours. Helme and Katz (1993) also noted that there was a tendency not to report pain, and they presented evidence of under-reporting of sensory and affective components of pain, e.g. in cases of myocardial infarction and peritonitis. Symptoms may be attributed to other concurrent disease states or not reported because of anxiety or denial. In addition, many individuals perceive pain as a natural part of ageing and do not report it. Compounding the effects of under-reporting by older people themselves, treating practitioners may also under-rate the significance of pain.

The results of these studies have implications for the care and treatment of the elderly. Kwentus *et al.* (1985) cautions against the possible effects of ageism. It may present a particularly prevalent barrier to the reporting and management of pain in older people and would indicate that specific education of health care providers and patients alike is required. As with other aspects of geriatric medicine, unless detailed inquiries are made about the specific symptoms of pain or its effects, problems will continue to be unidentified or misdiagnosed.

Impact of co-morbidity and chronic pain

Pathological load is considered by gerontologists to be the overriding factor contributing to increased pain complaints with age. As mentioned earlier in this chapter, many illnesses increase in prevalence with advancing age. The interplay and impact of multiple diseases in an individual case is the hallmark of geriatric medicine (Helme and Gibson, 1996). Thus survival into the later years brings increasing frailty and morbidity of chronic health problems as well as issues of co-morbidity (Harkins, 1988). Helme and Gibson (1996) emphasize that major clinical issues in aged care could be compounded by pain, further complicating the clinical picture. How then does co-morbidity compound the impact of pain?

Of all the patients in the referred population at the pain clinic for older people in Melbourne, two-thirds were female and over 70 years of age, and 90 per cent lived in their own homes, although many were receiving social and community support. Of the patients who were attending the clinic, 75 per cent presented with significant co-morbidity, that is, with more than two active medical problems, mostly of musculoskeletal or cardiovascular origin. Documentation of the physical and psychological co-morbidity clearly indicated that patients with high levels of co-morbidity, expressed as the number of disease states, presented with significantly higher levels of depression, physical impact and trait anxiety. The effects of co-morbidity appear to be largely additive. The presence of multiple medical problems was associated with a concomitant increase in self-reported depression and physical impact, regardless of whether the pain was mild, moderate or severe (Farrell et al., 1995). In addition, the nature of the co-morbidity complicates the presentation. Farrell et al. (1995) demonstrated that older people with chronic pain suffering from arthritis displayed a 38 per cent reduction in activity levels compared to chronic pain patients with post-herpetic neuralgia. They concluded that both the amount and the type of pathology contribute to the frequency and impact of pain on the overall level of functioning. Thus in the older patient it can be concluded that the development of a chronic pain complaint of mild intensity can have a major impact on mood and physical function, if it is accompanied by high levels of co-morbidity.

Recent empirical research has demonstrated the validity of these conclusions. Several studies examined whether patients with chronic pain could be empirically differentiated on the basis of their pain description, mood state and psychosocial status (Turk and Rudy, 1990; Klapow et al., 1995; Williams et al., 1995). The identification of such relatively homogeneous subgroups has important implications for the design and implementation of tailored cognitive-behavioural intervention programmes. Most recently, Klapow et al. (1995) described three empirically derived clusters or groups based on the outcomes of pain, impact of pain, and mood state. The first group included patients presenting with a 'chronic pain syndrome', and consisted of people with high levels of pain, functional impact and mood disturbance. The second group was described as having 'good pain control' and these patients had relatively low levels of pain, functional impact and mood disturbance. The third group was labelled 'positive adaptors', and these patients had relatively high levels of pain but low levels of functional impact and mood disturbance.

These results were replicated, with one exception, when the combined data from two pain clinics in Melbourne, Australia, were analysed. The two clinics have different age populations: one is a general pain clinic treating few older people and the other is a pain clinic treating predominantly older people (Corran *et al.*, 1994). Data from the older patients produced two similar groups, replicating 'the positive adaptors' and 'good pain control groups'. However, a third group identified by the data indicated a qualitatively different presentation. The patients in this group had high levels of mood disturbance, low levels of pain and high levels of pain impact. This group was termed the 'high impact group'. The mean age of the 'chronic pain syndrome group' (51.5 years) was significantly lower than that of the 'high impact' group (64.7 years), although there were a number of younger people in the latter group. These results were replicated when the samples were combined, with four groups being identified. The age distributions of the two groups, 'chronic pain syndrome' and 'high impact', are presented in Figures 18.2 and 18.3, respectively.

These findings point to the fact that at least one group of older patients, namely those in the 'high impact' group, presents with a unique profile of clinical symptoms, and this profile is not typically identified in young adult or middle-aged chronic pain patients. The 'high impact' group has a much higher level of comorbid disease when psychiatric illness is excluded. Farrell *et al.* (1995) suggest that factors such as coping skills, medical diagnosis and social circumstances may also be important for the emergence of this 'high impact' cluster. Ferrell (1991) notes the consequences of pain and related consequences for the person's quality of life. It leads to (or is associated with) depression, decreased socialization, sleep disturbance, impaired ambulation, increased health care utilization and increased cost. The results of co-morbidity studies confirm that major clinical issues can arise when co-morbidity and chronic pain occur concurrently.

Chronic pain syndromes and predominantly psychological conditions

The findings reported above indicate the existence of age differences in individual responses to the experience of chronic or persistent pain, particularly when co-morbidity is included in the analysis. A chronic pain syndrome refers to high levels of suffering, pain and impact, and is common to all age groups. Harkins *et al.* (1990) have indicated that chronicity is a key characteristic of pain, discomfort and suffering in the elderly. Depression may be a relevant factor, but the actual manner in which depression is involved has not been empirically demonstrated. Reports of an association between depression and pain indicate that 59 per cent of depressed people requesting treatment have chronic benign

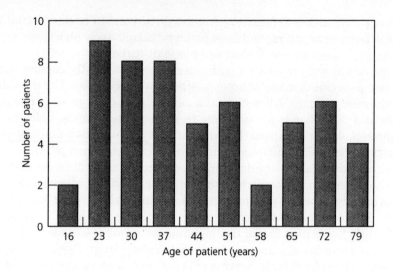

Figure 18.2   Frequency histogram for age: chronic pain syndrome cluster

pain, and 80 per cent of people attending pain clinics have been reported as suffering from depression (Kwentus *et al.*, 1985). Melding's (1995) later research on mood states and their relationship with pain found a 20 to 35 per cent incidence of depressive symptoms existing concurrently with physical disorders and chronic pain. Gibson *et al.* (1994) also reported that the frequency of depression in pain patients published in the literature ranged between 30 and 80 per cent.

Empirical classification of patients according to the levels of reported pain, mood and pain impact was not differentiated by diagnosis of the presenting problem. That is, whilst the 'chronic pain syndrome' group had a high number

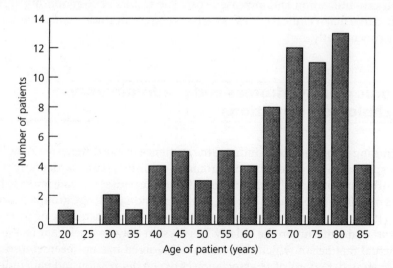

Figure 18.3   Frequency histogram for age: high-impact cluster

of subjects with a predominantly psychological cause of their pain, other subjects with a clearly identifiable physical pathology were also included.

A clinical assessment of a predominantly psychological cause of pain includes a primary depressive illness or a somatoform pain disorder in which there is preoccupation with pain not attributable to any other mental or physical disorder, or for which complaints of pain are grossly in excess of what would be expected from any physical findings (American Psychiatric Association, 1994). These represented approximately 9 per cent of patients attending the multidisciplinary pain clinic for the elderly in Melbourne. The differences between the diagnostic categories with regard to measures of pain, mood and pain impact are highlighted in Table 18.1. No statistically significant differences were found in reported pain levels between the three diagnostic groups. However, the predominantly psychological group of patients was significantly more depressed and reported greater psychosocial impact due to pain. The group of patients diagnosed with post-herpetic neuralgia reported less impact on physical activities due to pain than either of the other two groups.

The extended model of chronic pain (suggested earlier), which expands on Price's (1988) model of parallel and sequential processing, has a cognitive-behavioural focus for interventions. Cognitive variables implicated in the presentation of the chronic pain patient include poor outcome expectancy, lower self-esteem with negative pain beliefs and decreased motivation as a result of depression (Melding, 1995). These variables have all been demonstrated to reduce mobility and induce disuse-syndrome and dysfunction and, consequently, to increase pain. Studies exploring these factors in relation to younger patients have been conducted but the model has yet to be shown to be pertinent to older people. Melding (1995) has postulated that these variables can suggest directions and strategies to be followed in the treatment of the older person with chronic pain. She considers various implications of coping strategies used by individuals in chronic pain as well as the significance of the locus of control

Table 18.1 Mean levels of pain, mood and pain impact by diagnosis[a]

	Osteoarthritis	Post-herpetic neuralgia	Predominantly psychological
Pain			
PRIS	13.1	13.2	10.3
PRIA	4.9	4.8	4.8
Mood			
GDS	11.9	11.4	19.2*
Impact			
SIP physical	26.1	16.6*	29.7
SIP psychosocial	18.8	19.8	38.1*

[a] Statistical differences by ANOVA ($n = 16$). * $P < 0.001$. PRIA, affective pain rating index McGill Pain Questionnaire (Melzack, 1975); PRIS, sensory pain rating index McGill Pain Questionnaire; GDS, Geriatric Depression Scale (Yesavage and Brink, 1983); SIP physical, physical dimension Sickness Impact Profile (Gilson et al., 1975); SIP psychosocial, psychosocial dimension Sickness Impact Profile.

construct. Its significance in the phenomenology of chronic pain in older people has been indicated by Walker *et al.* (1989). Styles of coping associated with internal locus of control result in improved psychological adjustment, enhanced personal growth and diminished the incidence of crises with which an individual may have to cope. The opposite situation is expected with people who have an external locus of control, resulting in low self-esteem and poor outcome expectancy.

Improved functioning may be a more important treatment goal than relief of pain (Helme and Katz, 1993). Psychological strategies have a role in the management of chronic pain, and the principles of chronic pain management for older people are the same as for younger adults. One must take into account the pathophysiological changes especially in relation to pharmacology, co-existent pathology and psychosocial factors. Other important factors in coping with chronic pain are the perception of social and community support, personal life philosophy, and whether the pain is attributed to age itself. The goal of therapy is to reduce disability and medication side-effects, when the pain itself cannot be eliminated or reduced. In summary, epidemiological evidence and studies of experimental and clinical pain support the hypothesis that pain experienced by older people is different, but that it can be treated as readily as in younger adults. Although Harkins (1988) and Sorkin *et al.* (1990) emphasize the similarities to encourage equal treatment, the contrasting view of Helme and Gibson (1996) is that, if differences are recognized, then treatment can be effective. The conclusion which can be drawn from the research seems to support the view that age differences in presentation do exist, and that the person's psychological presentation is a particularly strong determinant of consideration for treatment.

When pain is refractory to the usual interventions, the benefits of a referral to a multidisciplinary pain clinic can be considered. In addition, when specific diseases are present, especially for older people, the role of a pain clinic with the availability of special expertise may be essential. Osteoarthritis, post-herpetic neuralgia and post-stroke pain are rare in the young, but they account for 60 per cent of the patients attending the pain clinic for the elderly in Melbourne. The benefits of psychological and multidisciplinary interventions for older people are demonstrated by the positive outcomes achieved by treating patients at one of the two Melbourne pain clinics. Patients from various diagnostic categories, including those with predominantly psychological causes of their pain, were treated at the second Melbourne clinic for older people and all of them showed an equal level of improvement.

Treatment of the 'oldest old' or the institutionalized old has been and continues to be neglected (Melding, 1995). The reasons for under-representation of older people at state-of-the-art treatment facilities are likely to be many and varied. Their exclusion may be directly due to age-related entry requirements, or they may be excluded because of age-related co-morbid conditions which would interfere with standard treatment protocols (Gibson *et al.*, 1996). Some older people are admitted to these facilities, but their numbers are small, the psychometric instruments used are not necessarily valid for that population, and factors such as cognitive status, functional measures and issues relating to co-morbidity, polypharmacy and social and community supports relevant to older people may not be measured. These factors are therefore not necessarily addressed in their treatment. Heterogeneity with regard to health and functional independence are known characteristics of the geriatric population, and multidisciplinary management is the key to successful geriatric medicine. This approach is used in the Melbourne multidisciplinary pain clinic for older people, and although the value of such clinics is known, appropriate funding is rarely achieved because of unfavourable priorities in health care policies. Helme and Gibson (1996) counsel on the benefits of multidisciplinary pain clinics for older people, including factors such as special treatment of diseases of the elderly, treatment focus, pace and outcome, particularly with regard to the 'oldest old'. The outcome data for geriatric care available to date, whilst sparse, are encouraging and indicate that even dependent and frail geriatric chronic pain patients can achieve substantial benefits from multidisciplinary interventions. Even a marginal improvement in pain and disability may make the difference between coping and not coping at home (Helme and Katz, 1993).

Although treatment at multidisciplinary pain facilities is recommended, the results obtained from these programmes suggest that they can be adopted for the less seriously dysfunctional older person with chronic pain. Indeed, Walker et al. (1989) highlighted the role of community-based professionals in the management of chronic pain, and their preventative role with the development of a chronic pain syndrome in the older person. Extrapolating from her own research findings, Walker captures the essence of cognitive, behavioural and environmental factors which impact upon and frustrate the older person in chronic pain.

Conclusions

Harkins et al. (1990) begin a chapter on pain in older people with four salient points gleaned from experimental, epidemiological and clinical studies. They pose the following five questions concerning the dimension of pain in older people.

1. What is the age-related epidemiology of pain problems?
2. Is age a predisposing factor for chronic pain?
3. Does the perception of pain decrease with age?
4. Does age affect the diagnosis and treatment of pain in the clinical setting?
5. In the light of the specific issues discussed in this chapter, there is a further question which should be raised: what other factors may influence the presentation of older people with chronic pain?

These five questions can now be answered as follows, and they summarize the dimensions of pain in later life.

1. Persistent or chronic pain is highly prevalent in older people. There is some evidence of a decrease in pain reported by the 'oldest old', but the majority of older people have adequate resources and support to cope in order to minimize the impact of pain in their lives.

2. Age is not a directly precipitating factor, but the increasing probability of disease or illness with age increases the likelihood of resultant pain.
3. At mild levels of painful stimuli, the perception and reporting of pain by older people are lower than the levels reported by younger people, but as the pain increases in severity, the differences between younger and older people are eliminated.
4. There is increasing evidence to suggest that multidisciplinary pain clinics and psychological treatment strategies are equally efficacious for those older people and younger individuals who have access to them. The major problem is a lack of availability of state-of-the-art treatment facilities for the older patient.
5. Psychosocial management of pain in the elderly is important. Appropriate and timely support can make a significant difference to the older person's ability to cope with pain. In addition, whilst the number of similarities exceeds the differences between younger and older adults' perception and experience of pain, important differences have been delineated. The most significant difference identified to date is the impact on the older person with chronic or persistent pain of other concurrent medical conditions. In summary, co-morbidity increases the risk of a disabling impairment for the older person in pain.

This chapter began with a pertinent quote from Farrell *et al.* (1996a). It can also end with another statement summarizing the status of research and its implications for the management of pain in the later years of life:

> The process of ageing is not without hazards, and the consequences of comorbidity for a significant proportion of older people should not be underestimated. Indeed, when we consider the burgeoning ranks of older people who suffer from chronic pain, it is most probably those with co-morbidity who are disproportionately represented.
>
> (Farrell *et al.*, 1996a, p.87)

References

All, A.C. 1994: Current concepts and management of cancer pain in older women. In Roberto, K.A. (ed.), *Older women with chronic pain*. New York: Harrington Park Press, 59–72.

American Psychiatric Association 1994: *Diagnostic and statistical manual of mental disorders*, 4th edn. Washington, DC: American Psychiatric Association.

Anderson, S. and Worm-Pederson, J. 1987: The prevalence of persistent pain in a Danish population. *Proceedings of the Fifth World Congress on Pain. Pain Supplement* **4**, S332.

Bauberger-Gateau, P., Chaslerie, A., Dartigues, J., Commenges, D., Gagnon, M. and Salamon, R. 1992: Health measure correlates in a French elderly community population: the PAQUID study. *Journal of Gerontology* **47**, S88–S95.

Beck, A.T. 1976: *Cognitive therapy and the emotional disorders*. New York: International University Press.

Bonica, J.J. 1990: *The management of pain*, 2nd edn. Philadelphia, PA: Lea and Febiger.

Brattberg, G., Thorslund, M. and Wikman, A. 1989: The prevalence of pain in a general population: the results of a postal survey in the country of Sweden. *Pain* 37, 215–22.

Corran, T.M., Gibson, S.J., Farrell, M.J. and Helme, R.D. 1994: Comparison of chronic pain experience between young and elderly patients. In Gebhart, G.F., Hammond, D.L. and Jensen, T.S. (eds), *Proceedings of the Seventh World Congress on Pain*. Seattle: IASP Press, 895–906.

Crook, J., Rideout, E. and Browne, G. 1984: The prevalence of pain complaints in a general population. *Pain* 18, 299–314.

Crook, J., Weir, R. and Tunks, E. 1989: An epidemiological follow-up survey of persistent pain sufferers in a group family practice and speciality pain clinic. *Pain* 36, 49–61.

Ellis, A. 1979: *Reason and emotion in psychotherapy*. New Jersey: Citadel Press.

Farrell, M.J. and Helme, R.D. 1995: The effect of medical status on the activity level of older pain clinic patients. *Journal of the American Geriatric Society* 43, 102–7.

Farrell, M.J., Gibson, S.J. and Helme, R.D. 1995: The effect of medical status on the activity level of older pain clinic patients. *Journal of the American Geriatric Society* 43, 102–7.

Farrell, M.J., Gibson, S.J. and Helme, R.D. 1996a: Chronic nonmalignant pain in older people. In Ferrell, B.R. and Ferrell, B.A. (eds), *Pain in the elderly*. Seattle: IASP Press, 81–9.

Farrell, M.J., Katz, B. and Helme, R.D. 1996b: The impact of dementia on the pain experience. *Pain* 67, 7–15.

Ferell, B.A. 1991: Pain management in elderly people. *Journal of the American Geriatric Society* 39, 64–73.

Ferrell, B.A., Ferrell, B.R. and Osterweil, D. 1990: Pain in the nursing home. *Journal of the American Geriatric Society* 38, 409–14.

Gibson, S.J. and Helme, R.D. 1995: Age differences in pain perception and report: a review of physiological, psychological, laboratory and clinical studies. In *Pain Reviews* 2. London: Edward Arnold, 111–37.

Gibson, S.J., Katz, B., Corran, T.M., Farrell, M.J. and Helme, R.D. 1994: Pain in the elderly. *Disability and Rehabilitation* 16, 127–39.

Gibson, S.J., Farrell, M.J., Katz, B. and Helme, R.D. 1996: Multidisciplinary management of chronic nonmalignant pain in older adults. In Ferrell, B.R. and Ferrell, B.A. (eds), *Pain in the elderly*. Seattle: IASP Press, 1–9.

Gilson, B.S., Gilson, J.S., Bergner, M. *et al.* 1975: The Sickness Impact Profile: development of an outcome measure of health care. *American Journal of Public Health* 65, 1304–10.

Harkins, S.W. 1988: Pain in the elderly. In Dubner, R., Gebhart, G.F. and Bond, M.R. (eds) *Pain research and clinical management. Vol. 3. Proceedings of the Fifth World Congress on Pain*. Amsterdam: Elsevier, 355–67.

Harkins, S.W. 1996: Geriatric pain: pain perceptions in the old. In Ferrell, B.A. (ed.), *Clinics in geriatric medicine*. Philadelphia, PA: W.B. Saunders Company, 435–59.

Harkins, S.W., Kwentus, J. and Price, D.D. 1990: Pain and suffering in the elderly. In Bonica, J. (ed.), *Management of pain*, 2nd edn. Philadelphia, PA: Lea and Febiger. 552–9.

Helme, R.D. and Allen, F. 1992: *Use of medications in a community-based elderly population: report to the Australian Council on the Ageing*. Melbourne: NARI Press.

Helme, R.D. and Gibson, S.J. 1996: *Pain in the elderly. Plenary address. Eighth World Congress on Pain,* Vancouver, 17–22 August 1996.

Helme, R.D. and Katz, B. 1993: Management of chronic pain. *The Medical Journal of Australia* **158**, 478–81.

Helme, R.D, Katz, B., Neufeld, M., Lachal, S., Herbert, J. and Corran, T. 1989: The establishment of a geriatric pain clinic: a preliminary report of the first 100 patients. *Australian Journal of Ageing* **8**, 27–30.

Hornsby, L. Katz, B., Helme, R.D., Gibson, S.J. and Corran, T.M. 1991: Outcome following discharge from a pain clinic for the elderly. *Australian and New Zealand Journal of Medicine* **21**, 585.

Jorm, A.F. and Henderson, A.S. 1993: *The problem of dementia in Australia.* Canberra: Australian Government Publishing Service.

Keefe, F.J. and Williams, D.A. 1990: A comparison of coping strategies in chronic pain patients in different age groups. *Journal of Gerontology* **45**, 161–5.

Klapow, J.C., Slater, M.A., Patterson, T.L., Doctor, J.N., Atkinson, J.H. and Garfin, S.R. 1995: An empirical evaluation of multidimensional clinical outcome in chronic low back pain patients. *Pain* **55**, 107–18.

Kwentus, J.A., Harkins, S.W., Lignon, N. and Silverman, J.J. 1985: Current concepts of geriatric pain and its treatment. *Geriatrics* **40**, 48–57.

McCormick, W.C., KuKill, W.A., Belle, G., Bowen, J.D., Teri, L. and Larson, E.B. 1994: Symptom patterns and comorbidity in the early stages of Alzheimer's disease. *Journal of the American Geriatric Society* **42**, 517–21.

Manetto, C. and McPherson, S.E. 1996: The behavioral-cognitive model of pain. In Ferrell, B.A. (ed.), *Clinics in geriatric medicine: pain management.* Philadelphia, PA: W.B. Saunders Company, 461–71.

Melding, P.S. 1991: Is there such a thing as geriatric pain? *Pain* **46**, 119–21.

Melding, P.S. 1995: How do older people respond to chronic pain? A review of coping with pain and illness in elders. In *Pain Reviews* 2. London: Edward Arnold, 65–75.

Melzack, R. 1973: *The puzzle of pain.* New York: Basic Books.

Melzack, R. 1975: The McGill Pain Questionnaire: major properties and scoring methods. *Pain* **1**, 277–99.

Melzack, R. and Casey, K.L. 1968: Sensory, motivational and central control determinants of pain: a new conceptual model. In Kenshalo, D. (ed.), *The skin senses.* Springfield, IL: Charles C. Thomas Publisher, 423–43.

Middaugh, S.J., Levin, R.B., Kee, W.G., Barchiesi, F.D. and Roberts, J.M. 1988: Chronic pain: its treatment in geriatric and younger patients. *Archives of Physical and Medical Rehabilitation* **69**, 1021–6.

Mobily, P.R., Herr, K.A., Clark, M.K. and Wallace, R.B. 1994: An epidemiologic analysis of pain in the elderly. *Journal of Ageing and Health* **6**, 139–54.

Parmelee, P.A. 1994: Assessment of pain in the elderly. In Lawton, M.P. and Tevesi, J.A. (eds), *Annual review of gerontology and geriatrics.* New York: Springer Publishing, 281–301.

Parmelee, P.A. 1996: Pain in cognitively impaired older persons. In Ferrell, B.A. (ed.), *Clinics in geriatric medicine: pain management.* Philadelphia, PA: W.B. Saunders Company, 473–87.

Parmelee, P.A., Smith, B. and Katz, I.R. 1993: Pain complaints and cognitive status among elderly institution residents. *Journal of the American Geriatric Society* **41**, 517–22.

Price, D.D. 1988: *Psychological and neural mechanisms of pain.* New York: Raven Press.

Roberto, K.A. 1994: The study of chronic pain in later life: where are the women? In Roberto, K.A. (ed.), *Older women with chronic pain*. New York: Harrington Park Press, 1–7.

Roy, R. and Thomas, M. 1986: A survey of chronic pain in an elderly population. *Canadian Family Physician* **32**, 513–16.

Roy, R. and Thomas, M.R. 1987: Elderly persons with and without pain: a comparative study. *Clinical Journal of Pain* **3**, 102–6.

Sengstaken, E.A. and King, S.A. 1993: The problems of pain and its detection among geriatric nursing home residents. *Journal of the American Geriatric Society* **41**, 541–4.

Sorkin, B.A., Rudy, T.E., Hanlon, R.B., Turk, D.C. and Steig, R.L. 1990: Chronic pain in old and young patients: differences appear less important than similarities. *Journal of Gerontology* **45**, 64–8.

Stein, W.M. and Ferrell, B.A. 1996: Pain in the nursing home. In Ferrell, B.A. (ed.), *Clinics in geriatric medicine: pain management*. Philadelphia, PA: W.B. Saunders Company, 601–13.

Suzman, R.M., Willis, D.P. and Manton, K.G. (eds) 1992: *The oldest old*. New York: Oxford University Press.

Turk, D.C. and Rudy, T.E. 1990: The robustness of an empirically derived taxonomy of chronic pain patients. *Pain* **43**, 27–35.

Turk, D.C, Okifuji, A. and Scharff, L. 1995: Chronic pain and depression: role of perceived impact and perceived control in different age cohorts. *Pain* **61**, 93–101.

Walker, J.M., Akinsanya, J.A., Davis, B.D. and Marcer, D.M. 1989: The nursing management of pain in the community: a theoretical framework. *Journal of Advanced Nursing* **14**, 240–7.

Williams, D.A., Urban, B., Keefe, F.J., Shutty, M.S. and France, R. 1995: Cluster analysis of pain patients' responses to the SCL-90R. *Pain* **61**, 81–91.

World Health Organization 1963: *Report of a seminar on the health protection of the elderly and aged and the prevention of premature ageing*. Copenhagen: World Health Organization Regional Offices in Europe.

Yesavage, J.A. and Brink, T.L. 1983: Development and validation of a geriatric depression screening scale. A preliminary report. *Journal of Psychiatric Research* **17**, 37–49.

Fibromyalgia and pain

Angela R. Vale

Introduction

Fibromyalgia is a chronic pain syndrome which has far-reaching consequences for the sufferer. The effects impact upon the person's family, relationships, work and social life (Baumstark and Buckelew, 1992; Henriksson *et al.*, 1992; Henriksson, 1994). Whilst pain is recognized as an essential element for the diagnosis of fibromyalgia, patients' pain has, until recently, been ignored or mismanaged. Within this chapter some of the reasons why fibromyalgia patients have received poor management and support will be addressed. Central to the debate will be issues relating to the management difficulties, both for professionals and for the patients, created by ongoing pain. Melzack and Wall (1988) claim that 'Pain is one of the most challenging problems in medicine and biology. It is a challenge to the sufferer who must often learn to live with pain for which no therapy has been found'. This challenge is one which would be recognized by many fibromyalgia patients.

The syndrome fibromyalgia was first described as fibrositis (Wolfe *et al.*, 1990), and was first cited by Gowers (1904). Lautenbacher *et al.* describe fibromyalgia as 'a chronic pain syndrome, characterized by diffuse, widespread pain and has multiple tender points at characteristic sites' (Lautenbacher *et al.*, 1994, p.45). The true prevalence of the condition is not known, since the studies that exist are not always comparable due to the variability in settings, methodology and rationale. McCain (1996) proposes that fibromyalgia has a prevalence of 2–5 per cent in the population and states that this would be a conservative estimate.

Fibromyalgia is complex and controversial, and has only recently been accepted as a legitimate syndrome (Powers, 1993). In the author's experience some medical staff have dismissed fibromyalgia patients as a waste of medical and nursing time since they are seen to be unwilling to help themselves. In the past this view was supported by a belief that fibromyalgia was a somatic expression of a psychiatric disorder rather than a physical illness. The roots of these beliefs often lie in the attitudes and belief systems of both medical and nursing staff. Indeed, assumptions may result in reductionist consideration of patients, with their pain being labelled as inappropriate and 'not respectable' or invalid – such a perspective is both simplistic and unprofitable (Fagerhaugh and Strauss, 1977; Weir and Crook, 1992).

These dismissive beliefs reflect professionals' own personal bias regarding pain, and particularly their perception and understanding (or rather lack of understanding) of patients suffering from fibromyalgia. Thus many doctors and nursing staff, to the intense frustration of patients, fail to appreciate the amount of pain experienced. The reciprocal nature of the relationship between nurse and patient influences both the decision-making and the behaviour of the nurse (Sternbach, 1978). Fibromyalgia often results in patients experiencing feelings of 'helplessness and lower self-efficacy' (Buckelew et al., 1995). This type of emotional vulnerability has been noted in patients with rheumatoid arthritis (Ryan, 1996). Tamler and Meerschaert (1996) report that patients often pick up on these negative feelings and behaviours and respond accordingly.

Within this chapter the complexities of fibromyalgia will be examined and the difficulties of diagnosing the syndrome will be explored. The ramifications of the medical uncertainty that accompanies the condition will be considered in relation to the ways in which this affects patients. Through addressing these issues it should be possible to encourage a more enlightened attitude from medical and nursing staff. If this happens then more supportive care should result.

Fibromyalgia: the condition and the road to diagnosis

Fibromyalgia occurs primarily in women aged 20–50 years, and the aetiology and pathophysiology of the disorder are unknown. After osteoarthritis, fibromyalgia is the second most common rheumatological disorder (Marder et al., 1991; Tamler and Meerschaert, 1996). Women are 20 times more likely to be affected than men. The condition tends to wax and wane, with patients having good days where they are able to be involved in more activities, and bad days when they are very restricted. Fibromyalgia is a chronic pain syndrome, and as such it has far-reaching effects on the patient. As with other types of chronic pain it is a 'dual phenomenon, one part being the perception of the sensation and the other the patients' psychological reaction to it. It follows that a person's pain threshold will vary according to mood, morale and meaning' (Twycross, 1978, p.496).

This view is broadly supported by Akinsanya (1985). The unique, individual, subjective nature of fibromyalgia pain must be borne in mind at all times when caring for the fibromyalgia patient.

One of the key needs of patients is for their pain to be believed and accepted – indeed this is a key reason for requesting medical help. After such belief has been established, it is important for patients to understand their diagnosis, its implications, why they have the condition and the treatment options. Fibromyalgia results in patients suffering from chronic pain, and despite the individuality of response there is a high degree of relative uniformity in the pattern of pain (Wolfe and Cathey, 1983). However, a longitudinal study of fibromyalgia patients undertaken by Hawley et al. suggests that 'patients with fibromyalgia differ significantly from each other. . . . Thus the picture of a stereotyped fibromyalgia patient with high levels of pain and psychological distress is not suggested by our research. Patients are different and individual'(Hawley *et al.*, 1988, p.1555).

The principal symptoms of fibromyalgia are predominantly neck and back pain, although pain may be experienced in many other parts of the body. A key characteristic of the condition is an inadequate amount of muscle endurance (Tamler and Meerschaert, 1996). Three key studies in the 1980s were primarily responsible for clarifying the clinical features of fibromyalgia (Yunus *et al.*, 1981; Campbell *et al.* 1983; and Wolfe *et al.*, 1985). Fibromyalgia pain is often aggravated by stress, cold and activity (Yunus *et al.*, 1989; Wolfe *et al.*, 1990). Many patients can identify an event that triggered the initial onset of symptoms, such as a car accident, a fall or some other stressor or illness (Wolfe, 1986). There are many associated symptoms (see Figure 19.1).

Non-restorative sleep is frequently identified in patients with fibromyalgia. Campbell *et al.* (1983) found a 95 per cent self-report of poor sleep. Non-restorative sleep has been associated with abnormalities in the non-REM sleep patterns of people with fibromyalgia (Modolfsky *et al.*, 1975). Research has highlighted another factor which can make fibromyalgia patients feel sleep deprived. Smeltzer states that 'fibromyalgia patients have more rapid eye movement (REM) sleep than normal so they have less restorative (non-REM) sleep and feel fatigued upon awakening'(Smeltzer, 1987, p.28).

This feeling of fatigue and general tiredness only enhances the sensation of pain and has been noted in many studies (Yunus *et al.*, 1981; McCain and Scudds, 1988). Goldenberg (1988) emphasizes the need to ensure that patients are able to experience improved levels of restorative sleep through the use of a short-acting tricyclic that does not have hangover effects. Serotonin deficiency may well be implicated in this poor sleep pattern, as serotonin is thought to be responsible for triggering stage IV sleep, inducing smooth muscle contraction. Serotonin mediates pain responses as well as preventing anxiety and depression (Tamler and Meerschaert, 1996).

- morning stiffness
- subjective swelling of extremities
- paraesthesia and dysaethesia of hands and feet
- headache – mainly occipital and bifrontal
- diffuse abdominal pain
- variable bowel habits
- urinary frequency
- urinary urgency – night and day
- dysmenorrhoea
- fatigue, often after minimal exertion
- non-restorative sleep and waking unrefreshed
- poor concentration and forgetfulness
- depressed
- irritable
- weepy

Figure 19.1 Principal symptoms of fibromyalgia (developed from Doherty and Jones, 1995)

Fibromyalgia results in functional impairment with the absence of demonstrable inflammatory, metabolic or structural abnormality. Although this is not emphasized in the literature, Hawley *et al.* (1988) found that functional disability was evident in fibromyalgia patients and that it contributed independently to the total severity of the individual's condition. This study also suggested that the symptoms of fibromyalgia are 'remarkably stable over time' (Hawley *et al.*, 1988, p.1554).

There are no specific laboratory tests or X-ray procedures that can detect fibromyalgia. Muscular abnormalities have been the focus of a number of studies, although no specific findings have been demonstrated. Diagnosis is based on medical history, the identification of tender points and the absence of other disease. Pain is located within the muscles themselves, as well as at the points where ligaments attach muscles to bones, and extreme tenderness is felt over many of these locations. These sites are called 'tender points' or 'trigger points'. The location of tender points is similar in all patients with fibromyalgia, and is therefore an important part of the diagnosis (see Figure 19.2). However, Powers identifies that 'the tender points may be largely unknown to the patient and often not even central to their areas of pain' (Powers, 1993, p.95). According to the American College of Rheumatology (1990), the criteria for the classification of fibromyalgia are: 'Pain on digital palpation must be present in at least 11 of the 18 tender sites' (Wolfe *et al.*, 1990).

Fibromyalgia is poorly understood and thus the disorder is difficult to diagnose, mainly due to the many differing symptoms. It is not unusual for the patient to seek help from many consultants and specialists before a firm diagnosis is made. The search for a diagnosis results in fibromyalgia sufferers feeling increasingly vulnerable and isolated. A comprehensive and skilled physical examination is crucial to making a diagnosis of fibromyalgia. This view is confirmed by Smeltzer (1987), who claims that fibromyalgia has been used as 'a waste-basket diagnosis' or seen in terms of it being a psychogenic disorder.

Many patients feel extremely frustrated by their experience of both the condition and the difficulty of obtaining a diagnosis. Mediating this frustration

- low cervical spine (C4-6 interspinous ligaments)
- low lumbar spine (L4-S1 interspinous ligaments)
- sub-occipital muscle (posterior base of spine)
- supraspinatus
- mid-point of upper trapezius
- skin roll tenderness of skin overlying mid-trapezius
- pectoralis insertion, maximal lateral to second costochondral junction
- lateral epicondyle, 'tennis elbow' site, 1–2 cm distal to epicondyle
- gluteus medius – upper, outer quadrant of buttock
- greater trochanter
- medial fat pad of knee

Figure 19.2 Common hyperalgesic tender sites (developed from Doherty, 1995)

is an important role for the nurse (Ryan, 1996). It is necessary to make absolutely sure that there are no underlying conditions that may present with widespread pain, weakness or fatigue, and these should be excluded by an investigational screen. Further tests may be warranted if a patient's history and examination suggest a predisposing or coexistent condition (Wolfe, 1995). Rothschild (1991) suggests that physiological alterations have been identified that allow an objective, rather than a subjective, report as confirmation of a clinical impression. Rothschild further states that 'Trigger points of fibromyalgia may manifest as focal alterations in electrical resistance and temperature. One approach to objective documentation therefore is thermography, a non-invasive technique without any known toxic effects' (Rothschild, 1991, p.11).

It is also important for medical and nursing staff to realize that patients may be concerned that they have a life-threatening condition, and that a firm diagnosis is highly desirable to help patients come to terms with the condition and ultimately start the treatment to help themselves.

Pathological or psychological? Belief and disbelief of patients' pain

A number of studies have documented the tensions between health care professionals and patients in relation to pain (Weir and Crook, 1992). Conflict can exist and frustration is evident in some relationships between professionals and patients, which can result in the patient's pain being inadequately addressed. Woodward (1995) proposes that, because many nurses assess patients' pain on the basis of their own personal beliefs, an accurate assessment is rarely achieved. Patients' belief systems and values need to be incorporated into the assessment if the latter is truly to reflect their experience.

With regard to fibromyalgia and pain, some medical and nursing staff find it difficult to shed their own values and accept that these patients are in genuine pain and have a genuine illness. Indeed, a number of studies have attempted to identify a psychiatric association for fibromyalgia. However, these studies have had methodological weaknesses. No such relationship has been fully established with a classically defined psychiatric disorder. Yunus *et al.* (1991) determined that the central features of fibromyalgia are most likely to relate to the fibromyalgia itself, rather than being dependent on psychological status. It is vitally important that patients know that the staff caring for them believe their pain is real. Most patients who suffer from fibromyalgia claim that they have felt as if they were going insane as a result of not being believed. Ryan goes on to discuss the issue of 'believing' and claims that 'They [patients] may be fearful that their credibility is in doubt because no abnormalities have been identified through traditional investigative procedures' (Ryan, 1995, p.26).

Whilst fibromyalgia is not classified as a psychiatric illness, it is obvious that *some* doctors feel that it is one. A study by Schaefer (1995) identified that the search for a diagnosis was often complex and involved patients having to negotiate their way through health care providers, convince other people that their pain was real, and deal with all of this whilst working with depleted financial, physical and psychological resources. Schaefer states that 'These women resented being told indirectly the symptoms had no scientific basis and that it was just their imagination. However, they had very little information about what it might be, and many began to think the physician was right' (Schaefer, 1995, p.98).

Patients often feel better when they are finally given a diagnosis of fibromyalgia, as this gives them a medical and therefore physical reason for their pain. A diagnostic label relieves their concerns that they have a psychological disorder, and it in some way validates their suffering in the eyes of certain professionals. However, despite the fact that fibromyalgia has a physical cause, there is inevitably a psychological component to this experience. Fishman and Greenberg argue that 'Persistent pain can change behaviour, also anxiety and depression are more common in patients with pain. It is also suggested that it is difficult to tell which came first – pain or psychologic dysfunction' (Fishman and Greenberg, 1996, p.379).

According to Clauw (1995), there has been considerable discussion about the relationship between fibromyalgia and psychiatric conditions. The statistics suggest that fibromyalgia patients have a higher than expected incidence of current (approximately 20 per cent) and lifetime (50 per cent) major depression, as well as of other affective disorders. The question is whether fibromyalgia is essentially a psychiatric condition producing a number of physical symptoms, or whether psychiatric complaints are just one more by-product of the pain, fatigue and disability experienced by individuals with fibromyalgia. Boissevain (1996) highlights the fact that, despite the preponderance of studies demonstrating that fibromyalgia patients are more depressed than comparable medical patients, there is 'rigorous disconfirming evidence' that this is not the case. Consistent levels of depression are not evident in fibromyalgia sufferers.

Two of the major difficulties that fibromyalgia patients have to contend with are either the scepticism of health care professionals or a lack of understanding of the ways in which fibromyalgia affects those experiencing it. Morrison (1991) believes that nurses need to question their own assumptions and become more self-aware. The same is true for all health professionals who interface with the client. The problem of self-awareness has to be tackled to enable reluctant staff to see that, to the patient, fibromyalgia is a devastating condition. The fact that the condition is not life-threatening and will not cause deformity is of little comfort to those patients in chronic pain. This knowledge on its own does not take away the pain. However, it does seem that doctors and nurses alike consider that this reassurance should make the patient 'feel better'. This type of approach is extremely unsupportive and reflects a real lack of understanding of the pain and devastation that the patient is experiencing. However, this reassurance may be seen by some health care professionals to be *the* treatment. In the author's experience there is almost the expectation that, after a 10-minute consultation with a doctor, the fibromyalgia patient is expected to conform, be well, pick up their bed and walk. This miracle is supposed to occur even though they are still in pain, and have received minimal information, support and education.

It is difficult to provide a rationale for the fact that some health care professionals may be so dismissive about the impact of fibromyalgia. However, some light may be shed on this when considering the psychological overlay to the condition which may make the patient 'unpopular'. Rogers and Rogers (1990) describe fibromyalgia patients as 'apprehensive, depressed, and agitated' (pp.39–40). This description suggests a picture of a person who is psychologically rather than physically ill and, although they do not state this – female. Schaefer (1995) claims that 'out of one hundred diagnosed with the syndrome, 73 to 88 are women' (p.95).

Some doctors suggest that fibromyalgia patients over-verbalize and tell great tales, especially with regard to how they are fighting the pain. Patients report disinterest by some medical staff who are seen to lose interest, switch off, lack listening skills and who respond with a reflex opinion and prescription at the end of the consultation. This kind of approach does not give the patient, who is already vulnerable and disempowered, the opportunity to relax and become involved in his or her own care. Schaefer (1995) highlights the misunderstanding of many doctors in relating to women with fibromyalgia. A typical response is related in which the doctor tells the woman 'she must be under stress and that she should make some changes in her life, provides her with an antidepressant because it will help her sleep, or sends her to a specialist because he or she has no idea what is happening' (Schaefer, 1995, p.95).

Although fibromyalgia is not life-threatening, a point which may often be used to reassure the patient, some fibromyalgia sufferers admit that they have sometimes contemplated suicide. Thus in reality the unremitting pain can become so unendurable that it can threaten the sufferer's life (Hacobian et al., 1996). It certainly impacts upon their quality of life and this may make the condition life-threatening. Hacobian et al. propose that 'patients may become suicidal. Suicidal ideation may represent a spectrum of intents, from self-harm to manipulation to reach a secondary gain' (Hacobian et al., 1996, p.405).

Managing fibromyalgia: options and opportunities

No cure has been found for fibromyalgia, and certainly few treatment modalities have been discovered to have a beneficial effect. According to Doherty and Jones 'The prognosis for fibromyalgia is poor. In one British study less than one in ten patients diagnosed in hospital lost their symptoms over five years' (Doherty and Jones, 1995, p.389).

Two main routes to treatment exist – pharmacological and non-pharmacological. Often pharmacological measures are used as adjunctive methods alongside non-pharmacological approaches. However, McCain warns that 'so far, only a minority of such [non-pharmacological] treatments has been studied using acceptable scientific methods' (McCain, 1996, p.20).

Treatment of fibromyalgia is generally seen to be unsatisfactory (Rothschild, 1991). Whilst this discussion does not intend to consider in any detail the medication used in the treatment of fibromyalgia patients, it is important to consider the conundrum that this can present. On the one hand, some doctors and nurses do not fully believe the amount of pain that the patient claims to have, but they still prescribe and administer analgesics, anti-inflammatory drugs and some form of night sedation or antidepressants. Amitriptyline is mainly used as a relaxant and analgesic, and is given at night to enhance the poor sleep pattern. Unfortunately, many patients find that it leaves them feeling unrefreshed with morning drowsiness. McCain (1996) comments that extreme sensitivity of the central nervous systems of fibromyalgia sufferers and the anticholinergic side-effects of even low doses of amitriptyline or cyclobenzaprine are responsible for these effects. Feeling that they have not slept well leads to further frustration, as patients claim that they would feel better if they could sleep, yet when they do sleep they feel no better when they wake up. A study by Carrette *et al.* (1986) identified a global improvement for patients at 5 and 9 weeks after the commencement of amitryptiline, although pain thresholds and morning stiffness were not clinically improved. Patients also reported a wide range of side-effects, including drowsiness, hallucinations, cardiac irritability and confusional states.

Non-pharmacological approaches do have value, and their specific potential benefits, according to Edwards, include:

> reducing or eliminating nociceptive aspects of pain, increasing patients' ability to participate in the activities of daily living, thus improving their self esteem and sense of control. Improving patients' ability to participate in physical therapy thus improving their overall health.
>
> (Edwards, 1996, pp.105–6)

Encouraging the involvement of family and friends in the patient's care reduces isolation and supports the patient's own coping skills. Woodward (1995) proposes the notion that 'well informed patients' are better able to be more involved in deciding which other non-pharmacological methods can assist in their pain management. It is interesting to record the notion that it requires a 'well informed patient' to instigate other treatments, rather than a well-informed nurse to offer them. This demonstrates that information can empower patients – a much better situation than one which gives the nurse power over patients by having control over what they know and limiting their access to resources.

Exercise is seen to be an important treatment modality, although the benefits of this approach are not always consistently demonstrated in the literature. One advantage of exercise is that it results in elevated serotonin levels, which will contribute to improved sleep patterns. A study by Nørregaard *et al.* (1997) aimed to demonstrate improvement in the patient's pain and fatigue as well as enhancement of muscle strength and physical capacity. However, the study was characterized by a low participation rate and poor compliance. Patients expressed fears of exacerbating their condition; indeed, those participants involved in the aerobic training reported that their symptoms did deteriorate. Nørregaard *et al.* highlight the difficulties of employing physical modalities in the treatment of fibromyalgia. Other studies demonstrate that cardiovascular fitness training can improve objective and subjective measurements of pain in fibromyalgia patients (McCain *et al.*, 1988). There were significant improvements in patients undergoing cardiovascular fitness training, in terms of pain threshold scores, compared to patients undergoing simple flexibility exercises. An emphasis is placed on the exercise continuing for a period greater than 3 months, since a shorter duration does not result in enhanced cardiovascular fitness.

However, such programmes of integrated, progressive exercise can create stressful situations for patients, especially during a period of hospitalization. This may be because, whilst in hospital, they are expected to follow an exercise regimen that coincides with the availability of the physiotherapist, rather than with the times when the patient feels best able to deal with it. Patients often state that they do not feel like doing exercises because of fatigue and pain. This cannot be seen to be the fault of the individual. Rather, it is a problem with the system of treatment, since too many patients have to be seen by too few physiotherapists. However, this reluctance to throw themselves into an exercise programme may add to the misguided assumption that these patients simply do not want to help themselves.

Other treatments available to the patients are mainly instigated by the doctors and carried out by the physiotherapists and nurses. These include the physiotherapy exercise regime, commencement of treatment with transcutaneous electrical nerve stimulation (TENS) machines (which work by transmission of small electrical pulses through the skin to the underlying peripheral nerves), hydrotherapy sessions, hot packs applied to tender areas, relaxation and aromatherapy massage. One of the recurrent themes both in the available literature regarding fibromyalgia and in reports by those who experience the condition is the need for education. This has mainly been patient education, although it should be realized that in many cases doctors, nurses and the whole multidisciplinary team need education to change their attitudes. Ryan states that:

> the nurse has an enormous role to play in enabling patients with chronic conditions, such as fibromyalgia, to develop effective coping mechanisms. We should be aiming for self-advocacy for patients by providing them with the knowledge they need to make informed decisions that suit their individual needs best.
>
> (Ryan, 1995, p.26)

An important aspect of care is to show the patient that you believe them and it is important that they know that you believe them, even if you cannot cure them. This is an important and necessary step to start effective systems to help the patient to develop coping strategies.

Ryan (1995) reports the development of a 6-week education programme that promotes understanding of fibromyalgia as a condition, and ways of mediating its effects. Each week of the programme focuses on different issues, such as coping with pain, exercise, relaxation and the psychosocial context of fibromyalgia. This programme has become part of a pain education programme involving chronic pain sufferers with a variety of pathologies (Ryan, 1997, personal communication). Rothschild (1991) suggests that hypnotic therapy would appear to offer a real alternative to the use of antidepressants for the management of fibromyalgia. Rothschild presents a brief review of 11 patients who had been unresponsive to other treatment modalities. He states that 'Hypnotic agent therapy in ten patients resulted in total resolution of symptoms within one to four weeks (mean three weeks)' (Rothschild, 1991, p.13). He also proposes that acupuncture, electroacupuncture and trigger point injection are other suitable methods of treatment.

Buckelew (1989) reiterates the list of treatments, but importantly places reassurance and an explanation of the nature of the illness at the top of the list as a major factor contributing to the rehabilitation of fibromyalgia sufferers. Reassurance and support before physical treatment is identified as the ideal, whilst in practice the patient often receives physical treatment and little if any reassurance and support. In later work, Buckelew et al. (1995) emphasized the importance to fibromyalgia patients of self-managing their pain and dysfunction. Self-efficacy can predict self-report of pain and physical scores over a number of other variables, such as disease severity, demographic variables and psychological distress. Other variables, such as other coping techniques and social support, were not addressed in this study but may have important implications for the findings.

Listening to patients and encouraging them to tell their stories is emphasized by Schaefer (1995), who sees this approach as one means of helping fibromyalgia sufferers to move on and to 'accept their new reality as their reality'. The importance of what patients have to say becomes apparent when professionals really start to listen.

In a small audit of practice, undertaken by the author, in-patients were asked for their comments about their pain during a stay in hospital. They were asked to locate and score their pain on a body outline chart that was divided into eight areas. A pain score of 0 to 5 was recorded for each of the eight areas, and thus it was possible for a patient to have a total score of 40 each time the chart was used (with a maximum possible total score of 80 for the whole day). The patients generally scored 2 to 3 (moderate to severe pain) for each of the areas during the day (total score of 16–24), increasing to 4 (very severe) at night (potential total score of 32). This would appear extreme for someone not supposedly in pain. According to the patients, analgesia was not withheld but was ineffective. The analgesia generally took up to 30 min to take effect, eased the pain for about 1 hour, and then pain levels increased back to the moderate to severe level until medication was due again. Within the weekly score sheet pain was always paramount, always present and always reducing the ability of the patient to carry out his or her activities of daily living.

One of the main problems identified was that patients felt that there was a lack of time to sit and talk to staff. The need for support was highlighted, and the fact that time to talk was needed within their programmes of care. One patient wrote 'When I got up, apart from very bad pain, I was also very depressed and down, very forgetful and my concentration was very bad'.

If this is not appreciated by staff, then it is difficult for the patient who is in pain, depressed and lacks the concentration to work through their pain.

Another patient wrote of her hospital experience 'I feel the rest, food and exercise has helped me cope better for the future. A lot of the black thoughts I have daily at home, I have not had for the past week'.

Obviously from comments such as these fibromyalgia sufferers require a great deal of support to help them cope with their illness. Evaluating an in-patient stay, one patient said 'When I was told about my illness, I thought for the last four years that rest was the only thing to help along with medication, but now I know better, good light exercise is good for you'.

Education and information are, therefore, essential – patients need to understand their condition and the strategies that will help them to cope with their illness.

Another major problem associated with fibromyalgia is loss of self-image and thus self-esteem. This has been demonstrated in associated work with patients with rheumatoid arthritis, where negative internal perception can be directly attributed to the physical limitations of the condition (Ryan, 1996). Loss of occupation is a fundamental blow, as is the changed role within the family and feelings of being different and a burden. All of these factors can impact negatively on patients, and self-esteem can be severely traumatized. Spencer claims that people may experience 'feelings of uselessness, isolation, boredom, guilt and depression' (Spencer, 1992, p.30). This also results in economic effects (Rothschild, 1991). Moreover, self-esteem can be damaged by changes in body image. Brennan proposes that altered body image has a strong effect 'particularly in interactions with others, but also in relation to patients' views of themselves' (Brennan, 1994, p.299). With fibromyalgia, self-esteem is 'knocked' even further if patients are not supported and helped to overcome their disability. The fact that the illness will not deform or kill them seems, in some cases, to make patients feel even more guilty. They feel that they have lost so much prior to the diagnosis yet they still have the pain, which they are told they must learn to live with. Brennan concludes that, in order to gain acceptance of their pain and condition: 'patients must be allowed to develop successful coping mechanisms, or psychological problems may intensify' (Brennan, 1994, p.299).

Conclusions

In conclusion, therefore fibromyalgia is an extremely debilitating disease. Sufferers need the help and support of friends, relatives, work colleagues, doctors and nurses. The illness needs to be understood by both the patient and the multidisciplinary team, and the patient must learn new coping strategies to enable him or her to live as normal a life as possible. Nurses must learn to believe the patient regarding the amount of pain experienced and try to re-develop their own belief systems concerning pain and its control. If a patient suffering from fibromyalgia is to improve and achieve a better quality of life, they must have support and help, and most of all they must be able to trust the people who claim to be there to help. Indeed, Tamler and Meerschaert go so far as to say that 'Because poor attitudes affect sound judgment, physicians who cannot tolerate patients with chronic pain should not be caring for them' (Tamler and Meerschaert, 1996, p.554).

It is apparent that, at present, the system for caring for patients is unsuccessful, and anything that nurses can do in the future to educate themselves and the patients can only improve both the care and the prognosis. Smeltzer (1987) states:

> Nurses must also make it clear to the patients that their pain is real and not just in their heads, and that although there is no known cause or cure for their ailment, treatment can be successful if the patient takes a positive outlook and learns to live with a certain degree of pain!
>
> (Smeltzer, 1987, p.29)

If the future for fibromyalgia sufferers is not to be bleak, they have the right to the best management available. This will involve pharmacological and non-pharmacological approaches. However, of paramount importance is the acceptance of their pain by health care professionals. If this occurs, then there is a real possibility of health care professionals working in a successful partnership with the patient.

References

Akinsanya, C.Y. 1985: The use of knowledge in the management of pain: the nurse's role. *Nurse Education Today* 5, 41–6.

Baumstark, K.E. and Buckelew, S.P. 1992: Fibromyalgia: clinical signs, research findings, treatment implications, and future directions. *Annals of Behavioral Medicine* 14, 282–91.

Boissevain, M.D. 1996: Psychological research in fibromyalgia: the search for explanatory phenomena. *Pain Research Management* 1, 51–7.

Brennan, J. 1994: A vital component of care: the nurse's role in recognising altered body image. *Professional Nurse* 9, 298–9.

Buckelew, S.P. 1989: Fibromyalgia: a rehabilitation approach. *American Journal of Physical Medicine and Rehabilitation* 68, 37–42.

Buckelew, S.P., Murray, S.E., Hewett, J.E., Johnson, J. and Huyser, B. 1995: Self-efficacy, pain and physical activity among fibromyalgia subjects. *Arthritis Care and Research* 8, 43–50.

Campbell, S.M., Clark, S., Tindall, E.A., Forehand, M.E. and Bennett, R.M. 1983: Clinical characteristics of fibrositis. I. A 'blinded', controlled study of symptoms and tender points. *Arthritis and Rheumatism* 26, 817–24.

Carette, S., McCain, G.A., Bell, D.A. *et al.* 1986: Evaluation of amitryptiline in primary fibrositis: a double-blind placebo-controlled study. *Arthritis and Rheumatism* 29, 655–9.

Clauw, D. 1995: *New insights into fibromyalgia*. Washington, DC: Fibromyalgia Association of Greater Washington.

Doherty, M. 1995: Practical problems and the fibromyalgia syndrome. In Butler, R.C. and Jayson, I.V. (eds), *Collected reports on the rheumatic diseases.*Chesterfield: Arthritis and Rheumatism Council for Research, 83–6.

Doherty, M. and Jones, A. 1995: Fibromyalgia syndrome. *British Medical Journal* **310**, 386–90.

Edwards, A. 1996: Nonpharmacologic treatment for pain. In Borsook, D., LeBel, A.A. and McPeek, B. (eds), *The Massachusetts General Hospital handbook for pain management.* London: Little, Brown and Company, 105–11.

Fagerhaugh, S.Z. and Strauss, A. 1977: *Politics of pain management: staff-patient interactions.* New York: Addison-Wesley Publishing Company.

Fishman, S.M. and Greenberg, D.B. 1996: Special problems in the treatment of pain. In Borsook, D., LeBel, A.A. and McPeek, B. (eds), *The Massachusetts General Hospital handbook for pain management.* London: Little, Brown and Company, 370–8.

Goldenberg, D.L. 1988: Research in fibromyalgia: past, present and future. *Journal of Rheumatology* **15**, 992–6.

Gowers, W.R. 1904: Lumbago: its lessons and analogues. *British Medical Journal* **1**, 117–21.

Hacobian, A., Stojanovic, M., Tribble, C.L. *et al.* 1996: Emergencies in pain management. In Borsook, D., LeBel, A.A. and McPeek, B. (eds), *The Massachusetts General Hospital handbook for pain management.* London: Little, Brown and Company, 370–8.

Hawley, D.J., Wolfe, F. and Cathey, M.A. 1988: Pain, functional disability and psychological status: a 12-month study of severity in fibromyalgia. *Journal of Rheumatology* **15**, 1551–6.

Henrickson, C. 1994: Long-term effects of fibromyalgia on everyday life: a study of 56 patients. *Scandinavian Journal of Rheumatology* **23**, 36–41.

Henrickson, C., Gundmark, I., Bengtsson, A. and Ek, A. 1992: Living with fibromyalgia: consequences for everyday life. *Clinical Journal of Pain* **8**, 138.

Lautenbacher, S., Rollman, G.B. and McCain, G.A. 1994: Multi-method assessment of experimental and clinical pain in patients with fibromyalgia. *Pain* **59**, 45–53.

McCain, G.A. 1996: A clinical overview of the fibromyalgia syndrome. *Journal of Musculoskeletal Pain* **4**, 9–34.

McCain, G.A. and Scudds, R.A. 1988: The concept of primary fibromyalgia (fibrositis): clinical value, relation and significance to other chronic musculoskeletal pain syndromes. *Pain* **33**, 273–87.

McCain, G.A., Bell, D.A., Mai, F.M. and Halliday, P.D. 1988: A controlled study of the effects of a supervised cardiovascular fitness training program on the manifestations of primary fibromyalgia. *Arthritis and Rheumatology* **31**, 1135–41.

Marder, W.D., Meenan, R.F., Felson, D. *et al.* 1991: The future and present adequacy of rheumatologic manpower. A study of health care needs and physician supply (Editorial). *Arthritis and Rheumatology* **34**, 1209–17.

Melzack, R. and Wall, P. 1988: *The challenge of pain.* Harmondsworth: Penguin.

Moldofsky, H., Scarisbrick, P. and England, R. 1975: Musculoskeletal symptoms and non-REM sleep disturbances in patients with 'fibrositic' syndromes and healthy subjects. *Psychosomatic Medicine* **37**, 341–51.

Morrison, P. 1991: Psychology of pain. *Surgical Nurse* **4**, 18–20.

Nørregaard, J., Lykengaard, J.J., Mehlsen, J. and Danneskiold-Samsoe, B. 1997: Exercise training in treatment of fibromyalgia. *Journal of Musculoskeletal Pain* **5**, 71–9.

Powers, R. 1993: Fibromyalgia: an age-old malady begging for respect. *Journal of General Internal Medicine* **8**, 94–105.

Rogers, E.J. and Rogers, R. 1990: Fibromyalgia and myofascial pain: either, neither or both. *Physician Assistant* **14**, 37–40.

Rothschild, B.M. 1991: Fibromyalgia: an explanation for the aches and pains of the nineties. *Comprehensive Therapy* **17**, 9–14.

Ryan, S. 1995: Fibromyalgia: what help can nurses give? *Nursing Standard* **9**, 25–8.

Ryan, S. 1996: Living with rheumatoid arthritis: a phenomenological exploration. *Nursing Standard* **10**, 45–8.

Schaefer, K.M. 1995: Struggling to maintain balance: a study of women living with fibromyalgia. *Journal of Advanced Nursing* **21**, 95–102.

Smeltzer, K.J. 1987: Fibromyalgia: the frustration of diagnosis and management. *Orthopaedic Nursing* **6**, 28–31.

Spencer, B. 1992: *Fibromyalgia: fighting back.* Toronto, Ontario: LRH Publications.

Sternbach, R. 1978: *The psychology of pain.* New York: Raven Press.

Tamler, M.S. and Meerschaert, J.R. 1996: Pain management of fibromyalgia and other chronic pain syndromes. *Physical Medicine and Rehabilitation Clinics of North America* **7**, 549–60.

Twycross, R.G. 1978: Pain and analgesics. *Current Medical Research and Opinion* **5**, 496–504.

Weir, R.E. and Crook, J.M. 1992: Chronic pain and the management of conflict. In Watt-Watson, J.H. and Donovan, M.I. (eds), *Pain management nursing perspectives.* Philadelphia, PA: Mosby Year Book, 426–53.

Wolfe, F. 1986: The clinical syndrome of fibrositis. *American Journal of Medicine* **81**, 7–14.

Wolfe, F. 1995: Editorial. *Pain* **60**, 349–52.

Wolfe, F. and Cathey, M.A. 1983: Prevalence of primary and secondary fibrositis. *Journal of Rheumatology* **10**, 965–8.

Wolfe, F., Hawley, D.J., Cathey, M.A., Caro, X. and Russell, I.J. 1985: Fibrositis: symptom frequency and criteria for diagnosis. An evaluation of 291 rheumatic disease patients and 58 normal individuals. *Journal of Rheumatology* **12**, 1159–63.

Wolfe, F., Smythe, H.A., Yunis, M.B. *et al.* 1990: The American College of Rheumatology 1990 criteria for classification of fibromyalgia: report of the Multicenter Criteria Committee. *Arthritis and Rheumatology* **3**, 160–72.

Woodward, S. 1995: Nurse and patient perceptions of pain. *Professional Nurse* **10**, 415–16.

Yunus, M.B., Masi, A.T., Calabro, J.J. *et al.* 1981: Primary fibromyalgia (fibrositis): clinical study of 50 patients with matched normal controls. *Seminars in Arthritis and Rheumatology* **11**, 151–71.

Yunus, M.B., Masi, A.T. and Aldag, J.C. 1989: Preliminary criteria for primary fibromyalgia syndrome (PFS): multivariate analysis of a consecutive series of PFS, other pain patients and normal subjects. *Clinical Experimental Rheumatology* **7**, 63–9.

Yunus, M.B., Ahles, T.A., Aldag, J.C. and Masi, A.T. 1991: Relationship of clinical features with psychological status in primary fibromyalgia. *Arthritis and Rheumatology* **34**, 15–21.

Shoulder pain in hemiplegia

Christine Elizabeth Brown

Introduction

Cerebral vascular accident constitutes a major cause of long-term physical disability and impairment. Shoulder pain is a problem frequently seen in stroke patients (Roy *et al.*, 1995) and reports of its incidence vary widely, from 5 per cent to 84 per cent (Roy, 1988; Zorowitz *et al.*, 1996). It is an important problem with a variety of causes which impact on the rehabilitation process, as it reduces the patient's ability to move and participate in activities. If left untreated or if it remains persistent, shoulder pain may result in reflex sympathetic dystrophy (van Ouwenaller *et al.*, 1986). Sodring (1980) reports that shoulder pain is more common in patients who have experienced severe strokes.

Shoulder pain can easily be overlooked by professionals concerned with the rehabilitation of the patient with hemiplegia. However, for the hemiplegic patient shoulder pain can create an additional burden. Shoulder pain is, arguably, a preventable pain. An individualized approach to support, care, prevention and management is vital if shoulder pain is to be addressed. To plan an effective treatment programme, the nature of the pain, and its precise anatomical location and duration, as well as the body position during the movement that causes the pain must be assessed (Ryerson and Levit, 1991). The treatment of shoulder pain is therefore related to the patient's pain itself, the range of movement, anatomy of the glenohumeral joint, associated reactions, spasticity and physiotherapists' knowledge of handling the patient. However, sound research into prevention of shoulder pain is limited (Roy *et al.*, 1995). In patients with hemiplegia there is always the possibility of this type of pain occurring. It should therefore be assumed that patients may be suffering from shoulder pain unless they have indicated otherwise and they should be handled accordingly.

Diagnosing shoulder pain

According to Griffin (1986), a major obstacle to determining the magnitude of the problem is the lack of an accepted set of diagnostic criteria. Pain is an elusive symptom that defies quantitative measurement. Diagnosis of shoulder pain is based on a combination of signs and symptoms. Griffin (1986) emphasizes the need for commonly agreed upon diagnostic criteria, as well as methods of measuring the pain and range of movement. Without these, it is impossible to compare different researchers' findings with regard to the incidence, efficacy, prophylaxis and treatment. This is possibly why researchers, clinicians and health professionals vary greatly in their views as to when shoulder pain commences and what causes it. The aetiological agents that are most commonly mentioned in the literature are subluxation, rotator cuff tears, severe paralysis, brachial plexus injuries, exacerbation of pre-existing pathological conditions and improper exercise or handling of the affected arm (Griffin, 1986). One single cause probably does not exist, and shoulder pain is probably multifactorial.

Ryerson and Levit (1991) have identified three categories of hemiplegic shoulder pain, namely joint pain, muscle pain and pain from altered sensitivity. Joint pain is caused when the joint is improperly aligned and normal rhythm is not maintained. It is perceived as a sharp and stabbing pain. Muscle pain has been described as a 'pulling sensation'. It occurs when a spastic or shortened muscle is lengthened too fast or beyond the range to which it is accustomed. Pain from altered sensitivity occurs as a result of altered sensory input to the central nervous system. It has been described as both diffuse and aching, and is usually localized just to the shoulder. It typically occurs in the acute stage of recovery. One explanation for its occurrence is that levels of 'tolerance' of the impaired central nervous system have been reached (Ryerson and Levit, 1991).

The onset of pain can either occur early on or several months into the stroke, in a flaccid or spastic arm, with or without subluxation. If it is not resolved as soon as possible, it develops from a sharp pain at the end of a range of movements, where the patient can point accurately to the painful localized area, to a diffuse pain in the arm as well as the shoulder, that can be present all the time (Davies, 1985). The patient now finds it difficult to describe the exact location of the pain. Many patients experience pain when the arm is in certain positions, or when lying in bed at night. This results in an immobile arm and a reluctance for it to be handled (Bukowski et al., 1986). Bukowski et al. (1986) express the view that pain can be directly related to the severity of the hemiplegia and also to the previous trauma that may be activated by the additional stress of paralysis.

Effects of shoulder pain

Pain itself can limit and halt recovery by inhibiting muscle activity, leaving the patient with an immobile arm. The patient becomes afraid to move, and this leads to difficulties in moving in bed, transferring, and in washing and dressing (Bukowski et al., 1986). Braun et al. (1971) found that patients with pain at rest usually withdraw from any active rehabilitation programme. Shoulder pain is accompanied by decreased motivation, mood changes and poor motor recovery, and also limits the patient's interests and desire to become socially active. It can lead to discouragement, anxiety and frustration (Davies, 1985).

The sequelae of shoulder pain are extensive. The patient cannot concentrate on learning new skills when he or she is distracted by the pain, and therefore rehabilitation is prolonged. Davies (1985) states that pain can inhibit muscle activity and that it is very difficult to stimulate the return of active movement in the hemiplegic arm whilst pain persists. Patients with shoulder pain display significantly less motor recovery in the upper limb and achieve less ambulatory success than comparable patients without shoulder pain.

The patient is afraid to move freely because of the pain, and is particularly reluctant to move the affected arm, so consequently balance reactions are prevented (Davies 1985). This can result in frequent falls, as the patient is unable to right him- or herself. Johnstone (1987) states that pain increases spasticity, the shoulder being one of the key points of control of spasticity. Patients have difficulty in regaining independence in daily living activities as pain and stiffness hinder washing, dressing and kitchen activities. Bukowski *et al.* (1986) found that morale becomes lowered due to the pain, inability to perform activities of daily living and lack of progress in rehabilitation. This results in the patient becoming increasingly anxious, discouraged and frustrated by their lack of progress. The pain also limits the patient's ability and desire to participate in social as well as physical activities (Griffin, 1986).

Shoulder pain has been linked to depression (Savage and Robertson, 1982), and a vicious pain cycle ensues. The patient is unable to sleep properly, becomes too tired to co-operate in therapy, and therefore makes little or no progress (Davies, 1985). Patients become more depressed through lack of progress, but the pain means that they are unable to take an active part in therapy, so they become even more depressed (Braun *et al.*, 1971). Davies (1985) suggests that such patients may withdraw from their surroundings, and even from family and friends, and can become aggressive.

Vulnerability of the shoulder

The shoulder joint is the most mobile joint in the body and extremely vulnerable to injury. The changes in muscle tone, posture and movement following a stroke contribute to its vulnerability (Borgman and Passarella, 1991). The shoulder joint actually consists of seven joints which normally move in a well co-ordinated manner to produce pain-free movement. The major site of movement is the glenohumeral joint, where the humerus fits into the shallow dish-like area of the scapula (glenoid fossa). The scapula is also maintained in proper alignment by the tone of the trapezius and serratus anterior muscles (Cailliet, 1991). The shoulder capsule is thin and composed of an outer layer of dense fibrous tissue which is poorly vascularized but richly innervated. The inner synovial layer is highly vascularized but poorly innervated, so is insensitive to pain but highly reactive to heat and cold (Cailliet, 1991). The joint depends upon mechanical and muscular support and adjustment in muscle action to allow the humerus free movement and prevent pinching or trapping of sensitive tissues (Borgman and Passarella, 1991). The scapula and humerus normally move together, and any interruption of this balance increases vulnerability to injury and pain.

Subluxation

Immediately following a stroke, muscle tone decreases and the arm becomes flaccid and unstable. The muscular support of the arm against gravity is lost. The gravitational pull, unsupported by flaccid muscle, produces painful stretching of the capsule or ligament (Wood, 1989). The humeral head subluxes downward and outward and the scapula rotates downward and forward due to loss of muscle tone. The humerus in this position is passively abducted (Cailliet, 1991). When the function of supporting muscle is lost, there is potential for joint damage, rotator cuff tears and general irritation resulting from disturbed joint mechanics (Bukowski *et al.*, 1986). Cailliet (1991) supports the theory that pain can start during the flaccid stage. He states that, in the flaccid shoulder, the added traction upon the joint capsule can be a source of pain, as may traction on the stretched supraspinous tendon.

Some experts believe that subluxation itself is not painful, but that improper handling of a subluxed shoulder can lead to pain (Wood, 1989). However, others disagree. Cailliet (1991) states that many clinicians and authorities in rehabilitation consider subluxation to be a cause of pain, disability and ultimately frozen shoulder. Subluxation may also cause traction injury to the upper trunk of the brachial plexus. Cerebral vascular accident constitutes a major cause of long-term physical disability and impairment. Shoulder pain is a problem frequently seen in stroke patients, and reports of its incidence vary widely, from 5 per cent to 84 per cent (Roy, 1988). It is an important problem with a variety of causes which impact on the rehabilitation process, as it reduces the patient's ability to move and participate in everyday activities.

Bobath (1978) discounts any importance of subluxation in relation to pain. Johnstone states: 'subluxation will not itself give pain but, badly handled, it is wide open to receive injuries' (Johnstone, 1991, p.75). Davies agrees, stating that the 'subluxed shoulder itself is not painful' (Davies, 1985, p. 207). Investigations conducted in 1976 at King's College Hospital found that all hemiplegic patients with total paralysis of the arm showed malalignment when X-rayed in an upright position within the first 3 weeks after the onset of stroke. Despite this, all patients had a full pain-free range of movement at the shoulder joint (Davies, 1985). According to Smith *et al.* (1982), 60 per cent of patients with total paralysis of the arm have malalignment of the shoulder. Ryerson and Levit (1991) conclude that the exact mechanism of pain has yet to be documented, in as much as there are many causes of subluxation with no pain, and many painful shoulders with no significant subluxation. A study by Zorowitz *et al.* (1996) found no association between shoulder pain and subluxation after stroke. However, others argue that subluxation is implicated in causing shoulder pain (Roy, 1988; Totta and Beneck, 1991; Roy *et al.*, 1994, 1995). Bohannon and Andrews (1990) report that, even though treatment of subluxation to reduce pain is not necessary, there are other reasons why the malalignment should be treated.

Spasticity

Many experts do not believe that pain becomes a problem until spasticity – high tone – develops (Wood, 1989). Work by van Ouwenaller *et al.* identified a close association of shoulder pain with spasticity which they proposed to be 'the prime factor . . . in the genesis of shoulder pain in the hemiplegic patient' (van Ouwenaller *et al.*, 1986, p. 26). Painful shoulder in the spastic phase has been attributed to spasm and contracture of the subscapularis muscle, the principal internal rotator and powerful adductor of the shoulder (Cailliet, 1991). With spasticity comes decreased movement, and muscle and soft tissue become pinched. The range of movement can contribute to shoulder pain caused by inadequate movement of the scapula (Wood, 1989). Spasticity tends to be mentioned more frequently as being associated with shoulder pain, perhaps because this is the predominant tone over time in chronic hemiplegia (Griffin, 1986). Borgman and Passarella (1991) agree that increased tone may result in painful shoulder. Spasticity was found to be associated – along with severe subluxation – with shoulder pain in a study by Poulin de Courval *et al.* (1990).

Davies (1985) states that pain is experienced at the site of compressed structures when there is insufficient scapula rotation. Delayed rotation is due to an increase in muscle tone which retracts and depresses the scapula. The pain indicates that the normal co-ordinated interaction of the joint has been disrupted by abnormal unbalanced muscle tone. However, if the tone is the same proximally as well as distally, the arm can be moved slowly and will give normal rotation – this applies to both a spastic and a flaccid arm (Davies, 1985). Davies goes on to say that pain is also caused by inadequate external rotation of the humerus, as the greater tuberosity impinges against the coracoacromial arch. The arm fails to rotate externally due to the spastic pull of the powerful internal rotation of the shoulder.

Other causes

Pain may also result from other causes, such as attrition, inflammation or previous trauma that has been latent but is now activated by the hemiplegia. It can occur as a result of degeneration of the joint, with tenderness and crepitations felt on movement (Cailliet, 1980). Griffin (1986) states that the painless movement of the shoulder normally decreases with age, partly due to postural changes such as dorsal kyphosis with resultant downward scapular rotation. Griffin (1986) further cites degeneration of articular surfaces due to age as a cause of pain.

Pain occurs as a result of one or more of the following: muscle imbalance with loss of joint range, impingement of the shoulder capsule, improper muscle stretching, tendonitis, hypersensitivity, hyposensitivity and sympathetic changes (Ryerson and Levit, 1991). Limited movement or spasticity can impair circulation, which may in turn impair the autonomic nervous system which can lead to a deep burning pain. In patients with left hemiplegia who have perceptual problems, there are difficulties in the proper interpretation of sensory input. This can produce a feeling of pain in the absence of the usual pathology (Cailliet, 1980).

Many activities can potentially cause pain through trauma. With the shoulder joint rendered vulnerable by hemiplegia, poorly aligned posture or positioning can lead to trauma and pain. The patient may lie incorrectly on the affected shoulder, or may 'nurse' the arm, affecting alignment of the arm and trunk as well as the shoulder (Bobath, 1978). Lifting the affected arm without controlling the scapula causes soft tissue compression and thus pain. Pain and fear increase flexar tone, so patients who have experienced pain under passive movement will show an increase in flexar tone even before the exercise is performed again (Davies, 1985). This leaves the scapula in depression and the arm internally rotated, and any attempt to force elevation of the arm will result in increasingly severe trauma.

Davies (1985) continues by saying that, by transferring or walking the patient by holding the arm, the trunk is unsupported and as the patient moves, the weight of the body forces abduction of the shoulder. If the patient is lifted by holding under the arms, the unprotected shoulder is forced into abduction by the weight of the body. Improper passive exercises by health professionals, family or patients themselves are a possible major cause of shoulder pain. This is due to failure to provide upward scapular rotation and lateral humeral rotation during passive abduction.

Neglect, communication difficulties and even obesity can lead to problems in achieving effective and therefore pain-free posture and positions (Bobath, 1978). Griffin (1986) is in agreement with this view, and develops it further by stating that the patients at highest risk of developing shoulder pain seem to be those with severe upper limb paralysis, particularly if sensory loss and mental confusion also exist. This is due to immobility of the arm and an increased likelihood of traction injury because the patient cannot protect him- or herself. Education of health professionals and family is imperative to prevent this happening. It is important to note that neurological deficits such as sensory loss, visual field deficits, communication disorders and loss of body image can affect the prognosis for upper limb function. These deficits, in combination with motor loss and abnormal muscle tone, may increase the risk of shoulder pain.

Prevention of shoulder pain

When the predisposing causes are carefully avoided, the vast majority of painful shoulders can also be avoided. Prevention must be the first consideration but, even so, some patients will develop shoulder pain. It is generally agreed that trauma can be avoided by proper handling and positioning of the patient (Borgman and Passarella, 1991). Attention should be paid to the patient's position when lying and sitting, and how he or she is assisted to move. All passive movements must be preceded by full mobilization of the scapula, and the scapula must then be supported so that the glenoid fossa continues to face upwards and forwards (Davies, 1985). When standing, the nurse must guide the patient's trunk forward by placing his or her hands over the scapular area. When positioning in bed, the shoulder must be forward and the affected arm placed in external rotation. When sitting, there must be a firm surface to support the affected arm and the arm should be brought forward away from the trunk (Bobath, 1978).

Davies (1985) emphasizes that any position or activity which causes pain must be altered immediately. Feedback from the patient, be it verbal or visual, is therefore extremely useful. If the patient experiences pain, they will hold their arm in flexion and be loath to move it – spasticity increases and fixes the scapula even more strongly. It is important to break this vicious circle or movement will become more painful each day (Davies, 1985).

Bobath (1978) and Johnstone (1987) both agree that it is important to involve patients and family as early as possible in accepting responsibility for position- ing of the arm as well as for correct self-assisting arm activity and active movement. Patients with neglect, sensory impairment and loss of body image allow their arm to hang down, causing retraction and abduction of the shoul- der (Johnstone, 1987). Health professionals and relatives must try to increase the patient's awareness of his or her affected side, one method being always to approach from that side and to keep the locker on that side. It helps to have the arm well supported and outstretched so that the patient can see his or her arm. The patient's attention must constantly be drawn to the affected arm. Pain must be prevented rather than just treated. 'Having suffered a stroke with all its devastating consequences, the patient should not have to live with pain as well' (Davies, 1985, p.207). Zorowitz *et al.* (1996) propose that maintenance of the integrity of the shoulder joint prevents complications such as pain, as this can be achieved by the use of a 'home range of motion exercise program' (Zorowitz *et al.*, 1996, p. 26).

Initial considerations: assessment and measurement

As already discussed, some shoulder pain is preventable, but some patients do develop pain. In the case of a patient who has already developed a stiff painful shoulder before the correct treatment programme was instituted, health pro- fessionals must gain the patient's trust. It is best not to move the arm, but to treat all other aspects of the patient's disability (Davies, 1985). The patient needs to experience some success in other aspects of rehabilitation. The patient must be given time – the painful shoulder did not develop overnight, so a week or two will not be detrimental to the end result. Davies (1985) expands on this, saying that, by initially leaving the arm alone, constantly reassuring the patient, correct positioning and working on other aspects of rehabilitation, the patient will, in general, allow his or her arm to be handled.

If the patient has an established stiff, painful shoulder, one of the first steps to be taken is to identify the cause. A detailed medical history is important to determine the history of any shoulder pathological conditions and to identify any trauma that occurred after the stroke, such as falls (Griffin, 1986). As previously stated, it can be assumed that the majority of patients will suffer shoulder pain if they have poor range of movement, spasticity, subluxation, and also have perceptual problems, neglect, an immobile arm or tend to neglect their affected arm, unless the patient indicates otherwise. It is difficult to assess pain if patients have language problems and/or cognitive impairment. Health professionals must look for signs of pain such as flinching, guarding, holding, restlessness, grimacing, moaning, rocking, pushing away and even aggression (Herr and Mobily, 1991).

Memory impairment, depression, communication difficulties and cognitive impairment make it difficult to measure pain and even to carry out adequate treatment. It is important to keep verbal questions and instructions to a minimum, and to make them simple to understand. Extraneous noises should be reduced, and health professionals must ensure that the patient is attentive (Herr and Mobily, 1991). Family, carers and friends can be a reliable source of information on changes of behaviour, function and activities that may lead one to believe that the patient is in pain. Herr and Mobily (1991) state that significant others may notice changes in sleep pattern, movement and interactions which may indicate that pain is present. As well as involving family, carers and friends in pain assessment/measurement, it is important to involve them in pain management. Not only is it beneficial for the patient, but also it allows significant others to be actively involved in the patient's care and comfort, and can help to minimize their feelings of helplessness.

A high proportion of stroke patients are elderly. Pain in this age group must be managed as it would be in any other age group. There is also an assumption that pain, sensitivity and perception decrease with age. However, there are conflicting data regarding age-associated changes in pain perception, sensitivity and tolerance (Herr and Mobily, 1991). Such assumptions must not be made, as this leaves the patient suffering needlessly and under-treated in terms of their pain and its cause. Herr and Mobily (1991) state that older patients may not complain of being in pain, for fear of what it may mean and what it will involve. This does not mean that they do not have pain. Herr and Mobily's findings showed that many elderly people believe that pain is something which they must live with, while others believe that it is unacceptable to show pain. Health professionals must work to dispel these beliefs.

Physical examination is very important in pain management, especially with regard to the alignment of the shoulder joint, range of movement and trigger points. A trigger point is an area sensitive to pressure of palpation that produces a pain sensation (Ferrell and Ferrell, 1992). This examination is probably best performed by the physiotherapist during their detailed assessment of the patient and their functional ability prior to planning and commencing a treatment programme. Evaluation of function is important, as pain can lead to functional impairment and severely hinder rehabilitation.

Psychological assessment and evaluation must be carried out, as the patient may be depressed or anxious due to pain, and there is a possibility of these symptoms causing an increase in pain. A clinical psychologist should conduct a thorough mental status assessment using a recognized assessment tool such as the Hospital Anxiety and Depression Scale or the Beck Depression Inventory (Ferrell and Ferrell, 1992). Both depression and anxiety need to be diagnosed and treated alongside the pain. Patients need to be involved in their care and rehabilitation, and in the prevention and management of their pain. They have lost control over their lives and bodies following a stroke, and they need to know that they have some control over their care and treatment. By involving them in decisions concerning treatment and giving them responsibilities, some locus of control is returned to them. Establishing a trusting and caring relationship is an important step towards pain management in the elderly stroke patient (Herr and Mobily, 1991).

Theory supporting treatment

The intensity of pain must be measured before treatment commences, and also during and after treatment in order to evaluate the effectiveness of the treatment. Pain intensity can be measured on categorical scales, numerical scales or visual analogue scales (VAS). The horizontal VAS is considered to be the best scale for research purposes, but some elderly patients have difficulty in understanding this scale (Herr and Mobily, 1991). For this group, Herr and Mobily (1991) suggest that a vertical scale is much easier to use. One such scale is a picture representative of a thermometer, showing pain climbing up the thermometer as the intensity increases. The scale is usually rated from 0 to 10, or colours can be used, ranging from blue (no or very little pain) through to red (most severe pain) (Herr and Mobily, 1991).

The gate control theory proposed by Melzack and Wall (1988) has implications for the treatment of pain – sensory and psychological as well as pharmacological. They identified the gating mechanism by which painful impulses are modulated in the dorsal horn of the spinal cord, and then travel to the thalamus and cortex, where they are recognized as pain. This theory recognizes the effects of cognitive and emotional processes within the cortex and midbrain on transmission of painful impulses. The theory also acknowledges that emotional states, learning, knowledge and thought processes help to determine whether the gating mechanism in the spinal cord allows or stops the transmission of pain impulses (Watt-Watson and Ivers Donovan, 1992). It can be seen from this theory that pain can be regulated or reduced at four points – first, at the peripheral site of pain, then at the spinal cord by stimulation of large nerve fibres, the next two areas being the brainstem and cortex (Watt-Watson and Ivers Donovan, 1992).

Cutaneous stimulation may help to relieve pain by activation of the large-diameter nerve fibres in the skin. The reticular system in the brainstem inhibits incoming stimuli. Therefore, if the patient is given normal or excessive sensory input, these impulses help to close the gate to pain impulses; inhibitory signals from the cerebral cortex and thalamus can alleviate pain. Thoughts, emotions and past experiences may affect pain impulse transmission. Pain can therefore be reduced by giving the patient a sense of control – providing information about the pain they are experiencing – and by alleviation or reduction of anxiety and depression (McCaffery and Beebe, 1989). A range of methods will result in more effective pain management than a single method approach.

Physiotherapy

The first approach to control of shoulder pain in hemiplegia is to prevent further trauma and to decrease pain by correct positioning and handling. The second step is physiotherapy treatment. This is important for reducing pain, as it helps to relax and strengthen muscles and reduce spasticity. Moving the affected arm under controlled conditions through normal-range movements can itself alleviate some of the pain. This also frees the shoulder and shows the patient and relatives that the arm can be moved. However, patients and relatives must be made aware that there will be some increase in pain when treatment commences, but that this will gradually decrease as treatment progresses. Analgesia is usually given 20 to 30 min, as appropriate, before a physiotherapy session in order to take this into account (Johnstone, 1987).

Pharmacological management

The effects of any previous pain relief and treatment must be taken into account, and can act as guidelines as to what is acceptable to the patient and what has been effective in the past. It is necessary to know how patients coped with pain in the past as an indication for future treatment. In the vast majority of cases of shoulder pain, analgesia is the next step in pain management. Aspirin and non-steroidal anti-inflammatory drugs (NSAIDs) are the most commonly used analgesics, having a general lack of serious side-effects and proven efficacy in pain relief. Analgesia must be given before pain occurs or increases. This means that appropriate doses can be administered, resulting in fewer side-effects, and the patient is not in as much pain, and their anxiety or fear of pain is reduced.

Non-steroidal anti-inflammatory drugs

Non-steroidal anti-inflammatory drugs have anti-inflammatory, analgesic and anti-pyretic effects. Damage caused to tissues by trauma results in the release of histamine, bradykinin and prostaglandins, all of which trigger inflammation and can produce pain (Watt-Watson and Ivers Donovan, 1992). These drugs prevent the synthesis of prostaglandins from arachidonic acid by inhibiting the cyclo-oxygenase enzyme that is necessary for the formation of endoperoxides (McCaffery and Beebe, 1989). They are particularly effective in relieving pain associated with inflammation in musculoskeletal disorders, and pain related to peripheral trauma. It is impossible to predict which NSAID the individual patient will respond to or tolerate best. It is a matter of trial and error, although Naproxen is generally better tolerated than Ibuprofen.

Side-effects can be a problem with any drug so the medical history of the patient must always be examined for any contraindications. By inhibiting prostaglandins, the protective mucous lining of gastric mucosa is reduced, and NSAIDs therefore predispose the patient to gastro-intestinal toxicity, which is enhanced by the fact that many NSAIDs can directly damage the gastric lining. To prevent this, NSAIDs should be taken with meals and an antacid should also be taken, or misoprastol, which is a prostaglandin analogue and which protects against NSAID ulcers, should be prescribed. Prostaglandins are vital for the production of thromboxane, which causes platelets to aggregate. NSAIDs reduce this aggregation, so prolonging bleeding time (Watt-Watson and Ivers Donovan, 1992).

With any drug therapy in the elderly, dosages may need to be altered due to changes in metabolism and elimination of drugs. An increase in the proportion of body fat may cause delayed onset and also accumulation with repeat doses of drugs such as diazepam that are fat soluble. Chronic disease, which often occurs in the elderly, contributes to reduced serum protein levels. Due to the reduced levels of circulating proteins, a proportion of the drug is left unbound, thus resulting in greater toxic effects. NSAIDs are protein bound and are likely to be associated with stronger pharmacological effects. Other side-effects include impaired renal function, memory loss, confusion and inability to concentrate. These cognitive dysfunctions clear after stopping the drug. Other drugs that the patient is taking must be taken into account, as they may interact with NSAIDs (McCaffery and Beebe, 1989).

Adjuvant analgesia

In some circumstances it is helpful to give a combination of drugs, and not just analgesics alone. This is known as adjuvant analgesia. These drugs are not intended for the treatment of pain, but can relieve pain as they have analgesic properties or enhance the effects of analgesics. Consideration must be given to the fact that they also have the potential for side-effects. Such drugs include antidepressants, tranquillizers and muscle relaxants. Muscle relaxants are for temporary use alongside physiotherapy, as they help to alleviate painful muscle spasm. Antidepressants are useful when pain is 'tingling' or 'burning'. They produce analgesia in doses below those necessary to alleviate depression. Obviously if the patient is also suffering from depression they are a good choice. They can also improve sleep. Side-effects can include dry mouth, sedation and orthostatic hypotension (McCaffery and Beebe, 1989).

The other drug therapy that is sometimes used in shoulder pain is intra-articular injection of the steroid dexamethasone phosphate (Decadron). Steroids halt all aspects of the inflammatory process, including pain. This drug is used when other methods do not appear to be successful. Relief can be obtained after just one injection, but up to three injections can be given. Full aseptic precautions are necessary, and the technique must be performed by medical staff who are familiar with it (Davies, 1985).

Non-pharmacological approaches

Pharmacological management of pain alone is often not adequate or even what the patient wants, and a combination of treatments or a different treatment may be required. Non-pharmacological intervention does not interfere with any ongoing treatment. Such methods that can be used on the stroke ward include superficial heat and cold, massage, relaxation and ultrasound.

Cutaneous stimulation involves stimulating the skin to relieve pain using heat, cold and massage. The treatment must be acceptable to the patient, and what is beneficial to one person is not necessarily so to another. The majority of stroke patients appear to prefer heat, as they feel that this is more relaxing. The site chosen for application is usually the painful shoulder itself, the opposite shoulder and the lower part of the affected area (Watt-Watson and Ivers Donovan, 1992).

Cooling can reduce the release of serotonin and histamine. It also decreases lymph production and cell permeability and so reduces oedema. Peripheral cold slows the conduction speed of the small unmyelinated nerve fibres that conduct pain impulses. It reduces muscle tone and spasticity, and is useful in muscle spasm but should not be used for patients with heart disease, peripheral vascular disease or hypersensitivity to cold (Watt-Watson and Ivers Donovan, 1992). It is therefore not suitable for all stroke patients. Cold packs should be sealed to prevent dripping, and must be flexible so as to conform to the body. Ice packs or frozen gel packs are used and placed on the site, wrapped in some gauze. Contact should be limited to 15 min at a time. Cooling effects on muscles last longer than heat (Johnstone, 1991).

Heat reduces pain through vasodilation, which increases blood flow and so also the elimination of cellular metabolites that stimulate pain impulses. It is thought that heat decreases the sensitivity of muscles to stretch and triggers pain-inhibiting reflexes through temperature receptors (Watt-Watson and Ivers Donovan, 1992). These actions are responsible for the relaxation of muscle spasms. Superficial heat also increases the pain threshold in the area to which it is applied, and decreases joint stiffness. It should only be used under supervision and with caution over areas with impaired sensation, or with patients who have communication problems. It should not be used where there is swelling or bleeding, or immediately following acute trauma. Heating packs are used to apply the heat.

Massage

Massage is an instinctive and natural response – we rub our aches and pains. Vickers (1966) identifies the fact that research shows various ways in which massage may relieve pain, either through gate-control mechanisms or release of endorphins, but states that no single explanation is likely to be satisfactory. The pressure of massage on superficial venous and lymphatic channels improves circulation and reduces the pain associated with oedema. It also causes capillary and, in some cases, arteriole dilation, thus further improving circulation. A study in 1989 by Kaada and Torsteinbo on 12 volunteers suffering from myalgia and other pain suggested that the analgesic action of massage may be mediated in part by the release of endorphins. There is little sound literature available on the ability of massage to reduce pain. There is evidence that if massage is combined with certain essential oils – the practice known as aromatherapy – then analgesia results (Price, 1993).

Other benefits of massage include distracting the patient from the pain, and improvement of the nurse–patient relationship. The nurse spends more 'quality' time with the patient and a bond of trust often builds up. The patient feels cared for and valued, and can use this quiet time to talk and express his or her feelings and worries. It can also allay patients' fears of having the affected arm handled. Touch in itself is therapeutic, and physical contact can improve body image. Family and carers can easily be taught how to massage. It is, of course, essential to obtain the consultant's and patient's consent before massage takes place (Tisserand, 1988).

Massage should not be performed over recent injury, skin lesions, lacerations or fractures, or immediately after surgery. In the case of stroke patients who experience muscle spasm, the unaffected arm is usually massaged and with good effect. In other cases, the affected hand is massaged, especially if the arm itself is sensitive to touch. In patients with severe muscle spasm, associated reactions or hypersensitivity of the affected arm, massage is not recommended (Johnstone, 1987).

Relaxation

Relaxation is a central control technique which exerts its effects through alteration of sensory and affective factors. It involves 'a state of relative freedom from both anxiety and skeletal muscle tension' (McCaffery and Beebe, 1989, p. 188). Relaxation allays anxiety and reduces tension and muscle spasm, thus decreasing pain. It can also reduce distressing thoughts and feelings, which is especially relevant for stroke patients. A large number of studies have demonstrated that relaxation is very effective for pain management (for example, Linton, 1982; Philips, 1988; Turner and Jensen, 1993). It can increase confidence, and a sense of self-control over pain, and it improves mood. It needs to be carried out with the patient in a comfortable and quiet environment, and it requires a passive attitude from the patient. In hemiplegic patients, only passive muscle relaxation must be taught or autogenic training – suggestions to make oneself feel warmer, lighter and floating (Watt-Watson and Ivers Donovan, 1992). Initial instructions are given by a clinical psychologist for the first three sessions. The patients are then provided with a tape that they can use themselves or under supervision. The technique involves slow rhythmical breathing and needs to be practised two or three times a week until the patient feels comfortable with it. Each session must end with a slow return to normal activities in order to prevent any dizziness.

Ultrasound

The last method of pain management in shoulder pain is ultrasound. This is carried out by physiotherapists after discussion with the consultant. Ultrasound consists of pressure waves that can be focused and beamed and are able to travel through water and soft tissues. It heats whatever absorbs it, e.g. bone, and as a result it is possible to warm gently the surface of bones and joints. It causes vasodilation, the increased blood flow removing histamine, bradykinin and prostaglandins. This appears to account for its pain-relieving properties. The second way in which it is effective is thought to be due to the fact that the heating of tissues generates nerve impulses which play a role in the afferent barrage and exert an inhibitory effect by closing the gate in the spinal cord (Melzack and Wall, 1988).

Conclusions

Some patients with shoulder pain require only physiotherapy, some need physiotherapy and analgesia, and some require all of the methods of pain management that have been mentioned. Pain is individual to each patient, and the effectiveness of all approaches to pain relief must be evaluated. One of the most important aspects in the care of the hemiplegic patient is prevention of shoulder pain, or minimization or alleviation of any pain that is present and prevention of further pain. Pain can seriously restrict a patient's ability to achieve independence in activities of daily living, and it is the responsibility of all members of the multidisciplinary team, as well as patients, relatives and carers, to ensure that maximum independence is achieved. This means that the whole team, as well as patients, relatives and carers, must be involved both in the prevention of pain and in pain management.

Whilst the ideal scenario would be to prevent shoulder pain from occurring, or to act to alleviate the pain, this is not always possible. Some patients still suffer from shoulder pain that cannot be alleviated. If pain is not relieved, patients must still be cared for and not just abandoned to their pain – it must be acknowledged that their pain has not been relieved. In these circumstances, patients, relatives and carers, must be offered help and emotional support.

References

Bobath, B. 1978: *Adult hemiplegia: evaluation and treatment.* London: Heinemann.

Bohannon, R.W. and Andrews, A.W. 1990: Shoulder subluxation and pain in stroke patients. *American Journal of Occupational Therapy* **44**, 501–9.

Borgman, M.F. and Passarella, P.M. 1991: Nursing care of the stroke patient using Bobath principles. An approach to altered movement. *Nursing Clinics of North America* **26**, 1019–35.

Braun, R.M., West, F., Mooney, V., Nickel, V., Roper, B. and Caldwell, C. 1971: Surgical treatment of the painful shoulder contracture in the stroke patient. *Bone and Joint Surgery* **53A**, 1307–12.

Bukowski, L., Bonavolonta, M., Keehn, M.J. and Morgan, A. 1986: Interdisciplinary roles in stroke care. *Nursing Clinics of North America* **21**, 359–74.

Cailliet, R. 1980: *The shoulder in hemiplegia*. Philadelphia, PA: F.A.Davis.

Cailliet, R. 1991: *Shoulder pain*. Philadelpia, PA: F.A.Davis.

Davies, P.M. 1985: *Steps to follow. A guide to the treatment of adult hemiplegia*. Berlin: Springer-Verlag.

Ferrell, B.R. and Ferrell, B. 1992: Pain in the elderly. In Watt-Watson, J.H. and Ivers Donovan, M.I. (eds), *Pain management: nursing perspectives*. St Louis, MO: Mosby Year Book, 349–69.

Griffin, J.W. 1986: Hemiplegic shoulder pain. *Physical Therapy* **66**, 1884–93.

Herr, K.A. and Mobily, P.R. 1991: Complexities of pain assessment in the elderly. Clinical considerations. *Journal of Gerontological Nursing* **17**, 12–19.

Johnstone, M. 1987: *Restoration of motor function in the stroke patient. A physiotherapist's approach*, 3rd edn. Edinburgh: Churchill Livingstone.

Johnstone, M. 1991: *Therapy for stroke. Building on experience*. Edinburgh: Churchill Livingstone.

Kaada, B. and Torsteinbo, O. 1989: Increase of plasma beta-endorphins in connective tissue massage. *General Pharmacology* **20**, 487–9.

Linton, S.J. 1982: Applied relaxation as a method of coping with chronic pain: a therapist's guide. *Scandinavian Journal of Behavior Therapy* **11**, 161–74.

McCaffery, M. and Beebe, A. 1989: *Pain. Clinical manual for nursing practice*. St Louis, MO: C.V. Mosby.

Melzack, R. and Wall, P. 1988: *The challenge of pain*, 2nd edn. Harmondsworth: Penguin.

Philips, H.C. 1988: Changing chronic pain experience. *Pain* **32**, 165–72.

Poulin de Courval, L., Barsauskas, A., Berenbaum, B. *et al*. 1990: Painful shoulder in the hemiplegic and unilateral neglect. *Archives of Physical Medicine and Rehabilitation* **68**, 673–8.

Price, S. 1993: *The aromatherapy workbook. Understanding essential oils from plant to bottle*. London: Thorsons.

Roy, C.W. 1988: Shoulder pain in hemiplegia: a literature review. *Clinical Rehabilitation* **3**, 35–44.

Roy, C.W., Sands, M.R. and Hill, L.D. 1994: Shoulder pain in acutely admitted hemiplegics. *Clinical Rehabilitation* **28**, 334–40.

Roy, C.W., Sands, M.R., Hill, L.D., Harrison, A. and Marshall, S. 1995: The effect of shoulder pain on outcome of acute hemiplegia. *Clinical Rehabilitation* **9**, 21–7.

Ryerson, S. and Levit, K. 1991: The shoulder in hemiplegia. In Donatelli, R.A. (ed.), *Physical therapy of the shoulder*, 2nd edn. New York: Churchill Livingstone, 117–49.

Savage, R. and Robertson, L. 1982: The relationship between adult hemiplegic shoulder pain and depression. *Physiotherapy Canada* **34**, 86–90.

Smith, R.G., Cruikshank, J. G., Dunbar, S. *et al*. 1982: Malalignment of the shoulder after stroke. *British Journal of Medicine* **284**, 1224–6.

Sodring, K.M. 1980: Upper extremity orthosis for stroke patients. *International Journal of Rehabilitation Research* **3**, 3–38.

Tisserand, R. 1988: *Aromatherapy for everyone*. London: Arkana.

Totta, M. and Beneck, S. 1991: Shoulder dysfunction in stroke hemiplegia. *Physical Medicine and Rehabilitation Clinics of North America* **2**, 627–41.

Turner, J.A. and Jensen, M.P. 1993: Efficacy of cognitive therapy for chronic low back pain. *Pain* **52**, 169–77.

van Ouwenaller, C., Laplace, P.M. and Chantraine, A. 1986: Painful shoulder in hemiplegia. *Archives of Physical Medicine and Rehabilitation* **67**, 23–6.

Vickers, A. 1996: *Massage and aromatherapy. A guide for health professionals.* London: Chapman and Hall.

Watt-Watson, J.H. and Ivers Donovan, M. 1992: *Pain management: nursing perspective.* St Louis, MO: Mosby Year Book.

Wood, C. 1989: Shoulder pain in stroke patients. *Nursing Times* **85**, 32–4.

Zorowitz, R.D., Hughes, M.B., Idank, D., Ikai, T. and Johnston, M.V. 1996: Shoulder pain and subluxation after stroke: correlation or coincidence? *American Journal of Occupational Therapy* **50**, 194–201.

Constructive management of cardiac pain

21

Michael Lappin

Introduction

Pain is a difficult concept to grasp. It cannot be measured directly, so it is never possible to know how much pain someone is suffering when he or she says it hurts (Townsend, 1988). Sofaer (1984) comments that this makes the nursing of a patient in pain a matter of subjective management. Pain is also worse when it is dwelt upon, when it is accompanied by anxiety, or if the pain is believed to be life-threatening.

Park and Fulton (1991) remark that numerous studies of hospital patients have confirmed that acute pain is often inadequately managed. Patients of all ages experience considerable pain despite the widespread availability of drugs and techniques to relieve suffering. The reasons for ineffective pain control in hospitals have been a source of much speculation and study. Some of the major reasons include a lack of understanding of the nature and pathophysiology of pain and control methods, a lack of pharmacological knowledge of opiates and of alternative methods of pain control. Additionally a dearth of practical efficiency frequently following a slender assessment, with the outcome often being no review of the adequacy of pain control or the effectiveness of analgesic drug regimes. The fear of addiction often leads medical and nursing staff to administer less analgesia to patients. Patients may also be concerned about this and as a consequence do not request sufficient analgesia to control their pain adequately. Again, this fear stems from a lack of knowledge of the true risks of addiction in the treatment of acute pain. Park and Fulton state that 'Addiction to opioids given for the management of acute pain is extremely rare' (Park and Fulton, 1991, p. 2). It is therefore appropriate to comment that fear of addiction should not be used as an excuse for withholding opioid analgesia.

Severe discomfort is a phenomenon that should be of great concern to nurses because of its significant impact on patient well-being. Pain and its assessment and management are fertile areas for nursing research (Puntillo, 1988). Predictably, critical-care nurses give pain research a high priority. Yet it is surprising to note the lack of nursing research on pain in critically ill patients. Within this chapter the writer seeks to develop a more thorough understanding of pain and its significance to patients with suspected acute myocardial infarction (MI), which would serve as a firm basis for nursing practice and future pain research in the area of coronary heart disease.

The case for better management

Acute myocardial infarction remains the leading cause of death in Western society (Second International Study of Infarct Survival, 1988). The greatest opportunities for improvement in mortality lie with improved and earlier treatment of this disease. Life-saving treatments such as early administration of thrombolysis and various quite simple medicines such as aspirin, ACE inhibitors and beta-blockers have produced substantial improvements in patient outcome. Emergency angioplasty is an alternative to thrombolysis, but is only available in specialist centres. Cardiac rehabilitation programmes that are hospital based have also been shown to improve mortality (O'Connor et al., 1989).

Pain, fear and apprehension are almost invariably present in patients suffering from acute MI. Willetts (1989) insists that prompt and adequate analgesia will relieve the pain and anxiety, and can reduce the risk of arrhythmias and ventricular fibrillation. Caunt (1996) comments that, as the benefits of early treatment and timely hospitalization for these patients have become apparent, admission rates to coronary care units have soared.

Many authors have expressed the opinion that nurses do not, in general, assess a patient's pain accurately, which leads to unacceptable delays in the initial treatment with painkillers (Davies and Seers, 1991; Gaston-Johansson et al., 1991; Caunt, 1996). Opioid analgesia is indicated for the severe pain associated with MI, as it has an effect on many systems. The pain, distress and anxiety that accompany myocardial ischaemia result in an increase in sympathetic tone and the release of catecholamines. Tachycardia, dysrhythmias, hypertension and increased myocardial workload may further embarrass the ischaemic myocardium, causing an extensive necrotic zone. Thus the use of opioid analgesics in these patients can improve cardiovascular function. The central effects of analgesics, by reducing the response to pain, will decrease sympathetic tone and catecholamine production. This will result in a reduction in the pre-load and after-load on the heart. The vasodilatory properties of morphine (resulting from histamine release) will further reduce the myocardial workload. The central mood-elevating effects of opioid drugs will also play an important role in alleviating anxiety in patients. The choice of analgesic agent depends upon the patient's level of pain, haemodynamic state and respiratory stability, and how the medication may be expected to modify these parameters.

Apart from the inadequate assessment of pain, there also remains an additional barrier to effective management, namely nurses' lack of knowledge about analgesic drugs, particularly opiates. Willetts (1989) comments that the efficient and intelligent use of these drugs is disastrously hampered not only by lack of understanding of their relief of both pain and anxiety, but also by fear of using them because of misinformation concerning their side-effects. Doctors and nurses are often criticized for their reluctance to use analgesia in sufficient doses when necessary. As a result, a patient's pain may go unchecked. Such reluctance arises from a failure to realize the duration of action of many drugs particularly morphine and diamorphine, which have a much more transient duration of action than is commonly assumed. There is also an exaggerated picture of the risk of addiction (Smith, 1985).

Another reason for withholding opioids is fear of potentially fatal respiratory depression. Misconceptions about addiction may account for the majority of under-treatment in acute pain. Dosages of analgesia and the intervals between them should be determined according to individual patient response. If a certain dose does not produce adequate pain relief, in general the dose should be increased. If it relieves the pain for a shorter period than the prescribed interval, then the interval should be reduced (McCaffery and Hart, 1976).

Willetts' (1989) study of pain on a coronary care unit (CCU) demonstrated that 30 per cent of nursing assessments underestimated the severity of the pain being experienced and 20 per cent overestimated its oppressive nature. Half of the patients in the sample received intramuscular (IM) diamorphine (which, incidentally, can interfere with cardiac enzyme results, causing a rise due to muscular injury) or oral medication such as nitrates and aspirin. Less than 50 per cent of the patients received adequate pain relief within 30 min of the administration of a pain-killer. Establishing a good nurse–patient relationship and patient education are of fundamental importance, and the nurse should always inform the patient of the significance of reporting pain. This study revealed that, although such communication was available, very few nurses actually explained the cause of pain and the availability of analgesia. It was found that 42 per cent of those nurses administering diamorphine feared inducing respiratory depression, and 16 per cent feared inducing an anaphylactic reaction. Although the staff in this trial were well aware that effective pain control does play an important role in limiting infarct size, their actual knowledge of the effects of diamorphine was relatively poor. It was found that 41 per cent knew that maximal respiratory depression is reached within 5–10 min of IV administration of diamorphine, and only 25 per cent knew that diamorphine's peak analgesic effect is reached within 20 min of IV administration. In total, 50 per cent of the nurses stated that if a patient who was experiencing pain requested diamorphine after receiving previous doses of the drug, they would be worried that the patient might be becoming dependent.

From the patient's viewpoint, 80 per cent said that their pain never really disappeared during their stay in the CCU. Over 50 per cent of the patients interviewed said that they had been in hospital for longer than 24 h before they were totally pain free, the longest time being 4 days. Interestingly, 40 per cent said that their level of anxiety about their condition increased during this time.

The study therefore suggests that the traditional treatment of pain in acute MI needs to be reconsidered, particularly with regard to the method of drug administration, the doses used, and sometimes the choice of drug. Over 50 per cent of the patients said that they felt they would have benefited from having pain-killers on a regular basis during the first 24 h of admission to hospital. In view of the reluctance of patients to report pain, and the difficulty in assessing the nature of such discomfort, there may be a place for low-dose diamorphine infusions or regular bolus injections during the first 24 h of admission to a CCU. This should reduce anxiety, circulating catecholamine levels and the risk of extending infarcted areas of myocardial tissue. Dysrhythmias caused by unstable (ischaemic) areas of heart muscle would also be limited.

Myocardial pain vs. descriptors of other chest pain

O'Connor (1995b) revealed in a later study that nurses underestimated the patient's pain in 46 per cent of myocardial infarction cases, particularly when the patients were in severe pain. Furthermore, Bondestam *et al.* (1987) found that even when myocardial infarction patients scored their pain between 7 and 8 on a numerical scale ranging from 0 (pain free) to 10 (worst pain possible), 20 per cent of them did not receive pain relief. As the primary symptom of acute MI, chest pain is often described by its sensory elements, e.g. aching, nagging, cramping, pressing and burning sensations. However, Gaston-Johansson *et al.* (1991) reported that the use of affective terms, such as 'suffocating', 'terrifying', 'killing' and 'torturing' in association with the sensory words, differentiated MI patients more clearly from non-MI patients than any other factor in the pain description. Thus, when pain is systematically described using both sensory and affective components, there appear to be unique characteristics which distinguish MI pain from other types of chest pain. Levine (1980) comments that if the differentiation of MI from other causes of chest pain could be improved, resources might be more effectively spent on high-risk and low-risk patients. Gaston and Johansson *et al.* (1991) discovered the affective component of pain to be greater than the sensory component of pain in the MI group of patients, whereas the non-MI patients reported the opposite situation. The MI and non-MI groups chose similar sensory words to describe their pain but, the MI group chose a higher number of words. The word 'squeezing' was used significantly more frequently ($P = 0.01$) by MI patients.

Another curious issue revealed by this study was that patients with anterior wall infarction reported higher pain scores for both sensory and affective component pain compared to the subjects with other infarct sites. They prompted accurate and careful assessment of the pain experience associated with MI as a basis for nursing action, and this is crucial in view of the importance of reducing myocardial injury. The authors also found it somewhat surprising that MI patients had such a high emotional component of pain, since there was an expectation that patients with physiological injury would experience more sensory pain. However, Melzack and Wall (1991) highlight the fact that anxiety can be associated with intense pain and experienced danger. This finding may add weight to the debate on the regime of drug therapy. In addition to giving opiates, for example, anxiety-relieving medication might also play a useful role.

The acute nature of myocardial pain

O'Connor (1995a) observes that pain is more than a sensation – it also has a distinctively unpleasant affective quality which can become overwhelming, especially for a patient with a suspected myocardial infarction. Pain can disrupt thought and ongoing behaviour because it demands immediate attention. Melzack and Wall (1991) propose that the characteristics of acute pain are a combination of tissue damage, pain and anxiety. Thus, by definition, myocardial infarction is acute pain.

Acute myocardial infarction pain and the discomfort associated with angina may be a signal for the individual to cease exercise and seek a medical opinion. Furthermore, chest pain that causes a restriction in activity may constitute the most alarming and anxiety-provoking symptom experienced by the patient. Gaston and Johansson et al. (1991) see pain as a complex multidimensional experience which should be measured as such. Billings et al. (1981) support this view by stating that the severity of acute MI pain is primarily determined by physiological and not psychological factors. However, psychological factors strongly influence patients' interpretation of their pain, the meaning that they attach to their pain, their behaviour and reaction to the pain.

Pain duration may be an indicator of infarct size, recurrent episodes of chest pain being a clear indicator of extension of infarct size. Herlitz et al. (1986), for instance, clearly demonstrated that a large proportion of patients with continuous chest pain experienced this as a result of perpetual ischaemia and, in some instances, infarct development. The study also demonstrated that patients with more severe pain had a higher 2-year mortality rate, and a higher incidence of ventricular fibrillation and congestive cardiac failure during their hospitalized period.

Using nursing models to guide assessment

The critical findings from such inquiries are important for all coronary care nurses if they are to prevent or relieve potential complications of myocardial ischaemia and infarction and to improve the outcome for patients. The solution, it would appear, is a definitive nursing assessment that could also facilitate indication of eventual diagnosis and prognosis. Although it has been suggested that holistic nursing models offer an ideal framework within which to assess and treat a patient in pain, O'Connor (1995a) has highlighted that pain assessment in nursing models was not considered to be a priority.

Activities of daily living (Roper et al., 1985)

O'Connor chose the model of Roper et al. (1985) as a theoretical framework to examine pain assessment. The majority of nurses in the UK are familiar with this model, which is based on the ability of a patient to perform everyday activities necessary for living. Nursing is viewed as helping people to prevent, alleviate, solve and cope with problems related to such activities. However, O'Connor cites Walker and Campbell (1989) who proposed that pain is not an activity of daily living and would therefore seem 'to present a theoretical difficulty for inclusion as a focus for primary assessment'. Roper et al. (1985) published a concise section on pain under the heading 'activity of communicating'. They acknowledge pain under the specific activities of daily living, e.g. eating and drinking, mobilizing, sleeping, and expressing sexuality, together with breathing. However, pain – like psychological distress – can influence any of the activities of living and the effects on those functions may overlap at times. Roper et al. observe that the nurse would normally chart the incidence of pain in relation to the activity of living if it was specific to the latter, but non-specific pain would then appropriately be included under the activity of communication.

Behavioural systems model (Johnson, 1980)

Consideration of other models of nursing would suggest that pain assessment could be embraced by most frameworks that are currently accessible to the nursing profession. For example, Johnson's Behavioural Systems Model (1980) encourages nurses to see individuals as having a set of interrelated behavioural subsystems, each of which is striving for balance and equilibrium within itself. Seven major subsystems are discussed, each of which motivates an individual's behaviour towards particular goals. A patient with chest pain due to myocardial infarction or angina would experience an imbalance in the subsystems of 'achievement' and 'dependency'. The goals of each behaviour would be towards control over oneself and one's environment (achievement) and towards conditions of security and dependency upon others (dependency). The individual's behavioural subsystems have been thrown into disequilibrium by the processes associated with physical disease – in this case, coronary artery occlusion or by atheromatous plaque formation resulting in a stenotic lesion. The model's emphasis upon observable behaviour shows a concern for people rather than their biological functioning. Thus nursing's distinctive contribution to patient care is through mechanisms which aim to facilitate optimal levels of behaviour. The role of the nurse becomes one of restoring balance within behavioural subsystems at times of psychological or physical crisis.

Adaptation model (Roy, 1980)

Roy (1980) presented an adaptive model of nursing which resembles Johnson's model, although she does not conceptualize the sets of interrelated systems in purely behavioural terms. Instead, she argues that people are best understood as sets of interconnected biological, psychological and social systems, all of which influence behaviour. Because of this emphasis, the model is described as a biopsychosocial model of nursing. Roy argues that each system exists in a state of constant interaction with the environment, striving to maintain relative balance both within itself and in its relationship to the outside world. In this way, each system within the person is motivated towards conditions of homeostasis and aims to achieve – within limits – a certain constancy of function. Roy discusses four principal systems of adaptation, namely the physiological, self-concept, role-function and interdependency systems. A patient presenting with cardiac-related discomfort could be reflected within any of the four adaptation modes, and potentially all of them, during their admission.

Roy suggests that, while doctors focus on biological systems and disease processes, the nurse's specific role is to promote adaptation in health and illness. The role of the nurse, therefore, is primarily that of manipulating stimuli so that they come to fall within the patient's zone of adaptation.

Riehl's symbolic interaction approach (Riehl, 1980)

Criticism of the models already mentioned implies an over-mechanistic approach to human needs. Aggleton and Chalmers (1986) use the analogy between a human being and a machine composed of parts and systems, and comment that it is likely to dehumanize the process of nursing itself. The shift of attention away from an examination of systems within the person to one that focuses on how people make sense of their immediate experiences has become more prevalent within health care over the past few years. An emphasis on human beings as 'givers of meaning' to the situations that they encounter runs parallel with an approach to explaining human behaviour developed by a group of social scientists called 'symbolic interactionists'. Mead (1934), cited in Aggleton and Chalmers (1986), believed that an important human quality is that associated with the capacity to understand the world in terms of symbols, where the word 'symbol' describes a word, image or action that represents something else. Human beings frequently spend their time communicating with each other via such symbols. Hence the expression 'symbolic interactionist' is used to identify someone who is particularly interested in analysing the ways in which symbolic interaction takes place.

The psychological concept of role-taking instituted by Mead is a mental or cognitive activity (not overt behaviour), and means taking into oneself another person's attitude, point of view or perceptual field. The term refers to the symbolic process whereby a person puts him- or herself in another's place in order to gain insight, to anticipate the other's behaviour, and to act accordingly.

Part of the nurse's role, therefore, involves an attempt to enter into the subjective world of patients in order to see things as they do. Through role-taking and attention to subjective components, the nurse can make an accurate assessment of an individual patient's needs, thus provoking a natural series of nursing actions. Assessment, like symbolic interactionism, is a dynamic process that is influenced by day-to-day input and, although the hospital nurse could identify long-term problems, they may be able to do very little about them personally (Riehl, 1980). Referral to rehabilitation facilities, pain specialists and other agencies then becomes a vital link in the health care chain. Nurses working with Riehl's model of nursing should aim to be empathetic and supportive towards their patients, and role-taking would seem to suggest that the nursing function should aim to complement that of the patient. This partnership fosters trust and equality, and the patient places faith in the nurse's judgement when a decision is made to organize multidisciplinary care.

Documenting pain assessment

One way of overcoming the difficulty associated with pain assessment is the use of a recognized assessment tool (Briggs, 1995). The simplest and fastest tools are visual analogue scores and verbal rating scales. In clinical practice, patients seem to find the verbal rating scale easier to use, and such scales have been shown to compare well with visual analogue scores. Maguire (1984) comments that the most reliable index of pain is the patient's verbal report, which would appear to correspond to the findings of the previously discussed study by Gaston-Johansson et al. (1991). Briggs (1995) advocates a written record, the main advantage being that it increases the likelihood of better communication between patient, nurse and doctor. Apart from the obvious legal implications, and the fact that continuity of care may be compromised if there is no effective documentation, such records would ensure that the patient is regularly asked about his or her pain.

A patient suffering an acute myocardial infarction would expect to have a period of at least 24 h of bed-rest prior to sitting out in a chair. Pain may therefore be underestimated when the patient is lying in bed. Physiological signs alone are not adequate criteria for the diagnosis of pain. Patients in acute pain show physiological signs such as increased pulse, pallor, sweating and increased blood pressure, but visceral pain may cause the blood pressure and pulse to fall rather than rise. However, these symptoms can occur in numerous situations that are not associated with pain. In addition, physiological adaptation can occur, so vital signs may return to normal soon after the initial onset of pain (McCaffery and Beebe, 1989). Thus despite all of the complex equipment available to the coronary care nurse for the measurement of the patient's physiological factors, it is equally important to assess behavioural signs of pain. Typical responses include rocking, rubbing of the affected area and changes in facial expression. Occasionally, such signs may be the only clues available, especially when the patient cannot or is reticent to acknowledge their pain verbally.

O'Connor (1995b) states that pain assessment and documentation are vital components of the care of a patient with acute MI, because communication of such information to other members of the multidisciplinary team is necessary to guide interventions in care. Fox (1982), cited by O'Connor (1995b), demonstrated a virtual absence of adequate pain assessment recorded by nurses. It was reported that nurses had condensed and rephrased patient's verbal reports (e.g. 'complaining of pain × 2'), and had failed to record the location, quality, quantity, pattern and intensity of pain. To record only the specific complaint of pain ('complained of pain') is meaningless, and indicative of inadequate pain assessment and subsequent management. The duration of pain is also a critical element, because of its significance to the already oxygen-depleted myocardium. Coronary care nurses must be urged to observe their patients constantly, to assess the real extent of their pain, and to note the effects of analgesia given. The presence of pain behaviour should also be evaluated regularly. Moreover, note should be made of the circumstances in which pain is reported, since some patients may admit to their relatives during visiting times that they are in pain, but be afraid to ask for pain-killers when they are isolated from their family and friends.

The impact of pain on the patient

Hosking and Welchew (1985) believe that the psychological impact of pain results in stress and anxiety, which in turn leads to more pain, slower recovery, longer hospital stay, increased distress and discomfort and an increase in physiological complications. The acute pain associated with myocardial infarction generates a high level of anxiety. Williams (1987) comments that this anxiety can lead to hypervigilance, whereby the patient makes a closer examination of bodily sensations and, by focusing on the latter, magnifies them, so further increasing their anxiety. While there may be an increase in somatization and hypochondriasis, patients are not usually depressed, as they have hope of a full recovery.

Angina sufferers, especially those who endure perpetual episodes of chest discomfort are most likely to experience depression. Patients fear and worry about their pain and suffer from anticipatory anxiety, e.g. fear that their pain will become intolerable at some point in the future. This can increase tension and reduce their tolerance of pain, and depression can then actually heighten their discomfort. Patients start to feel helpless and hopeless, and become increasingly submissive, thereby decreasing their desire for active collaboration in any therapeutic intervention. Thus any chance of a treatment alliance is lost.

On a cognitive level, the patient's perception of their pain is important – what their pain means to them, whether they feel that their life is threatened, whether they are thinking in a very negative way, whether their self-esteem is affected because of role loss or their employment status or position as family breadwinner. Cornock (1996) describes a small study which attempted to determine the value of adopting a psychological approach for patients with acute MI pain. He refers to the strong association between stress and anxiety and increased incidence of pain in heart patients. Consequently, he decided to focus on stress reduction techniques that incorporated the provision of information about the patient's condition and the cause of the pain, relaxation exercises and support at times of chest discomfort. Comprehensive information was provided to half of the subjects in relation to their diagnosis, symptoms, management, care, pain and their duration of stay in the CCU.

The findings of this small study revealed that the amount of pain experienced by all subjects was fairly constant. However, the main difference between the two groups of patients was in the way in which they perceived their pain. The experimental group felt in control of their pain, as they could alleviate it by asking for medication before the pain had reached an unbearable level. The psychological techniques did not relieve the pain, but did help to relieve the anxiety and stress associated with the pain of an ischaemic incident. The patient's pain tolerance and pain threshold appeared to be enhanced by reducing stress and anxiety. Cornock (1996) comments that, while pharmaceutical and medical treatments are indicated for patients with acute myocardial pain, psychological techniques play a supporting role in the overall care of the patient.

Leibesland and Melzack (1977), cited in Wilkinson (1996), comment that the psychological management of pain should enable nurses to control the pain experience of individuals. Many factors, including time constraints and manpower level, prevent all of the methods from being used for all of the time. Nevertheless, freedom from pain should be regarded as a patient's right, and delivery of pain control should not be limited by resources.

Conclusions

Williams (1987) observes that pain is a burden for the patient, but that pain patients are also exhausting, arouse anxiety and guilt, and drain the resources of all of the staff who are trying to manage and treat their pain. This is especially true for nurses, who have greater and longer contact with cardiac patients than other health professionals. A number of recommendations to enhance the care of these patients can be proposed.

Nurses can do a great deal not only to alleviate the pain but also to help the patient to cope with their pain. An understanding of how damaging pain can be to the patient's physical and mental status can help the nurse to assess patients accurately and facilitate the establishment of a treatment alliance. The result of this would be to give patients a feeling of being more in control. Many of the skills mentioned within this chapter are not presently employed. However, by utilizing the skills considered in this chapter nurses should become more confident and enabled to ease the burden of pain for their patients. Education is the first step towards good pain management, with an empathetic approach to care included. Empathy together with knowledge would allow for a deliberative nursing assessment (Hiscock, 1993).

References

Aggleton, P. and Chalmers, H. 1986: *Nursing models and nursing process*. Macmillan: London.

Billings, R., Kearns, P. and Levene, D. 1981: The influence of psychological factors on chest pain associated with myocardial infarction. *Acta Medica Scandinavica* **Suppl. 644**, 46–8.

Bondestam, E., Hogren, K., Gaston-Johansson, F., Jern, S., Herlitz, J. and Holmberg, S. 1987: Pain assessment by patients and nurses in the early phase of acute myocardial infarction. *American Journal of Nursing* **12**, 677–82.

Briggs, M. 1995: Principles of acute pain assessment. *Nursing Times* **9**, 23–7.

Caunt, J. 1996: The advanced nurse practitioner in CCU. *Care of the Critically Ill* **12**, 136–9.

Cornock, M.A. 1996: Psychological approaches to cardiac pain. *Nursing Standard* **11**, 34–8.

Davies, P. and Seers, K. 1991: Teaching nurses about managing pain. *Nursing Standard* **5**, 30–2.

Gaston-Johansson, F., Hofgren, C., Watson, P. and Herlitzm, J. 1991: Myocardial infarction pain: systematic description and analysis. *Intensive Care Nursing* **7**, 3–10.

Herlitz, J., Hjarmlson, A. and Holmberg, S. 1986: Variability, prediction and prognostic significance of chest pain in acute myocardial infarction. *Cardiology* **73**, 13–21.

Hiscock, M. 1993: Complex reactions requiring empathy and knowledge. Psychological aspects of acute pain. *Professional Nurse* **9**, 158–60.

Hosking, J. and Welchew, E. 1985: *Postoperative pain – understanding its nature and how to treat it*. London: Faber and Faber.

Johnson, D. 1980: The behavioral system model for nursing. In Riehl, J.P. and Roy, C. (eds), *Conceptual models for nursing practice*. New York: Appleton Century Crofts, 207–16.

Levine, H. 1980: Difficult problems in the diagnosis of chest pain. *American Heart Journal* **100**, 108–18.

McCaffery, M. and Hart, L. 1976: Undertreatment of acute pain with narcotic analgesia. *American Journal of Nursing* **76**, 1586–91.

McCaffery, M. and Beebe, A. 1989: *Pain – clinical manual for nursing practice*. Boston, MA: C.V. Mosby.

Maguire, D.B. 1984: The management of clinical pain. *Nursing Research* **33**, 152–6.

Melzack, R. and Wall, P. 1991: *The challenge of pain*. Harmondsworth: Penguin.

O'Connor, G.T., Buring, J.E. and Yusurf, S. 1989: An overview of randomised trials of rehabilitation with exercise after myocardial infarction. *Circulation* **80**, 234–44.

O'Connor, L. 1995a: Pain assessment by patients and nurses, and nurses' notes on it, in early acute myocardial infarction. Part 1. *Intensive and Critical Care Nursing* **11**, 183–91.

O'Connor, L. 1995b: Pain assessment by patients and nurses, and nurses' notes on it, in early acute myocardial infarction. Part 2. *Intensive and Critical Care Nursing* **11**, 283–92.

Park, G. and Fulton, B. (1991) *The management of acute pain*. Oxford: Oxford University Press.

Puntillo, K.A. 1988: The phenomenon of pain and critical care nursing. *Heart and Lung* 17, 262–71.

Riehl, J.P. 1980: The Riehl interactive model. In Riehl, J.P. and Roy, C. (eds), *Conceptual models for nursing practice*. New York: Appleton-Century-Crofts, 350–6.

Roper, N., Logan, W.W. and Tierney, A.J. 1985: *The elements of nursing*, 2nd edn. Edinburgh: Churchill Livingstone.

Roy, C. 1980: The Roy adaptation model. In Riehl, J.P. and Roy, C. (eds), *Conceptual models for nursing practice*. New York: Appleton-Century-Crofts, 179–88.

Second International Study of Infarct Survival 1988: Collaborative group randomized trial of intravenous streptokinase, oral aspirin, both or neither among 17 178 cases of suspected myocardial infarction. *Lancet* **8607**, 349–60.

Smith, S. 1985: How drugs act. *Nursing Times* **81**, 36–7.

Sofaer, B. 1984: *Pain: a handbook for nurses*. London: Harper & Row.

Townsend, A. 1988: Management of pain in patients with myocardial infarction. *Intensive Care Nursing* **4**, 18–24.

Wilkinson, R. 1996: A non-pharmacological approach to pain relief. *Professional Nurse* **1**, 222–4.

Willetts, K. 1989: Assessing cardiac pain. *Nursing Times* **8**, 52–4.

Williams, M. 1987: Some psychological aspects of pain. In Latham, J. (ed.), *Pain control*. London: Austen Cornish, 37–53.

The pain of withdrawing from illicit heroin use

22

Stephen Cromey

Introduction

Opiate withdrawal has been appropriately described as subjectively severe but objectively mild, and is one of the longest studied and most well-described withdrawal syndromes (Farrell, 1994). Edwards *et al.* (1981) have made a distinction between illicit heroin dependence, and physiological dependence as a consequence of pain management. Indeed, Ward *et al.* (1992) have suggested that it is useful to distinguish conceptually between those client types who neither wish nor intend to continue taking opioids and those whose compulsive drug-seeking behaviour characterizes heroin dependence. This chapter is concerned with the latter client group and will consider the pain of withdrawing from illicit heroin use.

A complex interplay of public perceptions of the opiate withdrawal syndrome has led to the idea that heroin withdrawal involves 'unbearable' pain. According to Gossop (1987a) there is a strong public appetite for voyeuristic titillation, evident within the media, relating to heroin use, and he suggests that the use of sensationalist accounts to describe the withdrawal process has led to the development of myths which fail to match up to the reality of opiate withdrawal (Gossop, 1987a). Indeed, the stereotypical account of heroin withdrawals, as portrayed by terms like 'cold turkey', provides a more animated version of withdrawal than the quiet, persistent and dull aching nature of withdrawal as witnessed on a day-to-day basis (Farrell, 1994).

In the light of these issues, this chapter will address pain management possibilities for those individuals who are coming off heroin. The physical aspects relating to pain experienced during withdrawal will form the focus of discussion, as opiate misuse, unlike the use of other illicit drugs (e.g. Ecstasy, amphetamines, LSD and cannabis) has the capacity to develop physical dependency (see Table 22.1). Indeed, among the factors that affect the likelihood of an opioid becoming an abuse problem is its capacity to produce physical dependence (Preston, 1991). The pain management strategies will be addressed in two stages. First, attention will be given to the techniques most

Table 22.1 Illicit drugs and their capability of causing physical dependency

Drug	Psychological dependency	Physical dependency	Effects
Heroin (Smack, Gear, Brown, Skag)	Yes	Yes	Reduced sensitivity and emotional reaction to pain. Drowsiness – 'nodding'. Feelings of euphoria – 'warmth' and 'intense rush' reported by users.
Amphetamine (Whizz, Billy, Speed, Uppers)	Yes	No	Increased alertness, diminishes fatigue, delays sleep, loss of appetite, mood elevation
Lysergic acid diethylamide (LSD) (Acid)	Yes	No	Distorted perceptions of sound/vision, intense feelings of dissociation, insight and elevation of mood
Cannabis (Blow, Dope, Draw, Weed, Grass)	Yes	No	Heightened appreciation of colours and sound, relaxation, drowsiness, loss of inhibitions
Ecstasy MDMA ('E')	Yes	No	Similar in nature to amphetamines, with hallucinogenic qualities plus feelings of empathy with others – the 'hug drug'

commonly used which do not involve the prescribing of substitute drugs such as methadone (Physeptone). The second section will focus mainly on the use of methadone, as it is around this approach that much of current UK treatment is centred.

Opiate use

Opiates such as morphine, named after Morpheus, the 'God of Sleep', are characterized by their ability to relieve pain and influence mood. The euphoric effects of morphine (described in Table 22.1) are uniquely powerful and have been used for hedonistic purposes throughout the history of mankind; references to the use of opiate-based substances can be dated as far back as 4000 BC, and such substances were described in Sumerian ideograms as the 'plant of joy' (Berridge and Edwards, 1991). Today consumption of illicit heroin (a potent semi-synthetic product of morphine) within the UK is increasing. Estimates of the exact numbers of heroin users are somewhat tentative, but statistics showing the rise in addicts registered at the Home Office are indicative of the increased level of heroin use within the UK. In 1989 there were 14 785 registered 'drug addicts', and by 1993 this number had increased to 27 976 (Baker and Marsden, 1994). A direct consequence of the increased prevalence of heroin use has been the demands placed upon health care settings such as Accident and Emergency (A&E) departments, primary health care teams and specialized drug dependency units.

Pain management approaches using non-opiate treatment/(self-detox)

According to Polkinghorne (1996), views differ considerably on the causes of drug misuse and how it should be defined. At the extremes, two conflicting paradigms are as follows:

- the disease model, in which drug misuse is seen as a disease of drug dependency, similar to other chronic diseases, with its own natural history and identifiable pattern;
- the drug-taking career model, which sees drug misuse in a more social context, with choices about drug-taking closely linked to culture and lifestyle (Polkinghorne, 1996).

The following pain management sections are explicitly linked to the latter model, in which individuals are seen as having responsibility for their own actions and choices with regard to the use/misuse of substances.

The development of problematic heroin use is concerned with two aspects: the development of tolerance (a physiological phenomenon), and the subsequent potential for dependence both mentally and physically (Dorn and South, 1987). Tolerance is characterized by the need to increase the dose of heroin in order to obtain the same effects that were previously obtained with a lower dose (Gossop, 1987a).

Individuals who have become physically and psychologically dependent upon heroin will experience discomfort ('withdrawal symptoms') if they reduce their heroin intake suddenly or stop using the drug altogether. This is caused by the imbalance of noradrenaline production which, during opiate use, is over-produced. According to Preston and Malinowski (1994), when opiate use is decreased or abruptly stopped, noradrenaline overstimulates the brain and nervous system, causing most of the withdrawal symptoms. Physical dependence upon heroin may contribute to sustained drug-seeking and drug use as opiate-dependent individuals attempt to prevent the onset of unpleasant withdrawal symptoms (Preston, 1991). The experience of opiate withdrawal symptoms is 'flu-like' and varies in intensity depending upon individual circumstances and levels of previous opiate use (Farrell, 1994) (see Table 22.2).

Two phrases of drug slang are derived from the above symptoms of withdrawal. 'Cold turkey' has been coined in reference to the appearance of the skin when it is affected by sweating, hot and cold flushes and piloerection (gooseflesh). A further withdrawal effect in some individuals results in slight tremors in certain limbs, with occasional twitching of the legs. This produces a sudden kicking movement, which has led to the phrase 'kicking the habit' (Gossop, 1987a). Other more esoteric withdrawal symptoms that have been identified are involuntary ejaculation in the male and spontaneous orgasms in the female dependent opiate user. Overall, with the exception of these curious symptoms, the effects of withdrawal from heroin are comparable to a bad dose of influenza (Gossop, 1987a).

Table 22.2   Symptoms of opiate withdrawal

Physical symptoms	• Sweating • Watery eyes • Dilated pupils • Goose pimples 'turkey' • Aching muscles and bones • Increased blood pressure, pulse and respiratory rate • Abdominal cramps • Fever • Vomiting and diarrhoea • Yawning and sneezing
Behavioural symptoms	• Opiate cravings • Abstinence phobia • Disturbed sleep • Irritability and mood swings • Drug-seeking behaviour • Criminal behaviour

According to Waller (1993), 'treatment does not always necessitate the prescribing of chemical substitutes (such as methadone), and indeed the avoidance of such prescribing is not likely to be medically disastrous unless the patient is pregnant'. Ghodse (1995) concurs with this sentiment, and suggests that opiate abstinence is a non-life-threatening condition and that the choice of treatment should be made according to what 'suits' individual clients, their particular circumstances and symptomatology. Indeed, the majority of heroin users come off heroin by themselves without the need for health care professionals or any form of substitute prescribing (Duncan, 1988).

The following pain management techniques/strategies are directed towards a heroin-dependent individual who is not abusing other substances such as benzodiazepines or alcohol.

• Set a date and time to commence self-detox, and expect the withdrawal process to last between 3 and 5 days. Withdrawal symptoms are usually at their worst on the second and third days after stopping all opiate use.
• A comfortable and supportive environment involving family members and/or friends is advantageous. If necessary, a 2-week break/holiday from work would give sufficient time to deal with the physical effects of withdrawal.
• Reduce the level of heroin intake gradually by reducing the amount and frequency of use before complete cessation.
• Be positive and pro-active by treating the symptoms as they arise in a similar fashion to treating a severe cold or flu: take plenty of fluids and rest, and avoid severe changes in temperature (Duncan, 1988).
• Warm baths and massage help to soothe muscle cramps.
• Diversional activities are also invaluable. Indeed, the use of distraction has generally been shown to be an effective strategy for pain management (Powell, 1996).

According to Duncan (1988) the above method of cutting down and withdrawal is the most commonly used technique for coming off heroin. For some individuals, however, relapse is a common experience and staying off heroin becomes much more difficult than the detox process itself. Many individuals learn from relapse situations and are able to build upon these in order to achieve complete abstinence from opiates.

Pain management using substitute opiate prescribing

For some individuals who are dependent on heroin there is a need to consider the treatment modality of prescribing a substitute (methadone). This is especially so for those who have tried unsuccessfully to become opiate free by themselves and are experiencing a current phase of chaotic drug misuse.

The introduction of methadone can help to stabilize chaotic clients, and has advantages in reducing crime, in decreasing injecting behaviours and in reducing illicit drug intake (Polkinghorne, 1996). These positive effects are also linked to a reduction in HIV/AIDS-related behaviours. Indeed, as a consequence of the emergence of AIDS, methadone has been proposed as a component of HIV 'harm reduction' programmes for intravenous opiate users. According to Waller (1993) it is these reasons (harm reduction measures), rather than the relief of physical withdrawal, that represent the main advantage of prescribing methadone. However, having acknowledged this, many clients request methadone treatment in order to overcome the pain of heroin withdrawals:

- '*The main reason* (for requesting methadone) *was to stop rattlin' . . . that really does your head in*';
- '(methadone) *stops the withdrawals which I really hate. I was fed up of having to worry all the time where my next score would be and if I didn't have the money I knew I'd be in agony again*';
- '*Needed it to stop aching all the time. . . . It got to the stage where heroin was doin' me in, I needed the meth' to keep me straight*'.

Indeed, many clients' views on the effectiveness of methadone treatment are seen in terms of stability, avoidance of withdrawals, and averting the panic of needing to 'score' (obtain drugs), rather than complete abstinence from heroin itself (Cromey, 1996).

Methadone detoxification can be implemented within specialist in-patient units and, more commonly, in the community via GPs and/or specialist drug services. The pain management of methadone detoxification incorporates all of the issues raised in the above self-detox section, in addition to the following guidelines.

Assessment for methadone treatment

A full history within the assessment process is of great importance, including a detailed account of the patient's drug history, phases of abstinence (if any) and treatment options that have previously been explored. Information should also be collected with regard to associated problems such as financial difficulties, family/relationship problems, housing, employment or legal issues.

Assessment should also attempt to understand a client's level of motivation and their desired goals of treatment. The initial assessment can screen clients who are unsuitable for methadone treatment. Indeed, the inappropriate use of methadone can have the counter-productive effect of reducing a client's motivation to want to come off opiates. George (1990) has suggested that methadone-prescribing may encourage opiate users to maintain their existing lifestyle, and thus prevent them from having the compelling incentive to try to stop using opiates.

A further aim of the assessment process is to filter out individuals who are requesting methadone for non-therapeutic reasons. Preston (1991) has noted that compounds such as methadone which have the ability to substitute for heroin and suppress withdrawal in physically dependent individuals may have considerable abuse potential. Some individuals intentionally abuse methadone and sell on their prescriptions in order to buy heroin, whilst others simply use methadone as an extra supply to their overall drug intake.

If methadone-prescribing is appropriate, a contract should be drawn up so that clients and practitioners have a mutual understanding of the goals and boundaries of the treatment protocol. This should ideally include specific dates on the duration of detoxification/treatment. Urinalysis should also be carried out during the assessment phase in order to ascertain a client's illicit drug intake. Further urinalysis monitoring during detoxification serves two important functions, first to ensure that clients are ingesting the methadone which is being dispensed, and secondly to detect whether they are taking any other non-prescribed substances (Ward *et al.*, 1992).

Conversion rates

Conversion of a client's heroin intake to methadone is not a precise science. The purity rates of heroin are variable, and factors such as how the heroin is taken (intravenously or orally) will influence the amounts of methadone required. Practitioners who wish to obtain guidelines for prescribing methadone should contact local drug agencies/services, as regional variations and patterns of heroin use differ considerably. Table 22.3 outlines the more common forms of methadone equivalents from street heroin.

Table 22.3 Methadone equivalent doses to street heroin[a]

Drug	Quantity (g)	Methadone equivalent (oral)
Street heroin (oral)	1 g (£60 approx.)	80 mg
	0.5 g (£35 approx.)	40–60 mg
	0.25 g (2 × £20 bags)	30–40 mg
	0.125 g (1 × £10 bag)	1–15 mg

[a] Methadone equivalents should be increased by 5–10 mg when heroin is used intravenously (Preston, 1996).

Many clients overestimate their use of heroin to practitioners out of fear that they will not receive enough methadone. It is often necessary therefore to commence methadone doses on the lower heroin–methadone ratio in order to minimize the likelihood of intoxication.

Detoxification regimes

The relationship between pain and psychological factors has been widely recognized, and it is clear that states of anxiety may promote or induce pain (Tyrer, 1992). Hall (1979) has described the notion of abstinence phobia or pathological detoxification fear in methadone maintenance clients who are attempting to withdraw from methadone as an exaggerated anxious reaction to comparatively mild withdrawal symptoms. Anxiety is a common feature of the opiate withdrawal syndrome, but for some individuals extreme levels of anxiety are observed that evoke phobic-like responses such as avoidance (i.e. refusal to proceed with the detoxification) (Hall, 1979). Hall suggests that this reaction is probably due to previous experiences of abrupt or involuntary withdrawal (such as may occur in prison), or to observing others experience severe withdrawal symptoms, or to inaccurate information about the severity of methadone withdrawal, such as that which circulates within the heroin-using subculture.

Davis (1988) has suggested that a key objective in dealing with pain management should be the reduction of the anxieties associated with detoxification. Indeed, most clients who undergo methadone detoxification will experience both psychological and physical withdrawal (Preston, 1996). Providing information about the possible feelings of discomfort is therefore of great importance in reducing client anxieties, thus enabling the withdrawal process to be managed more effectively. Ward et al. (1992) have further suggested the use of cognitive behavioural interventions, including the explicit use of cognitive restructuring of withdrawal symptoms, for those clients who display phobic-type reactions to the implementation of detoxification schedules.

On initiation of the methadone prescription, the starting dose should be maintained for 7 to 10 days. This is in order to assess the client's reaction to methadone and to adjust the initial dose as necessary. The minimum starting dose should keep the client free of withdrawal symptoms, thus enabling the detoxification process to commence.

According to Waller (1993) the rate of detoxification should be negotiated between client and practitioner, and is best tailored to the individual, rather than one particular detoxification schedule being rigidly enforced. Detoxification regimes should be gradual, and when the dose is reduced to less than 20 mg the tapering of the dose should be slowed down (Ward et al., 1992). The actual duration of the detoxification regime is also a matter of individuality. For those clients who have abused opiates for under 12 months the detoxification may be as short as 2 to 3 weeks. However, for clients who have abused opiates for longer than 12 months, a detoxification may last for up to 2 or 3 months. Extremely chaotic clients would need a period of stabilization/maintenance before considering a detoxification protocol. Gossop (1987a) has further suggested that for many long-term heroin abusers the prospect of becoming opiate-free is 'terrifying', and that the prospect of learning to live without a 'chemical crutch' can make the goal of complete abstinence seemingly unobtainable. According to Ward *et al.* (1992), the distress associated with withdrawal from methadone is better tolerated by some individuals than others. When it is considered that problematic users of heroin may have a deeply ambivalent attitude towards their approach to withdrawal, in addition to all of the lay 'knowledge' they have acquired through various means, the subsequent terrors and anxieties are not difficult to comprehend. Thus a significant aspect of managing the pain of withdrawals relates to the provision of information about what can be expected, together with an enabling supportive relationship with professional workers who can both listen and encourage a positive approach.

Staying off heroin on completion of detoxification

The length of time for which physical withdrawals last differs from one individual to another. The production of noradrenaline, which is over-produced during opiate abuse, is normally back in balance after 7 to 14 days, which is usually when most of the physical symptoms fade completely. However, sleep disturbance is a further side-effect experienced by many individuals on completion of their detoxification. According to Preston and Malinowski (1994) this may be related to endorphin production, which is diminished by the use of illicit opiates – and once stopped, endorphin production can take up to 6 months to return to normal levels.

A significant feature of methadone detoxification is the residual symptoms, which can last up to 40 days after the initiation of the detoxification process, thus causing a long and protracted withdrawal (Gossop *et al.*, 1987b). Farrell (1994) has noted that if the pain of withdrawal is spread over 2 months instead of 10 days, then clients may not be able to endure it: '. . . it is not the intensity but the duration of pain that breaks the will to resist'. The issuing of methadone can thus be seen as a two-edged sword – initially bringing relief from withdrawals, but consequently causing the pain to be protracted in duration. Users' accounts succinctly portray the dilemmas posed by methadone withdrawals. Methadone users have made the following comments:

- *'I know it's (methadone) more addictive than gear (herion), which does put you off it a bit. Your turkey lasts for ages . . . it really gets into your bones'.*
- *'I can't get off methadone, it really is a bad one . . . going on meth' was the worst thing I did. You rattle for months when you're locked up, whereas with brown (heroin) it's finished after a week'* (Cromey, 1996).

Preston and Malinowski (1994) have noted how withdrawal symptoms may indeed be worse and last longer than those experienced when coming off heroin itself. It is for these reasons that adjuncts to methadone detoxification have been introduced. The emergence of treatments such as clonidine and lofexidine (BritLofex) in complementing methadone detoxification is gaining popularity. Lofexidine, for example, is not an opiate and therefore does not have the dependency potential of opiates (Preston, 1996). However, its usefulness in reducing all symptoms of withdrawal is somewhat limited. Further information on the use and implementation of clonidine/lofexidine protocols is obtainable from local specialist drug agencies/services.

According to Meystre-Agustoni et al. (1990), the relapse rate is high in drug dependence. Indeed, on completion of the methadone detoxification process many individuals experience a return to illicit opiate use. Ward et al. (1992) echo this sentiment, and posit that former methadone clients who experience a protracted withdrawal syndrome also have to contend with a renewed desire to use heroin in response to environmental cues and emotional states that arise as they attempt to lead a heroin-free lifestyle. Relapse management and relapse prevention counselling are thus of prime importance during and after a client's detoxification.

Putting the pain of withdrawals in perspective

The myths that surround opiate withdrawals often cause great anxiety not only for those experiencing difficulties in coming off opiates, but also for health care professionals responding to this particular client group. The exaggerated fear of withdrawal (withdrawal phobia) for many heroin users often serves as a justification for continuing to use illicit drugs and/or prescribed substitutes (Gossop, 1987a). Similarly, many health care professionals readily implement the use of methadone in reaction to a client's presenting opiate problem. Methadone has now become a highly visible form of treatment which attracts large numbers of clients and could be perceived as 'doing something constructive about the presenting heroin problem' (Shannon, 1992). However, Mandleburg (1988) has suggested that such a response (issuing methadone) is essentially reductionist in nature – a very complex problem being reduced to the most simplistic element. He reasons that:

> When the community is confronted by the urgent distress of addicts we sometimes feel like the beleaguered mother who can only calm the screaming baby by feeding. It seems that the need is so urgent that the infant cannot wait for the mother to work out what is troubling the child. An excessive reliance can be developed on the milk itself. Methadone can enable the addict to put their pain out of their minds and its use can enable us to put them out of ours.
>
> (Mandleburg, 1988)

In concluding this chapter it can be appreciated that methadone plays a key role in the management of opiate dependence. However, it is only one strand of the pain management possibilities for the process of heroin withdrawal. There are several further options for assisted opiate withdrawal, including electro-acupuncture, the use of general anaesthetics, and (perhaps the most invasive) sleep-inducing procedures (Farrell, 1994). For many heroin-dependent individuals the idea of a totally pain-free detoxification would be very attractive. However, all forms of detoxification (with the possible exception of sleep-inducing procedures) incur some discomfort and include many withdrawal symptoms. It could thus be argued that there is importance in valuing the experience of pain. By allowing the body's own defence mechanisms to deal with the ensuing symptoms of withdrawal (the self-detox method), the individual may come to feel the sense of achievement alluded to earlier. Attempts to put off the inevitable withdrawals through the use of methadone or other prescribed treatments could perhaps be seen as 'delaying the agony', causing a protracted experience of withdrawal (Farrell, 1994). Indeed, this seeking a 'pill for every ill' approach is an option frequently pursued by many who are opiate dependent. This approach is ultimately disempowering, with the potential to create more difficulties in the long term, as adaptive coping strategies for autonomous pain relief are not being developed. Thus when considering pain management options in relation to withdrawing from opiates, it may be worth bearing in mind that – ultimately – there is no gain without pain.

It is beyond the remit of this chapter to consider in any depth the psychological/emotional pain associated with withdrawing from heroin, yet the two are inextricably linked within the experience of the individual. The sense of achievement that is felt after having been through the physical discomfort of withdrawal is often placed in perspective by the subsequent psychosocial stressors (e.g. cravings, unresolved interpersonal conflicts) in preventing relapse from occurring. In fact, upon reflection, many ex-users of heroin feel that the physical detoxification process (including all the 'aches and pains') was indeed the 'easiest bit'.

References

Baker, O. and Marsden, J. 1994; *Drug misuse in Britain*. London: Institute for the Study of Drug Dependence.

Berridge, V. and Edwards, G. 1991: *Opium and the people: opiate use in nineteenth-century England*. London: Yale University Press.

Cromey, S. 1996: *The efficacy of methadone treatment within a community drug team setting – a client's perspective*. Unpublished thesis, Manchester Metropolitan University, Manchester.

Davis, S.P. 1988: 'Changing nursing practice for more effective control of post-operative pain through a staff-initiated educational programme. *Nurse Education Today* 8, 325–31.

Dorn, N. and South, N. 1987: *A land fit for heroin? Drug policies, prevention and practice*. London: MacMillan Education.

Duncan, R. 1988: *How to stop: a do-it-yourself guide to opiate withdrawal*. London: The Blenheim Project.

Edwards, G., Arif, A. and Hodgson, R. 1981: Nomenclature and classification of drug and alcohol-related problems: a WHO memorandum. *Bulletin of the World Health Organization* 59, 225–42.

Farrell, M. 1994: Opiate withdrawal. *Addiction* 89, 1471–5.

George M. 1990: Methadone screws you up. *International Journal on Drug Policy* 1, 24–5.

Ghodse, H. 1995: *Drugs and addictive behaviour: a guide to treatment.* Oxford: Blackwell Science.

Gossop, M. 1987a: *Living with drugs,* 2nd edn. London: Wildwood House.

Gossop, M., Bradley, B. and Phillips, G.T. 1987b: An investigation of withdrawal symptoms shown by opiate addicts during and subsequent to a 21-day in-patient methadone detoxification procedure. *Addictive Behaviours* 12, 1–6.

Hall, S.M. 1979: The abstinence phobia. In *Behavioural analysis of substance abuse.* NIDA Research Monograph 25. Rockville, MD: National Institute on Drug Abuse, 196–201.

Mandleburg, T. 1988: Methadone: magic or madness? *Drug and Alcohol Review* 7, 209–15.

Meystre-Agustoni, G., Wietlisbach, J.M. and Haller-Maslov, E. 1990: Methadone treatment in medical private practice: outcome according to the number of courses followed. *British Journal of Addiction* 85, 537–45.

Polkinghorne, J. 1996: *The task force to review services for drug misusers: Report of an independent review of drug treatment services in England.* London: Department of Health.

Powell, T. 1996: *The mental health handbook.* Oxford: Winslow.

Preston, A. 1996: *The methadone briefing.* London: Institute for the Study of Drug Dependence.

Preston, A. and Malinowski, A. 1994: *The detox handbook: a user's guide to getting off opiates.* London: Institute for the Study of Drug Dependence.

Preston, K.L. 1991: Drug abstinence effects: opioids. *British Journal of Addiction* 86, 1641–6.

Shannon, P. 1992: Methadone treatment: the therapeutic mirage. *International Journal on Drug Policy* 3, 91–8.

Tyrer, S.P. 1992: *Psychology, psychiatry and chronic pain.* Oxford: Butterworth-Heinemann.

Waller, T. 1993: *Working with GPs.* London: Institute for the Study of Drug Dependence.

Ward, J., Mattick, R. and Hall, W. 1992: *Key issues in methadone maintenance treatment.* New South Wales: New South Wales University Press.

Index

Page numbers printed in **bold** type refer to figures; those in *italic* to tables.

abdominal pain 252, 252–3
Accident and Emergency departments 31–2
acting-in and acting-out 98–9, 106
activities of daily living model 299
acupuncture 12, 16, 72
acute pain 186, 190–1, 248
  definition 187
  in young people 233–7
acute pain services (APS) 153–4, 160–1
  children's hospitals 164
  clinical nurse specialists (CNS) 164–6
  continuous audit 161
  pre-acute pain services 154–5
  standard protocols 161
  UK development 153, 162–4
  see also analgesia; management of pain
adaptation model 300
addiction
  analgesic-induced 156
  to opioids 294, 296
adjuvant analgesia, for shoulder pain 288–9
Adolescent Pediatric Pain Tool (APPT) 236, **238–9**
adolescents *see* young people
age-related differences 249, 252
  see also older people
amitriptyline, for fibromyalgia 271
amphetamine, effects *307*
anaesthesiology-based post-operative pain management service (APS) 160–1
anaesthetic consultants 153–4
analgesia
  administration methods 157–8
  effectiveness in fibromyalgia 273
  epidural infusion (EIA) 157–8
  for hemiplegic shoulder pain 287–9
  inadequate 53, 55, 58, 294
  opioid administration 156–8
  Post-Operative Audit Chart **159**
  young people 236, 237–40

  see also opioids; patient-controlled analgesia
angina 302
anti-emetics, and patient-controlled analgesia 160
anticipatory pain 2
antidepressants, in hemiplegic shoulder pain 288
anxiety 31–2
  and myocardial infarction 295, 298, 302–3
  in opiate withdrawal 312
  young people 234, 235
  see also depression; fear; stress
aromatherapy 290
arthritis 254
artificial limb, a personal experience 18–25
aspirin 287, 296
assent *see* child assent
assessment of pain 46, 80, 155–6, 157
  assessment tools 176–8
  children 215
  documentation 157, 301–2
  nursing models as guide to 298–301
  rating scales **237**, 286, 301
  young people 236, **237**
audit 150–1, 161
Australia, pain clinics 246–7, 254, 255

The Back Book 189
back pain 187, 187–8, 190, 252, 253
background pain 2, 5, 22
Behavioral Approach-Avoidance and Distress Scale (BAADS) 219
behavioural systems model 299
behaviour
  behavioural signs 301–2
  consulting behaviour 188–9, 193
  cultural perspectives 35–6
  illness behaviour 32, 188, 193
  middle-aged women 139–40
  pain influences on 110

benchmarking 174–6, 183–4
  comparison and sharing 181–3
  continuum examples **176, 178–9, 179, 180–1**
  re-scoring 183
  scoring graphs **182, 183**
best practice
  benchmark of 174–6
  identifying 171, 173–6
  patient-focused 172, 173, 173–4, 180
  professionals' experience 174
  research-based 173
  sharing 171, 172–3, 181–3, 184
biobehavioural model of children's pain 211, **212**
biomedical model of care 186, 187, 191
biopsychosocial model of care 109–10, 186, 187, 191
bioscience domain 94
body/mind dualism *see* mind/body dualism
bone marrow biopsies 3–4
Bristol Cancer Help Centre 11, 15–16
British Association of Counselling 110–11
BritLofex 313–14
Buddhism 130

cancer 244
cannabis, effects *307*
cardiac pain *see* myocardial pain
care planning, collaborative 172, 180
Centre for Reviews and Dissemination 173, 174, 185
chemotherapy 6, 6–7, 17
chest pain 252, 252–3
  see also myocardial pain
child assent, consent and refusal 195–205
  age and decision-making 196, 197–8, 199
  best interests test 197
  consent vs. refusal 197–9
  definitions 195–6
  key questions about 200
  legal issues 199–200
  New Zealand 199, 202–3
  rights of children 198–9, 202, 203–4
children
  analgesia/anaesthesia 201
  biobehavioural model 211, **212**
  birth order and pain 216–17

with chronic pain 211, 214
cognitive development level 213
coping strategies 201, 218–24
culture 217–18
developmental stages *214*
experience of pain 206–7, 210–12
factors affecting pain 210, **211**
family influences 216–17, 221–4
gender differences in pain response 215
historical attitudes towards pain 207–10
misconceptions and evidence about pain *209*
need to be listened to 224
negative experiences 201–2
'novice to expert shift' 213
pain vocabulary 213–15
parental support 201
parents' influence on attitude to pain 73–5, 76, 77, 201, 221
personal characteristics and experience of pain 213–15
preparation for painful procedures 200–1
previous experience of pain 215–16
recognition of pain *214*
social and cultural influences 215
undertreatment 207–10
visual/graphic pain scales 215
see also child assent; young people
Children and Pain (leaflet) 173
children's hospitals, acute pain services 164
Chinese cosmology 130
Chinese medicine 72–3
chronic pain 5–7
  biology and psychology model 250, **251**
  children with 211, 214
  complexity of 186
  coping strategies 188
  definition 187, 248
  early activation 190–1
  in later life 243–4, 254–5
  management 109–11, 116, 189–90
  prevention 186–94
chronic pain syndromes 254, 255–9
clinical effectiveness 171
clinical nurse specialists (CNSs) 164–6
Clinical Outcomes Group 174, 185

Clinical Standards Advisory Group 189
clonidine 313–14
co-operative enquiry 93
Cochrane Centre database 173, 185
cognitive-behavioural programmes 250,
    254, 257
cognitive impairment 247
'cold turkey' 308
communication 29, 178
    between adults and young people 233
    benefit of recounting pain experiences
    42
    with and between professionals 28–30,
    31, 36–8, 107–8
    see also information; language;
        vocabulary
community, pain in the 244–5, 259
co-morbidity 254–5
complementary therapies 14, 15–17
    see also pain relief
complications of pain 46
confidence, in professionals 4–5, 15
consent see child assent
constructivism 92
consulting behaviour 188–9, 193
context mediators, of empathy 54–5
Continuing Professional Development
    (CPD) credits 146
cooling, for shoulder pain 289
coping strategies 10–13
    categories and definitions 220, 222–3
    children 201, 218–24
    chronic pain 188
    older people 250, 257–8
coping with pain
    active vs. avoidant 220
    age and 220–1
    appraisal of stressor 219
    assessing styles of 219
    cognitive/intrapsychic 218
    direct action 218–19
    individuality in 221
    and information 219–20
    stages 219
cosmetic surgery 121–2, 122–4
cosmology, Chinese and Western 130
counselling 109–17
    case examples 112–14, 114–16
    Code of Ethics and Practice 111–12
    description 111–12
    non-directive 112

in pain management 112–14
person-centred 112
supervision of 109–10
training courses 109
CPD (Continuing Professional
    Development) credits 146
critical theory 92
culturally congruent care, definition 79
culture 66–83
    approaches to 68–70
    and children's pain 217–18
    definitions and meanings 68, 80
    ethnic groups 69
    and health 70–3
    influence on nurses 78
    integration into main group 76
    and language 35–6, 72, 73
    and nurse training 80–1
    and nursing management of pain 78
    and pain 73–5
    research evidence 75–7
    subgroups 69, 70
    transcultural nursing 69–70, 78–81
    young people 234
Culyer Report 151
cutaneous stimulation, for shoulder pain
    289
cyclobenzaprine 271

Decadron 288–9
delayed pain 9–10
dementia 247
dental pain 252
depression
    and angina 302
    in fibromyalgia patients 269, 270
    and the menopause 135, 137
    older people 246, 255–6, 257
    young people 235
Descartes, René 129–32
detoxification 312–13
    abstinence phobia 312
    cognitive behavioural interventions
        312
    on completion of 313–14
    pathological detoxification fear 312
    relapse management 314
    self-detox 308–10, 315
    withdrawal symptoms in 315
dexamethasone phosphate 288–9
diamorphine 157–8, 296

diazepam 288
disease, definition 71
distraction 240
doctor–patient communication 29, 36–8
doctor–nurse communication 29
documentation 157, 178–80, 301–2
drug dependency 240
drug misuse 308
dualism
  and alienation 122–4
  and the body 120, 124–5
  see also mind/body dualism
duration of pain, myocardial infarction
    298, 302

Ecstasy, effects 307
education and training 71, 142–52
  analgesia 156
  change, ideas for 146
  conclusions 152
  Continuing Professional Development
    (CPD) credits 146
  counselling 108
  cultural aspects of care 80–81
  Curriculum for Professional Education in
    Pain 144–5
  distance learning 149
  in empathy 53–5, 58
  fibromyalgia 272–3, 274
  medical students' history-taking 29
  organizations offering 142–3, 144–6,
    146
  'pain days' 149
  pain management 142–52
  of pain-management specialists 148–9
  political pressure 150, 152
  postgraduate curricula 144–6, 146–7
  of professionals 149
  Royal College of Anaesthetists 144–6
  Royal College of Psychiatrists 144–5
  undergraduate curricula 143–4
  USA 144, 146–8
elderly see older people
emotional state, young people 234, 235
Empathic Understanding Scale 56, 57
empathy 46–65
  as a behaviour 56
  conceptualization 49–50, 51, 55
  and counselling 111, 112
  definitions 50, 56–7
  measures of 54–5, 56–7

mediators of see empathy mediators
nurses' responses 58
nursing models 51–3
and pain management 55–8, 59–60
as a personal characteristic 57
phases 51–2, 52
as a process 57
vs. sympathy 50, 51
and therapeutic outcomes 58–60
training in 53–4, 55, 59
Empathy Construct Rating Scale (ECRS)
    55, 56
empathy mediators 51–3
  context mediators 54–5
  nurse mediators 53–4
  patient mediators 54
Empathy Scale 57
empowerment 11–12
epidural infusion analgesia (EIA) 157–8
Episcopalians 76
ethnic groups 69
  see also culture
exercise, for fibromyalgia 271–2

facial pain 252, 252–3
families
  and children's pain 216–17, 221–4
  model of dysfunctional adaption to
    pediatric pain 212
  support for 223–4
  see also parents
fear 19–20
feminism 118–26
  perspective on pain 118–20
  perspective or epistemology? 119
  see also women
fetal memory 99–100, 104–7
  Hugh's story 100–4, 107–8
fibromyalgia 264–77
  analgesia, effectiveness 273
  depression 269, 270
  description 264, 265
  diagnosis 267–8
  education programme 272–3, 274
  exercise 271–2
  functional impairment 267
  and gender 265, 270
  hypnotic therapy 273
  information for patients 271, 272, 273,
    274
  management 270–4

medical and nursing attitudes 264–5, 268–70, 272, 274–5
non-pharmacological treatments 270, 271, 272, 273
pathological or psychological? 268–70
prognosis 270
reassurance and support 273–4
and self-esteem 274
self-management 273
and sleep 266, 271
symptoms 266, **266**
tender (trigger) points 267, **267**, 268
treatment 270–3
folk medicine 74
folk-ways 79
Freud, Sigmund, on dynamic psychology 129
frozen shoulder 281

gate control theory (GCT) 47–8, 66–7, 71, 74, 88–9, 130, 243, 286
gender differences in pain response 215, 233–4, 244
generalized pain 2, 5
Gillick v West Norfolk and Wisbech Area Health Authority (1985) 198–9
guided imagery 114, 115–16, 240
guidelines 173

headache 135–6, 252, 252–3
health
  concepts 70
  cultural perceptions 71–3
  lay models 79–80
heat, for shoulder pain 289
hemiplegia, shoulder pain in see shoulder pain
herbal medicine 72–3
heroin
  conversion rates to methadone 311–12
  dependence 308
  effects 307
  illicit vs. physiological dependence 306
  increasing illicit use 307
  pain management 309–10
  staying off 313–14
  tolerance 308
  withdrawal symptoms 308–9
  see also detoxification; opiates
history-taking, by medical students 29
hook-swinging 73–4

hormone deficiency 139–40
hot flushes, and the menopause 135, 137
hypnotic therapy, for fibromyalgia 273

Ibuprofen 288
identity, fear of loss of 10, 14, 15
illness
  cultural perceptions 71–3
  definition 71
  explanatory models 71–2
  sources of 71
illness behaviour 32, 188, 193
information
  alleviating pain and distress 30
  conveying diagrammatically 27
  see also communication; language
informed consent 196
intense pain 2–5
interactive model 300–1
interdisciplinary care teams 172, 180–1
International Association for the Study of Pain (IASP) 85, 142–3, 144
isolation 113

joint pain 252, 279

'kicking the habit' 308
King's Fund 174, 185

La Monica Empathy Profile 55
Lake, Dr Frank 101–2
language 26–8
  for conveying information 26–7, 28, 37
  and culture 35–6, 72, 73
  and experience 27–8
  indexicality of 128
  and mind/body dualism 132–3
  models of 72
  spatial information 27, 28
  and suffering 30–2, 38
  see also communication; vocabulary; voice
learned responses 5
leg pain 252
limb, loss of, a personal experience 18–25
Lock, M. 129–30, 131, 133, 140
locus of control 188, 257–8
lofexidine 313–14
lysergic acid diethylamide (LSD), effects 307

McGill Pain Questionnaire (MPQ) 29, 39–42, 236
management of pain 46
    anaesthesiology-based post-operative pain management service (APS) 160–1
    audit and research 150–2
    chronic pain 108–10, 116, 189–90
    counselling 111–13
    and culture 78
    education and training 142–52
    and empathy 55–8, 58–9
    guidelines 173
    and interpersonal process 47–9
    nurse-based anaesthesiologist-supervised model 161
    in opiate withdrawal 308–14
    pain management units 109
    post-operative 154–5, 156
    post-operative, working party report 161–2, 167–8
    Post-Operative Audit Chart **159**
    pre-chronic pain 192–3
    protocols, benchmarking continuum **181**
    summary 167–8
    the way forward 166–7, 168
    young people 237–40
    see also acute pain services; analgesia; education and training
Marx, Karl, on human labour 129
massage 289–90
mastectomy vs. menopause 133–4
maturation 234
measurement of pain see assessment of pain
medical students, history-taking 29
memory, for painful experiences 234
menopause 128–9
    gradations of suffering 138
    vs. mastectomy 133–4
    and mind/body dualism 132–3
    normal 134–9
    and pre-menstrual tension 138
mental pain 2, 7–9
    on losing a child 6, 7–9
methadone 309, 310, 314
    abuse 311
    assessment for treatment 310–11
    conversion rates from heroin 311–12

detoxification regimes/symptoms 312–13
    see also detoxification
migraine 12
mind/body dualism 33–5, 127–8
    Descartes' theories 129–33
    and language usage 132–3
    and the menopause 132–3
morphine 157, 295, 296
muscle pain, shoulder 279
muscle relaxants, shoulder pain 288
Muslims 76
myocardial pain 294–305
    acute nature of 298
    and anxiety 295, 296–7, 298, 302–3
    assessment 301–2
    duration of pain 298, 302
    impact on patient 302–3
    management 295–7
    vs. other chest pain 297–8
    patients' experience of 296–7, 297–8
    perception of pain 303

Naproxen 288
National Centre for Clinical Audit 174, 185
neonatal studies 216
New Zealand, child assent and refusal 199, 202–3
nitrates, for myocardial pain 296
non-steroidal anti-inflammatory drugs (NSAIDs) 287–8
noradrenaline, and opiate use 308, 313
Northwest Paediatric Benchmarking Group 175–6
nurse–doctor communication 30
nurse–patient communication 29–30, 31
nurse–patient interaction 48–9
nurses
    attitudes to patients' pain 48, 49, 53–4, 155
    as empathy mediators 53–5
    as 'pain managers' 156, 166–7
    prescribing 167
nursing, transcultural 69–70, 78
nursing homes 245–6
nursing models
    empathy 51–3
    as guides to pain assessment 298–301

Oedipus complex 104
Offer Self-Image Questionnaire 234

older people
  age groups 244
  in the community 244–5
  coping strategies 250, 257–8
  depression 246, 255–6, 257
  dimensions of pain 259–60
  in nursing homes 245–6
  and pain clinics 246–7
  pain locations 252–3
  perception of pain 248–52, 253, 285
  sensory changes 248–9
  under-reporting 253
opiate withdrawal 306–7
  assisted withdrawal options 314–15
  non-opiate treatment 308–10
  pain of 314–15
  relapse rate 314
  substitute opiate prescribing 310–14
  symptoms 308, 309
opiates
  effects 307
  nurses' lack of knowledge 295–6
  use 307
  see also detoxification; heroin; opiate
    withdrawal
opioids 295
  addiction to 294, 296
  administration 156–8
  and respiratory depression 296
  routes of administration 157, 158, 160,
    163
osteoarthritis 257, 258

pain
  categories 2, 187
  definitions 33, 47, 86, 87, 187
  description 33
  domains of 95
  multidimensionality of 243
  personal stories 1–17, 18–25
  private vs. public 73
  understanding cause of 5–6
  see also management of pain
pain clinics, Australia 246–7, 254, 255
pain control groups, benchmarking
    continuum 180, 182
'pain days' 149
pain intensity measurement 286
pain reduction techniques 13–17
pain relief, non-pharmacological 240,
    246

fibromyalgia 270, 271, 272, 273
  shoulder pain in hemiplegia 289–91
Pain Society of Great Britain and Ireland
    142, 146
papaveretum 157
paradigms see research paradigms
parents
  decision-making for child 197–9, 200
  influence on children's attitudes to
    pain 74–5, 76, 77, 201, 221
  information for 235–6
  see also children; families
participative reality 93
patient-controlled analgesia (PCA) 32,
    158–60
  young people 238–9
patient–doctor communication 29, 36–8
Patient Information Leaflets 15
patient–nurse communication 29–30, 31
patient–nurse interaction 48–9
patients
  active or passive role? 29, 37
  best practice focus on 172, 173, 173–4,
    180
  as empathy mediators 54
  empowerment 11–12
  mood and empathy 55
  pain management and empathy 55–8,
    58–9
  relevance of views 34
phantom pain 22–3, 115
philosophy, vs. science 84
physical pain 2
physiotherapy, for hemiplegic shoulder
    pain 287
planning, benchmarking continuum
    181
political domain 95
positivism 90–1, 131
post-herpetic neuralgia 257, 258
Post-Operative Audit Chart 159
postpositivism 91–2
practice see best practice
pre-acute pain services 154–5
pre-chronic pain 187, 191–3
pre-menstrual tension, and the
    menopause 138
pregnancy 105–6
prescription, by nurses 167
primary care, role of 189
privacy 13

professionals
confidence in 4–5, 15
need for explanations from 107
support needed from 19–20, 21, 24
psychological aspects of pain 33, 66–8,
255–9
psychosocial domain 95
psychotherapy principles 98–9
punishment, pain as 214
purchaser specifications 172

Questionnaire Measure of Emotional
Empathy (QMEE) 57

race 69
see also culture
record-keeping *see* documentation
reductionism 88
refusal *see* child assent
regression 102
Relationship Inventory, Empathy
Subscale 56
relaxation 114, 115, 290–1
religion, vs. science 84
research 84–6, 150–2
access to 173
domains 94–5
the future 96
interdisciplinary 96
methodologies 89–90
qualitative vs. quantitative 89–90
research question 86
research paradigms 85, 87–8
constructivism 92
critical theory 92
definition 90
differing disciplines 89–90
growth or conflict? 93–4
key questions 91
paradigm shifts 85, 88–9
participative reality 93
positivism 91–2, 131
postpositivism 91–2
respiratory depression, and opioids
296
Riehl interactive model 300–1
Roy adaptation model 300
Royal College of Anaesthetists 144–6
Royal College of Psychiatrists 144–5

science, vs. philosophy and religion 84
scientific revolutions 85, 88

self-detox 308–10, 315
self-hypnosis 16
sensory changes, with age 248–9
serotonin deficiency, and fibromyalgia
266
shoulder pain, in hemiplegia 278–93
adjuvant analgesia 288–9
assessment 284–6
categories 279
causes 280–3
diagnosis 278–9
effects of 279–80
family involvement 284, 285, 291
management, non-pharmacological
289–91
management, pharmacological 287–9
massage 289–90
measurement 286–7
non-steroidal anti-inflammatory drugs
287–8
physical examination 285
physiotherapy 287
prevention 283–4
psychological assessment 286
relaxation 290–1
signs 285
spasticity 282
subluxation 281
treatment theory 286–7
trigger points 285
ultrasound 291
vulnerability of shoulder 280–3
sick role 189
sickness, definition 71
sleep 266, 271, 313
social aspects of pain 66–8, 77
sociology of the body 120
spiritual pain 99–100
Spiritualists 75–6
splitting 98
Staff Patient Interaction Response Scale
(SPIRS) 54–5, 57, 58
stomach pain 252
stress 7, 218, 303
see also anxiety; fear
stress migraine 12
stroke *see* shoulder pain
subjectivity, of pain 47–8, **86**
suffering
definition 30
and language 30–33, 38

vs. pain 85, 127–8, 131, 134
typology 31, **32**
support
  from family 21
  needed from professionals 19–20, 21, 24
sympathy, vs. empathy 50, 51

tender (trigger) points 267, **267**, 268, 285
terminology *see* vocabulary
therapeutic outcomes, and empathy 55–8
threshold, levels 75
tolerance 36–7
training *see* education and training
tranquillizers, in hemiplegic shoulder pain 288
treatment, lay models 79–80
trepanning 74
trigger (tender) points 267, **267**, 268, 285

ultrasound, for shoulder pain 291
United Nations Convention on the Rights of the Child 195
United States of America (USA)
  anaesthesiology-based postoperative pain management service (APS) 160–1
  clinical nurse specialists 165
  education in 144, 146–8

visceral pain 252–3
visualization 15–16
vocabulary 38–42
  children 213–15
  descriptive 28–9
  differing meanings of words 75
  myocardial pain 297

voice, importance of 28–30, 31, 38

Welsh Spiritualists 75–6
Williams, S. 130–2, 140
womb memory *see* fetal memory
women
  bodies associated with pain 118, 120, 123
  'the body beautiful' 121–2
  cosmetic surgery 121–2, 122–4
  disenfranchised from healing 124
  middle-aged, behavioural theories 139–40
  pain as life-enhancing experience 119, 121
  patriarchal femininity 125
  self-abnegation 121
  womanliness 122–4
  see also feminism; menopause
words *see* vocabulary
Working Party Report, post-operative pain management 161–2, 167–8

York, acute pain team 163
young people 231–42
  acute pain 233–7
  analgesics 236, 237–40
  attitudes of health professionals 236
  culture 234
  definition 231, 232
  emotional state 234, 235
  gender differences in pain response 233–4
  pain assessment 236, **237**
  pain management 237–40
  postoperative pain 237
  preoperative preparation 235
  see also children